PROGRESS IN FOOD CHEMISTRY

PROGRESS IN FOOD CHEMISTRY

ERNST N. KOEFFER
EDITOR

Nova Science Publishers, Inc.
New York

For permission to use material from this book please contact us:
Telephone 631-231-7269; Fax 631-231-8175
Web Site: http://www.novapublishers.com

LIBRARY OF CONGRESS CATALOGING-IN-PUBLICATION DATA

Progress in food chemistry / Ernst N. Koeffer (editor)
p. cm.
Includes bibliographical references and index.
ISBN: 978-1-60456-303-0 (hardcover)
1. Food—Analysis. 2. Food—Consumption. I. Koeffer, Ernst N.
TX541.F653752 2008
664'.07—dc22

2008003658

Published by Nova Science Publishers, Inc. ✢ New York

CONTENTS

PREFACE

Food chemistry is the study of chemical processes and interactions of all biological and non-biological components of foods. The biological substances include such items as meat, poultry, lettuce, beer, and milk as examples. It is similar to biochemistry in its main components such as carbohydrates, lipids, and protein, but it also includes areas such as water, vitamins, minerals, enzymes, food additives, flavors, and colors. This discipline also encompasses how products change under certain food processing techniques and ways either to enhance or to prevent them from happening. An example of enhancing a process would be to encourage fermentation of dairy products with lactic acid; an example of a preventing process would be stopping the Maillard reaction on the surface of freshly cut Red Delicious apples whether by hand or mechanical methods. This new book presents the latest selected research from around the world.

Chapter 1 - Phenolic compounds are natural metabolites widely represented in plants which have recently gained special attention for their beneficial effects on human health. Polyphenols show antioxidant activity due to their ability to scavenge free radicals and to act as metal chelators. As a result of their antioxidant activity these compounds are able to protect tissues from oxidative stress thus preventing cell damage as in the case of neurodegenerative and cardiovascular diseases.

The numerous phenolic compounds that mainly derive from secondary plant metabolism of the shikimate pathway can be subdivided into nonflavonoids, flavonoids, tannins and lignins, according to the variety of simple phenolic units. Moreover, basic structure can be substituted with various groups giving mainly glycosylated or acylated derivatives, or more complex molecules. Many scientific studies have been conducted in order to characterize phenolic compounds and to correlate their antioxidant activity with their medical benefits. Chemical characterization of phenolic compounds usually requires as a first step the extraction from food and later the use of more sophisticated techniques, mainly liquid chromatographic methods such as LC-MS, LC-MS/MS, LC-NMR.

The main source of polyphenols is nutritional, since they are found in a wide array of edible products such as fruit (apples, blackberries, cherries, citrus, cranberries, grapes, pears, plums, raspberries, and strawberries), vegetables (broccoli, cabbage, celery, onion and parsley), honey, wine, chocolate, green tea, olive oil, and so forth. Polyphenols strongly affect the sensory properties of food such as color, taste (astringency and bitterness) and smell. The type of polyphenols contained in plant-derived foods and beverages depends on which raw material is used for their production. Their identification allows the tracing of the vegetable source and this can be extremely important in food characterization. However, the original phenolic pattern can be modified by the extraction process or following chemical and biochemical reactions. Anthocyanins, for instance, show only limited stability as they are affected by a number of factors such as pH, light, water activity, enzymes, oxygen, temperature, duration of processing and storage conditions.

Chapter 2 - Foods of animal origin, such as honey, milk and offal, are able to accumulate toxic metals posing a risk to health of general consumers and more vulnerable groups. For this reason, the European Commission Regulation No. 1881/2006 recommended maximum levels for metals as contaminants in food matrices. On this basis, the development of quantification methods supported by validation figures and uncertainty associated with each quantity become the central point to assure the quality and comparability of the final data. In this work, procedures based on microwave digestion with oxidizing agents followed by detection with sector field inductively coupled plasma mass spectrometry were developed and validated to measure arsenic, cadmium and lead in honey, cow milk, infant formulas and offal. Limits of detection and quantification, sensitivity, specificity, linearity range, trueness/recovery, repeatability, within-laboratory reproducibility and robustness were the main issues of the validation process. The analytical information obtained from the validation study was then used to calculate the method uncertainty without no extra work to be done. The benefit of this approach lies in its conceptual simplicity, low cost and application to routine analysis. The methods were applied to a number of marketed samples so as to contribute to the knowledge of the daily human exposure to metals from stable and special foods.

Chapter 3 - Pulsed electric field (PEF) technology has been used to preserve fruit juice and to delay spoilage by microorganisms. In vinification, sulphur dioxide (SO_2) is used as antimicrobial and as antioxidant. The aim of this study was to assess the effect of the sulphur dioxide content on the nitrogen metabolism (consumption of amino acids and formation of biogenic amines) and the production of volatile compounds throughout the alcoholic fermentation of must processed by PEF. Taking advantage of the fact that PEF treatments allow reducing the level of sulphur dioxide and, at the same time, guarantee the biochemical and microbiological stability of the must this study could be a starting point leading to an effective reduction of the sulphur dioxide content in wines. For this purpose, must of *Vitis vinífera* var. *Parellada* was stabilized by a PEF treatment and inoculated with *Saccharomyces cerevisiae* Na33 strain. The fermentations were carried out with and without SO_2.

From the results obtained, it was observed that the PEF treatment led to four logarithmic reductions of the microbial population of *Parellada* must without modifying the content of fatty acids and free amino acids of *Parellada* grape juice, which are essential for the development of the yeast during fermentation. As far as the development of the wine alcoholic fermentation is concerned, results showed that yeast consumed preferably the amino acids in the first half of fermentation in presence of SO_2. The final concentration of amino acids in the wines obtained using PEF was greater when the must fermented without SO_2 than when the latter compound was present. Therefore, it could be stated that the presence of SO_2 facilitated the consumption of amino acids and, hence, the wine may have higher microbiological stability than that obtained from fermentation without SO_2. Regarding the biogenic amines, they were mainly synthesized after the consumption of the first 25% of sugars and their formation was qualitative and quantitatively low. The SO_2 concentration did not affect the formation of biogenic amines during the alcoholic fermentation. On the other hand, the evolution of the volatile compounds profile throughout the fermentations with and without SO_2 was similar. The content of volatile acids in the wine obtained using SO_2 was not significantly different than that fermented without adding this compound. However, the final content of total alcohols and esters were different even thought the differences were small.

Consequently, when grape must was treated by PEF, the SO_2 concentration usually used in winemaking could be reduced to safer levels or even eliminated without an important effect on the volatile compounds content of the final product. Therefore absence of SO_2 should not have a negative impact on sensory characteristics of wine.

Chapter 4 - The term "coffee" is usually employed in reference to the consumable beverage obtained by extracting roasted coffee with hot water, but it actually comprises a wide range of intermediate products, starting from the freshly harvested fruit (coffee cherries), then to green beans and to the final product of consumption (roasted coffee). Green coffee beans are the main item of international trade, and their quality is evaluated according to a wide variety of criteria, including bean size, color, and shape, processing method, crop year and flavor (cup quality). Among these, flavor is the most important criterion, and it is directly affected by the presence of the so-called defective coffee beans. The presence of defective beans is usually a consequence of problems that occur during harvesting and pre-processing operations. The most important defects are black, sour or brown, immature, bored or insect-damaged, and broken beans. Both black and sour defects are associated with bean fermentation and play a major role in downgrading coffee flavor. Immature beans (from immature fruits) contribute to beverage astringency. Such defective beans are usually present in the coffee produced in Brazil, due to the strip-picking harvesting and processing practices adopted by the coffee producers. They are separated (color sorting) from the non-defective beans prior to commercialization in external markets, and the majority of these beans are dumped on the Brazilian internal market. Thus, the roasting industry in Brazil has been using these defective beans in blends with healthy ones, and, overall, a low-grade roasted coffee is consumed in the country. Currently there are no analytical methodologies that allow for detection and quantification of defective beans in roasted coffee, and thus an assessment of chemical attributes that could provide differentiation between defective and healthy coffee beans is of relevance. Thus, a review on physical and chemical attributes of defective coffee beans in comparison to healthy ones is herein provided, for both green and roasted coffees. Physical attributes include bean size, volume, density, color and water activity. Chemical attributes include proximate composition, acidity, pH, sucrose levels, caffeine, trigonelline, chlorogenic acids, amines and volatile substances. The evaluation of such attributes indicates that, in the case of green coffee, it is possible to differentiate defective and non-defective (healthy) beans by color, size, acidity levels, sucrose levels, and the presence of histamine. In the case of roasted coffee, only an evaluation of the volatile profile will effectively provide the means for differentiation.

Chapter 5 - Carotenoids are an important class of micronutrients in tomato and tomato-based products, which are widely studied due to their beneficial effects in the prevention of chronic diseases such as cardiovascular disease and various types of cancers. However, carotenoids are susceptible to isomerization and/or oxidative degradation during processing and storage. The degradation of carotenoids and change in their isomeric forms has been reported to cause variation in biological activity. This chapter intends to review the recent studies dealing with the stability of tomato carotenoids during processing and storage. Typical thermal processing condition of boiling in water for a short period of time increased the yield of lycopene due to disruption of tomato cell matrix. However, high temperature along with long duration treatment caused detrimental effect on carotenoids. Lycopene, γ-carotene and δ-carotene were relatively stable to isomerization, while lutein and β-carotene were more prone to isomerization, which may be accounted for by the difference in the structural characteristics of carotenoids and their localization/accumulation in tomatoes. The lycopene loss under various house-hold cooking conditions followed the order: frying > baking > boiling > microwaving, and soaking tomato slices in vinegar retained more lycopene than in oil or oil/vinegar mixture. The stability of dehydrated tomato products was affected by various factors such as temperature, oxygen permeability, water activity and sample texture (fine or coarse). Dehydration to intermediate moisture content (20-40%) with a water activity at 0.69-0.86 and storage temperature at $\leq 18^0$ could minimize carotenoid loss in tomato products. Complete inactivation of natural enzymes by blanching may prevent carotenoid degradation in tomatoes during frozen storage. The higher the storage temperature, the faster the degradation rate, and the lycopene degradation under different storage conditions followed the order: air and light > air and dark > vacuum and dark. From the commercial point of view, the post-harvest life span of tomatoes could be extended under controlled-atmosphere storage of high CO_2 and low O_2 level. Treating tomatoes with osmotic solution (sucrose or high dextrose equivalent maltodextrin) prior to processing or storage minimized the carotenoid loss. By subjecting the tomato sample to high hydrostatic pressure before storage, carotenoid degradation might be minimized by complete inactivation of enzymes.

Chapter 6 - Microwaves have been employed as a heat source since the 1940s, with applications in the food and chemical processing industries. The inherent complexity of microwave heating itself, associated to the coupled transport phenomena that occur as a result of microwave application, has led several researchers to develop models and present simulation studies describing heat and mass transfer occurring during microwave processing of food products. The discretization techniques employed for model solution include finite differences (FD), finite volume (FV) and the finite element method (FEM). Even though with model complexity and simulation results accuracy increasing over the past years, there are still issues to be addressed in terms of modeling and simulation applied to microwave processing. In view of the above, the objective of the present study was to present an overview of the mathematical models that describe transport phenomena occurring during microwave treatment of food products and comment on the discretization techniques that have been employed to solve such models, in order to pinpoint the modeling and simulation issues that need to be addressed in future studies.

Chapter 7 - An extracellular low molecular weight (LMW) protease from the intestine of smooth hound (*Mustelus mustelus*) was purified and characterized. The enzyme was purified to homogeneity by fractionation with ammonium sulphate, Sephadex G-100 gel filtration and DEAE-cellulose anion exchange chromatography with a 10.7-fold increase in specific activity and 22.6% recovery. The molecular weight of the purified enzyme was estimated to be 14,800 Da by SDS-PAGE and gel filtration. *Mustelus mustelus* protease appeared as a single band in native-PAGE. The optimum pH and temperature for the enzyme activity were pH 8.0 and 60 °C, respectively. The relative activity at pH 9.0 was 80.5% and the enzyme showed high pH stability between 6.0 and 9.0.

The enzyme showed extreme stability towards oxidizing agents, retaining more than 80% of its initial activity after 1 h incubation at 30 °C in the presence of 1% H_2O_2 and 2% sodium perborate. Furthermore, the purified enzyme showed relative stability and compatibility with commercial liquid detergents. The enzyme retained more than 75 and 61% of its initial activity after preincubation 60 min at 30 °C in the presence of Dixan and Ariel.

The purified enzyme was strongly inhibited by soybean trypsin inhibitor (SBTI) and phenylmethylsulphonyl fluoride (PMSF) a serine-protease inhibitor. The kinetic protease constants K_m and k_{cat} of the purified enzyme for casein were 0.313 mM and 0.088 s^{-1}, respectively, while the catalytic efficiency k_{cat}/K_m was 0.281 s^{-1} mM^{-1}.

Chapter 8 - Quantitative structure-activity relationships (QSAR) represent an attempt to correlate structural or property descriptors of compounds with several types of biological activities. These physicochemical descriptors, which include parameters, related with hydrophobicity, topology, electronic properties, and steric effects are determined empirically or, more recently, by computational methods. Activities used in QSAR studies (the dependent parameters) include chemical measurements and biological assays. QSAR software programs generate equations (models) by statistically identifying molecular descriptors and/or substructural molecular attributes that are correlated with dependent parameter. These programs are capable of identifying similar structural alerts associated with activity in a test compound and through a computer-aided method to predict how a chemical behaves based on its structure. QSAR is a theoretical method widely used in medicinal chemistry and recently was found to be appropriate to be employed either in food research. This method increasing interest in the mid-1980, and was implemented in a computer-aided rational approaches in drug design, representing an attractive method to estimate theoretical data as well to validation of any statistical model that seems to be reasonable in describing an interaction between a bioactive chemical constituent and the respective biological activity. The technique can be used to investigate toxicity, potency, stability and functionalities of food ingredients. One of the principal applications of QSAR method in food research is to understand better toxicology data, in order to inform risk assessments and to support risk management decisions that are protective of human health. Ideally, a risk assessor would have available all of the relevant information about the toxicity of the compound; their interactions with living systems; and the possible exposure conditions. Advances in the development of computational methods have available additional resources for safety assessment such as structure similarity searching and quantitative structure - activity relationship models. The purpose of this chapter is to discuss how a QSAR analysis can be used to predict important information from chemical structure and to review the application of this technique in food research.

In: Progress in Food Chemistry
Editor: E. N. Koeffer, pp. 1-45
ISBN: 978-1-60456-303-0

Chapter 1

PHENOLIC COMPOUNDS IN FOOD

***Carlo I. G. Tuberoso*[1] *and Christina D. Orrù*[2]**
[1] Department of Toxicology, University of Cagliari,
Via Ospedale 72, 09124 Cagliari, Italy
[2] Department of Biomedical Sciences and Technology, University of Cagliari,
Cittadella Universitaria, 09042 Monserrato, Italy

ABSTRACT

Phenolic compounds are natural metabolites widely represented in plants which have recently gained special attention for their beneficial effects on human health. Polyphenols show antioxidant activity due to their ability to scavenge free radicals and to act as metal chelators. As a result of their antioxidant activity these compounds are able to protect tissues from oxidative stress thus preventing cell damage as in the case of neurodegenerative and cardiovascular diseases.

The numerous phenolic compounds that mainly derive from secondary plant metabolism of the shikimate pathway can be subdivided into nonflavonoids, flavonoids, tannins and lignins, according to the variety of simple phenolic units. Moreover, basic structure can be substituted with various groups giving mainly glycosylated or acylated derivatives, or more complex molecules. Many scientific studies have been conducted in order to characterize phenolic compounds and to correlate their antioxidant activity with their medical benefits. Chemical characterization of phenolic compounds usually requires as a first step the extraction from food and later the use of more sophisticated techniques, mainly liquid chromatographic methods such as LC-MS, LC-MS/MS, LC-NMR.

The main source of polyphenols is nutritional, since they are found in a wide array of edible products such as fruit (apples, blackberries, cherries, citrus, cranberries, grapes, pears, plums, raspberries, and strawberries), vegetables (broccoli, cabbage, celery, onion and parsley), honey, wine, chocolate, green tea, olive oil, and so forth. Polyphenols strongly affect the sensory properties of food such as color, taste (astringency and bitterness) and smell. The type of polyphenols contained in plant-derived foods and beverages depends on which raw material is used for their production. Their identification allows the tracing of the vegetable source and this can be extremely important in food characterization. However, the original phenolic pattern can be modified by the extraction process or following chemical and biochemical reactions.

Anthocyanins, for instance, show only limited stability as they are affected by a number of factors such as pH, light, water activity, enzymes, oxygen, temperature, duration of processing and storage conditions.

1. Introduction

Phenols consist of almost 10000 known structures. They are secondary metabolites ubiquitous from roots to aerial parts, in all plants. The most common classification of phenolic compounds is in non-flavonoids, flavonoids, lignans, neolignans $(C_6\text{-}C_3)_2$ and lignins $(C_6\text{-}C_3)_n$. The first class can be subdivided into phenolic acids, stilbenes and gallotannins; while flavonoids are subdivided into flavanones, flavones, flavonols, flavan-3ols, isoflavonoids and anthocyanins [1-5].

Interestingly, qualitative and quantitative composition of phenolic compounds in plants varies according to species or families or even to environmental conditions. Phenolic compounds are important for plant physiology as they are involved in growth and development pathways; in defense mechanisms and influence the color of flowers and fruits. Phenols are able to affect several biological activities in human beings, which cannot synthesize them, but can introduce them through the food chain.

1.1. The Phenolic Compounds

The extreme variability in phenolic compounds structures is connected with their different ways of production. Their biosynthesis starts from the two basic pathways of the shikimate and acetate-malonate pathway, but many phenolic compounds derive from the breakdown or different rearrangements of both phenols and other organic molecules. Figures 1.1.a. show how the main classes of phenolic compounds are synthesized.

Simple phenols are very common in fruits and they can be obtained by the shikimate pathway [6], but also from the degradation of hydroxycinnamic acids. Benzoic acids $(C_6\text{-}C_1)$ are colorless, but they can be involved in oxidation reactions and produce yellowish derivatives. Moreover they are precursors of volatile phenols like ethyl and vinyl phenol and guaiacol.

Hydroxycinnamic acids $(C_6\text{-}C_3)$ can be found in a free form, glycosylated or esterified with acids. Moreover, hydroxycinnamic acids can combine with sugar moieties of anthocyanin glucosides (acylated anthocyanins). *p*-Hydroxyphenyl acids are key molecules for the biosynthesis of lignins because *p*-coumaric, ferulic and sinapic acids are converted through CoA derivatives into aldehydes, alcohol and finally to lignins [7] (figure 1.1.b.). Additionally, *trans*-cinnamic acid is a key molecule in coumarins biosynthesis. Coumarins are lactones that show strong biological activities. Umbelliferone, esculetin and scopoletin are the most widespread coumarins in nature.

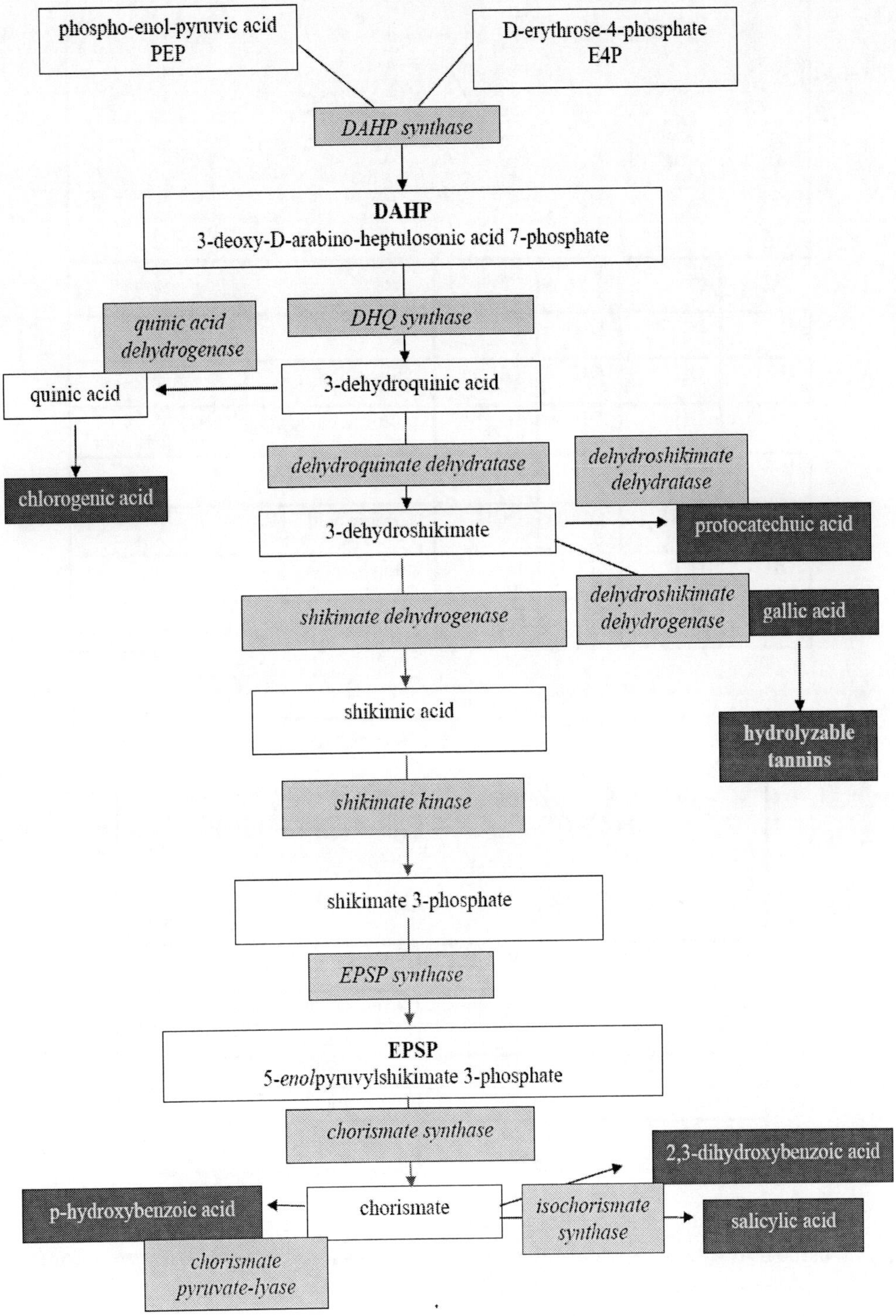

Figure 1.1.a. Shikimic and chorismic acids pathway.

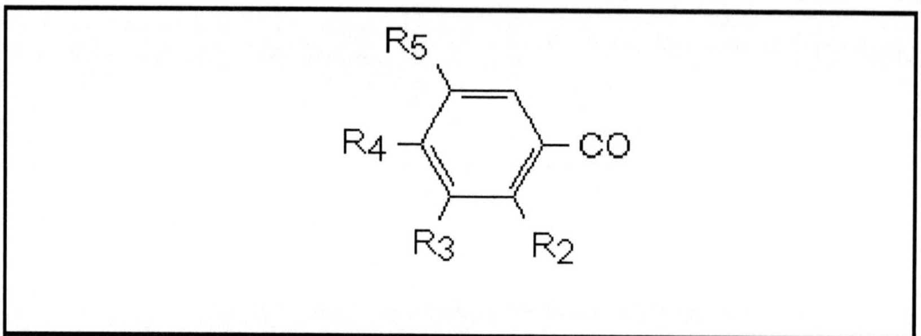

R_2	R_3	R_4	R_5	
H	H	OH	H	*p*-hydroxybenzoic acid
H	OH	OH	OH	gallic acid
H	OH	OH	H	protocatechuic acid
H	OCH_3	OH	H	vanillic acid
H	OCH_3	OH	OCH_3	syringic acid
OH	H	H	H	salicylic acid
OH	H	H	OH	gentisic acid

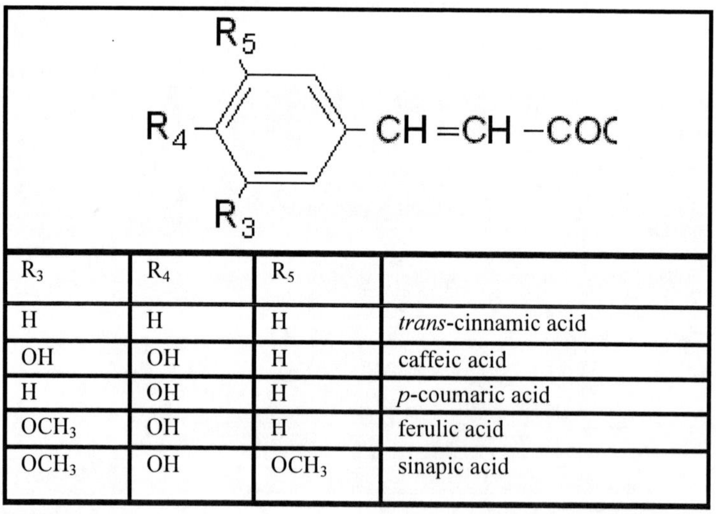

R_3	R_4	R_5	
H	H	H	*trans*-cinnamic acid
OH	OH	H	caffeic acid
H	OH	H	*p*-coumaric acid
OCH_3	OH	H	ferulic acid
OCH_3	OH	OCH_3	sinapic acid

Stilbenes (C_6-C_2-C_6) are non-flavonoids phenolics that are produced in response to stress such as pathogens attack (phytoalexin). One of the most studied is *trans*-resveratrol (3,5,4'-trihydroxystilbene) that was initially found in grapes and wines and later in peanuts and tea. Further studies reported also *cis*-configurations and glucosides.

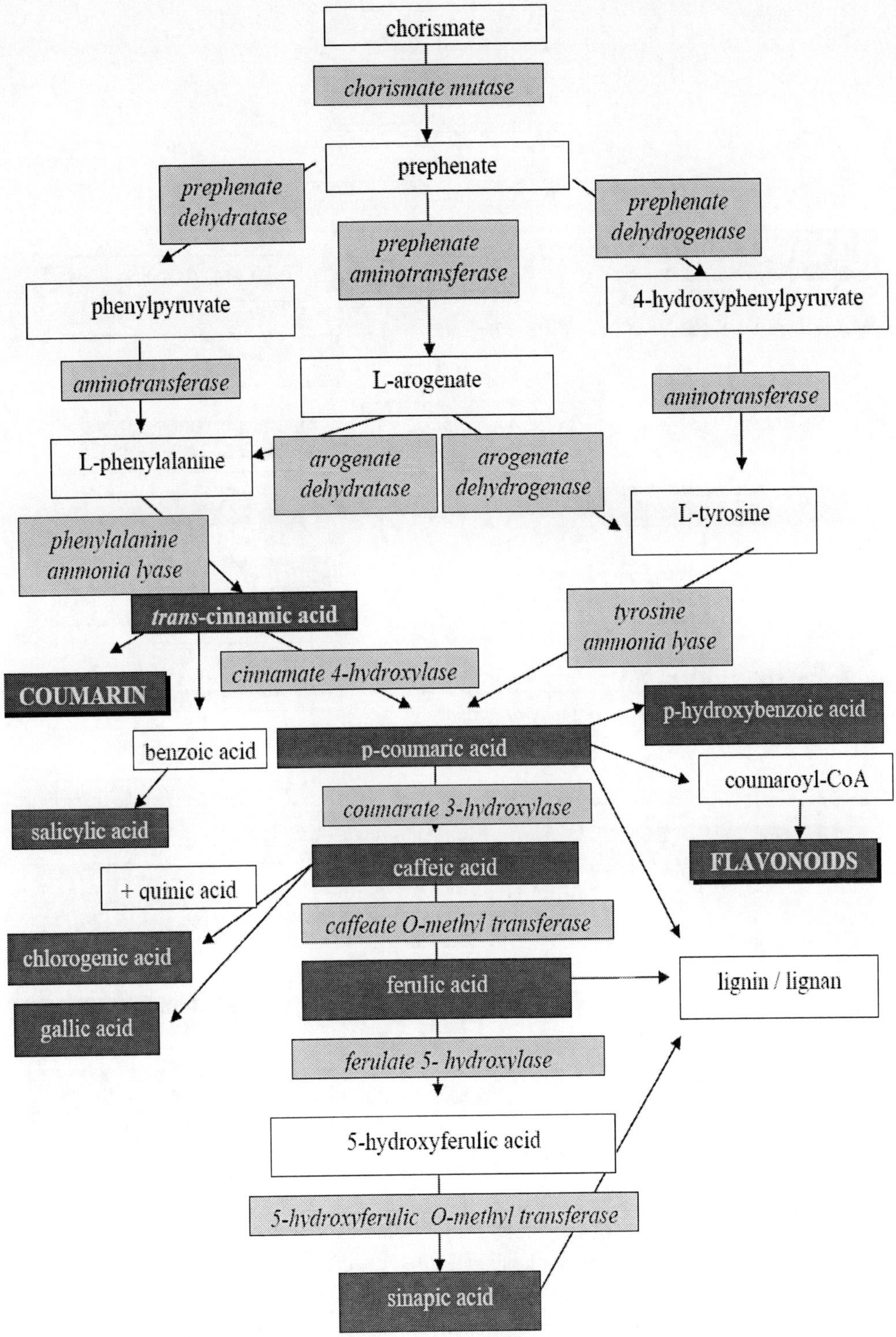

Figure 1.1.b. Phenylpropanoid compounds pathway.

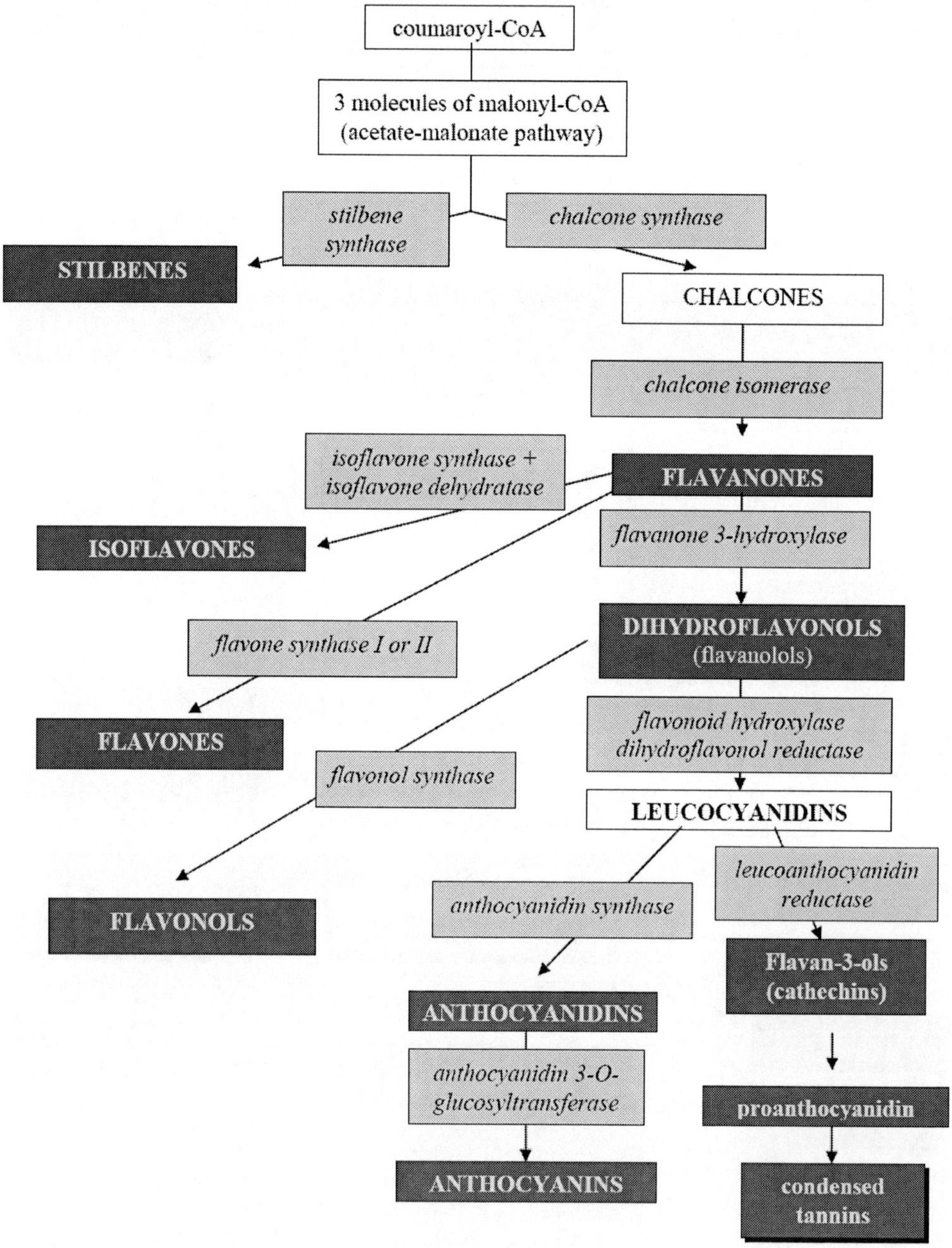

Figure 1.1.c. Biosynthesis of flavonoids.

Flavonoids represent one of the most studied classes of phenolic compounds. They are derivatives of the chalcones biosynthesis (figure 1.1.c.) and have a 15-carbon skeleton consisting of 2 phenolic rings and an oxygenated ring (C_6-C_3-C_6) (figure 1.1.2). It is common to find them as basic structures (aglycon) or with sugar moieties (glycoside) [8,9].

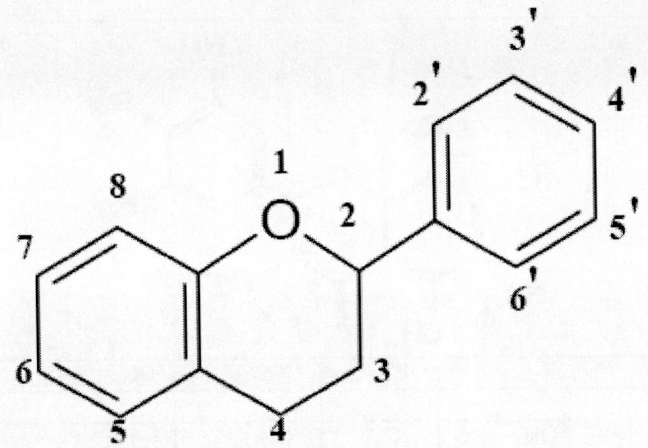

Figure 1.1.2. Basic flavonoid structure.

Flavones are one of the largest flavonoid subgroups and include aglycons, *O* and *C*-glycosides. Furthermore, methyl ethers are very common and also isoprenylated flavones have been reported. Flavones sugars go from monosaccharides to disaccharides and trisaccharides: pentose like xylose, rhamnose, arabinose; hexose like glucose, galactose, and cellobiose have been found. They are common in herbs and grains and less frequent in fruit. Flavones biosynthesis is catalyzed by two different flavone synthase proteins: the FSN I is a soluble dioxygenase whereas the FSN II is a membrane bound cytochrome P450 enzyme [10]. Flavonols are yellow pigments widespread in plants, and their glycosides are characterized by the same sugars found in flavones. Flavanones show an asymmetric carbon at C-2 and, when the optical rotation was measured, the (2S)-configuration resulted the most common. They are very common in citrus (hesperidin, narirutin, eriocitrin, neohesperidin,) and they contribute to their bitter flavor (i.e. naringin in grapefruit) [11]. Dihydroflavonols (flavanolols) show a pale yellow color and are a key step in the flavonols, flavan-3-ols and anthocyanins biosynthesis (figure 1.1.c).

Flavan-3-ols are represented by molecules such as (+)-catechin and (-)-epicatechin and their esters with gallic acid like gallocatechin or epigallocatechin. Catechin and epigallocatechin can polymerize and produce procyanidins by reaction between carbon C4 (C ring) and carbons C6 and C8 (A ring). Dimeric procyanidins are divided into type-B and type-A, while trimeric are divided into type-C and type-D. Such compounds are very common in many herbs and plants.

Isoflavones are characterized by the benzenoid substitution at the 3 position of C ring. They have an estrogen-like activity in mammals. Genistein, daidzein and biochanin-A are the most common. Soybeans and soy products are the richest sources of isoflavones in human diet.

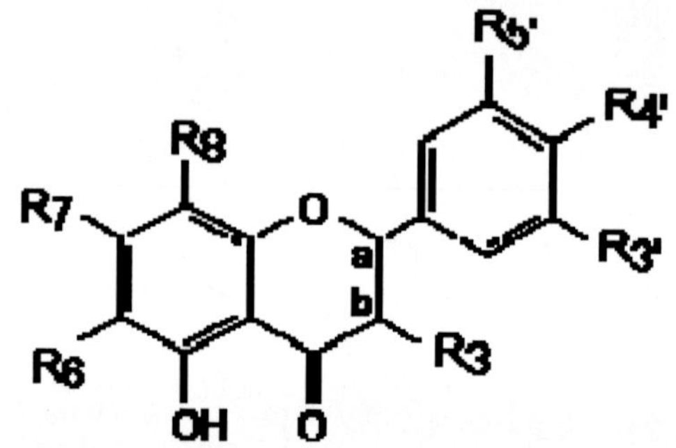

a-b*	R_3	R_7	$R_{3'}$	$R_{4'}$	$R_{5'}$	
d	H					Flavones
		OH	H	OH	H	apigenin
		OH	OH	OH	H	luteolin
		OH	H	H	H	chrysin
		OCH_3	H	H	H	tectochrysin
d	OH					Flavonols
		OH	OH	OH	H	quercetin
		OH	OH	OH	OH	myricetin
		OH	H	OH	H	kaempferol
		OH	H	H	H	galangin
s	H					Flavanones
		OH	H	OH	H	naringenin
		OH	H	OCH_3	OH	hesperetin
		OH	H	OH	H	liquiritigenin
		OH	H	H	H	pinocembrina
s	OH					Flavanolols
		OH	OH	OH	H	taxifolin
		OH	H	H	H	pinobanksin
		OH	H	OH	OH	fustin

a-b bond: double (d) or single (s).

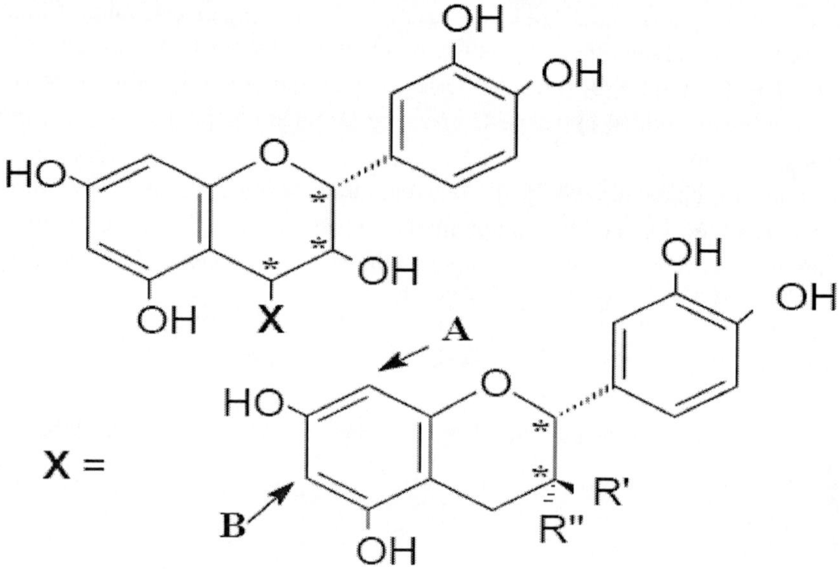

Anthocyanidins are obtained from leucoanthocyanin by means of a synthase that converts the C ring to the flavylium cation. There are 17 known natural anthocyanidins, but only six of them are widely distributed. Anthocyanidins can be aglycons or glycosides (anthocyanins), or have acylated groups on the sugar moieties. The most common sugars are glucose, galactose, xylose, arabinose, rhamnose, rutinose, while the most frequent acids are gallic, *p*-coumaric, up to now over 600 natural anthocyanins have been reported [12]. These compounds give orange-red-purple-blue color to vegetables, promoting insect attraction and thus pollen or seed dispersal; and also have antioxidant, antifungal and antimicrobial activity [13]. The color of anthocyanins is influenced by pH and cations (mainly Cu^{2+}, Mg^{2+}, Fe^{3+}, Al^{3+}). Recent studies have tried to estimate the daily consumption of anthocyanins. For instance, in the United States a mean consumption of 12.5 mg/day/person was estimated, 77% of which consists of non-acylated anthocyanins and among the acylated, monoglycosides and cyanidin derivatives are predominant [12].

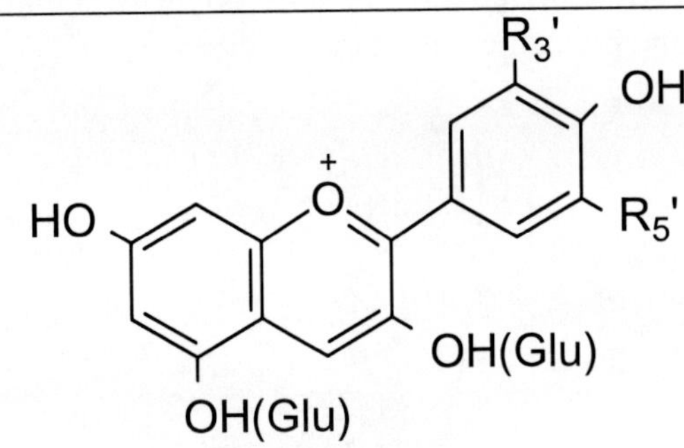

$R_{3'}$	$R_{5'}$	
OH	H	cyanidin
OH	OH	delphinidin
OCH_3	OCH_3	malvidin
H	H	pelargonidin
OCH_3	H	peonidin
OCH_3	OH	petunidin

Tannins are higher molecular weigh phenols (molecular weights > 500 up to 30,000) and are usually subdivided into two groups, the condensed and the hydrolyzable tannins. Condensed tannins are oligomers derivatives of flavan-3-ol units linked by carbon-carbon bonds and not susceptible to cleavage by hydrolysis. Hydrolyzable tannins are characterized by gallic or ellagic acid unit esterified to sugars, mainly glucose, and they can easily be hydrolyzed by enzymes or acids and alkalis or heat. Tannins are characterized by their interaction with proteins.

1.2. Biological Activities

Epidemiological and experimental data indicate that phenols have numerous biological activities. These compounds appear to be able to prevent cardiovascular diseases and cancer, and many researches suggest that they could be useful for example in the therapeutic treatment of neurodegenerative and infectious diseases. The various biological activities of polyphenols derive from their antioxidant, anti-inflammatory and hormonal activity and from their ability to influence enzymatic processes, cell growth and genes expression (figure 1.2.1).

There is a vast body of literature concerning the biological effects of polyphenols. What follows is a synthetic overview of some of the most studied properties of these compounds and their potential role in the prevention of many diseases.

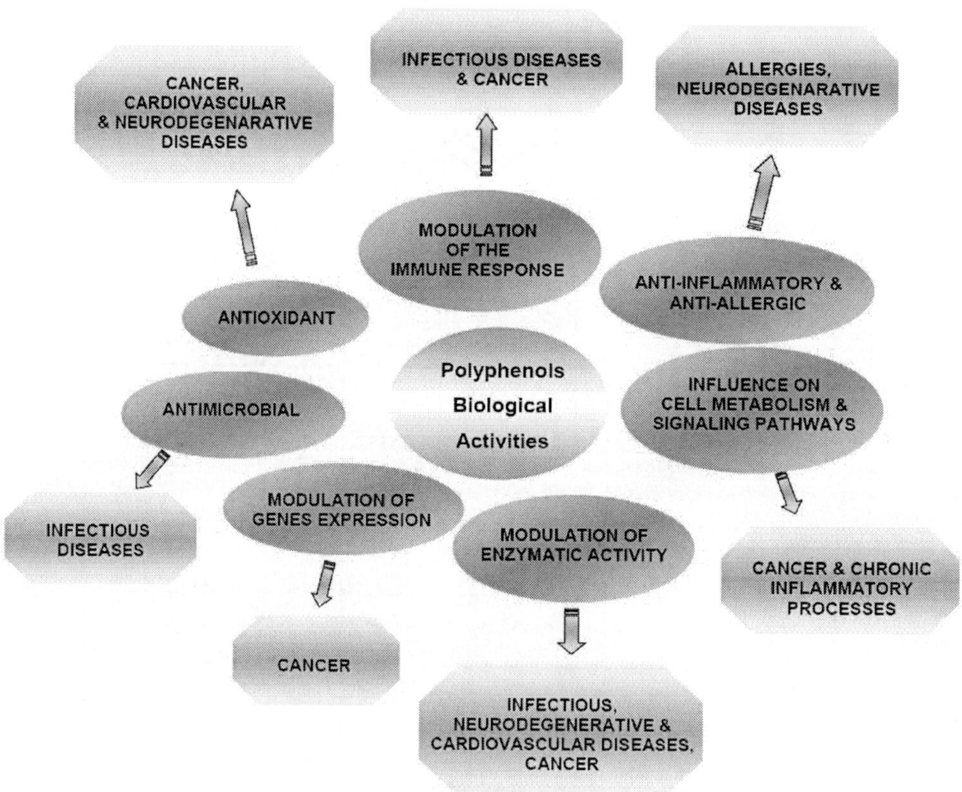

Figure 1.2.1. Polyphenols Biological Activities.

Antioxidant Activity

Cell metabolism produces small quantities of free radicals and other oxygenated compounds also known as highly Reactive Oxygen Species (ROS) which are eliminated by the catalytic activity of enzymes such as superoxide dismutase (SOD), catalases and

Glutatione reductase, and by endogenous reductants, such as glutathione (GSH), ascorbate, tocopherols (vitamin E), and ubiquinol (figure 1.2.2).

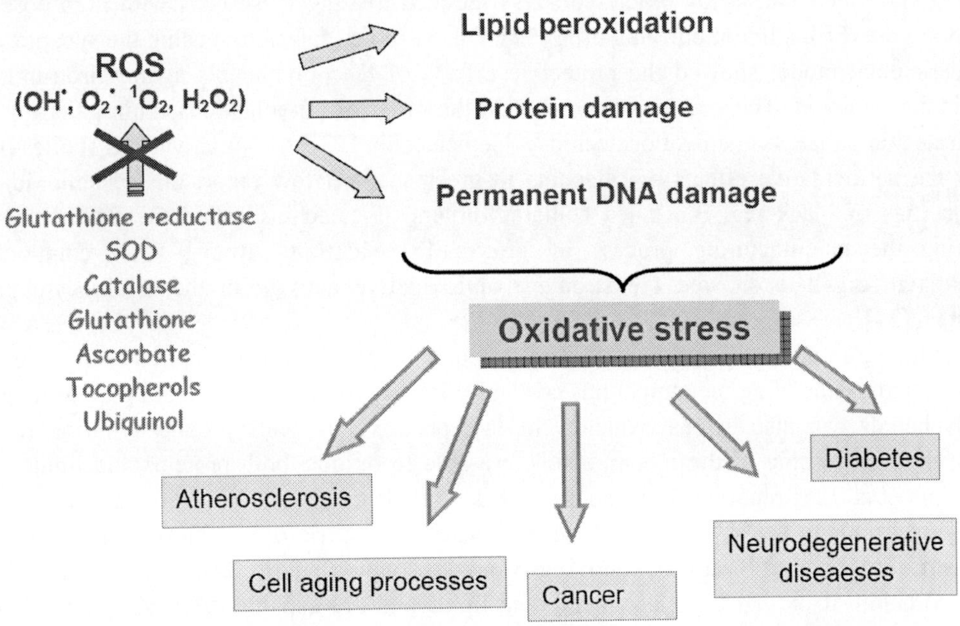

Figure 1.2.2. Oxidative stress mechanisms and their role in progressive diseases.

Despite this complex network of antioxidant molecules and enzymes that work together to prevent oxidative damage, during several pathological processes ROS production can significantly increase leading to oxidative stress. As a consequence of this imbalance between oxidative and anti-oxidative processes fundamental cell components such as DNA, proteins and lipids can be permanently damaged.

Owing to their chemical structure, polyphenolic compounds have the ability to protect tissues from these aggressive substances. Probably the main antioxidant activity that has been associated with polyphenols is the ability to scavenge free radicals. This activity is reduced by the presence of a sugar moiety in the molecule. Polyphenols antioxidant activity is also connected to their ability to induce phase II enzymes such as glutathione transferase (GST) that will enhance the excretion of oxidizing species [14,15], or induce antioxidant enzymes such as metallothionein (a metal-binding protein with antioxidant properties). These compounds may also inhibit cytochrome P450s (CYPs) [16,17] or enzymes such as cyclooxygenase [18,19] or lipoxygenase [20] that have oxidant activities.

Anthocyanins have several positive therapeutic effects mainly correlated to their strong antioxidant properties. In particular, cyanidin-3-*O*-glucoside, which represents about 80% of the total anthocyanins content in blackberry extract, is a good scavenger of peroxynitrite that inhibits multiple peroxynitrite-induced oxidative processes therefore preventing vascular hyporeactivity, and endothelial dysfunction [21].

Catechins are another group of phenolic compounds that act as strong scavengers of superoxide, hydrogen peroxide, hydroxyl radicals, and nitric oxide produced by various chemical reactions. By means of their catechol structure they chelate with metals therefore preventing metal-catalyzed free radical formation [3]. The antioxidant activities of tea catechins have been studied using various *in vitro* and *in vivo* methods. Using human hepatoma cells (HepG2) Jiao H. et al. showed that green tea polyphenols partially prevented cytotoxic effects caused by oxidative stress induced treating these cells with high doses of Fenofibrate (FF), a lipidmodifying drug [22]. Other studies carried out using the synaptosome experimental model showed the protective effects of tea polyphenols against iron-induced lipid peroxidation. These effects decreased in the order of (-)-epigallocatechin gallate > (-)-epicatechin gallate > (-)epigallocatechin > (-)epicatechin [23]. Although various studies point out the antioxidative effects of catechins in green tea, yet few report on the antioxidative properties of black tea. Black tea contains dimers of catechins called theaflavins formed during the manufacturing process by enzymatic oxidation. Among these compounds, theaflavin digallate showed the strongest antioxidative activity in the erythrocyte ghost system [24].

Although many experimental data support the antioxidant activity of phenolic compounds, depending on compounds concentration or environmental conditions, some plant polyphenols can also act as oxidants. In fact phenoxyl radicals produced during radical scavenging by some of these compounds, are able to oxidize both proteins and lipids [25]. Oshima et al. [26] reported that a number of flavonoids otherwise considered as antioxidants may occasionally act as prooxidants in the presence of nitric oxide (NO). It has also been shown that hydroxyl radicals deriving from flavonoids morin and naringenin, initiate peroxidation of oxidized nuclear membrane lipids and are capable of causing DNA strand breaks in isolated rat liver nuclei [27]. Therefore it is important to note that polyphenols can improve cell survival by means of their antioxidant activity, protecting DNA, proteins and lipids from oxidative damage. Nevertheless these compounds can also show negative effects owing to their prooxidant activity [28].

Anticancer Activity

Polyphenols, and particularly flavonoids, are able to influence a large number of cell regulatory pathways, such as those of growth [29], apoptosis [30,31], DNA damage repair, energy metabolism [32,33], hormonal activity [34], genes expression [32,35], inflammation, and response to oxidative stress acting as antioxidants and free-radical scavengers, as enzyme inhibitors, hormones or anti-hormones, and modulators of genes expression. Thus these compounds have been extensively studied for their ability to inhibit tumor proliferation or rather prevent the development of cancer.

Cell growth metabolism, including cell division, can be slowed by flavonoids which are able to inhibit tyrosine-specific protein kinases, topoisomerases I and II, as well as the cell division control protein kinases. This could be particularly important in cancer prevention because the reduction of cell proliferation lowers the concentration of toxic tumor catabolites which will not exceed the capacity of the hepatic detoxification mechanisms. Experimental results by Shoij and coworkers have shown that procyanidins, which represent about 50% of the apple polyphenols, have a strong inhibitory effect on melanogenesis. According to their studies these compounds inhibit the biosynthesis as well as the activity of tyrosinase, a key enzyme in melanogenesis [36].

The ability to promote cell death by inducing apoptosis is a common feature of many polyphenols with anticancer activity. It has been reported that lauryl gallate, a gallic acid derivative with antioxidant activity, has a proapoptotic effect on the mouse B-cell lymphoma line Wehi 231 [37]. This compound also acts as a potent antiproliferative agent by inducing cell cycle alterations and apoptosis in three human breast cancer cell lines displaying a multidrug-resistant phenotype [38].

Experimental data indicate that polyphenols anticancer activity is generally correlated to more then one biological effect. Navindra P. S. et al., for example demonstrated that the *in vitro* anticancer activity of pomegranate juice polyphenols is associated with the antiproliferative, apoptotic and antioxidant activity of polyphenols [39]. Meiers et al. also reported that the aglycones of the food anthocyanins, cyanidin and delphinidin, show the ability to inhibit human tumor cells growth *in vitro* [29]. Recently clinical efficacy of various EGCG and green tea preparations on human cervical lesions and prostate cancer chemoprevention were investigated, the results support some of the potential heath benefits that have be ascribed to the consumption of green tea and EGCG [40].

DNA damage is normally repaired by specific enzymes, however when these physiological mechanisms fail to restore normal conditions, permanent DNA alterations can induce tumors development. There is limited evidence for the protective role of polyphenols against DNA damage. Nevertheless a study showed that among the various anthocyanins investigated, cyanidin and delphinidin were the most effective molecules in preventing single-strand breakage (SSB) formation of DNA. DNA damage was reduced by 56% in rat smooth muscle cells (SMC), and by 40% in hepatoma tumor cells (MH1C1). Other anthocyanins exerted a less protective effect, never exceeding 30% [41].

An important mechanism of cancer prevention by polyphenols regards their ability to modulate xenobiotic metabolising enzymes (XME) expression, thus having profound effects on both the activation and excretion of exogenous carcinogens. For example a number of dietary polyphenols inhibit specific cytochrome P450s (CYPs) [42], protecting against mutagenesis by this mechanism.

Although the majority of experimental data suggest that polyphenols are able to protect from cancer over the past years some researchers have pointed out that they could also have mutagenic effects. Mariko Murata et al. suggested that oxidative damage induced by isoflavone metabolites plays a role in tumor initiation [43]. Other studies report on the potential link between the development of some types infant leukemia and the ingestion of flavonoids by pregnant women [44,45]. Recently Bandele O J et al., have investigated the chemopreventive but also genotoxic properties of three classes of flavonoids: flavones, flavonols and isoflavones, showing that these compounds which are well known topoisomerase poisons enhanced DNA cleavage by affecting human topoisomerase II activity [46].

Among the various food and beverages that have been investigated for their anticancer activity, wine is one of the most studied. Many epidemiological studies have pointed out a reduced incidence of cancer within regular wine drinkers. These anticancer effects seem related for example to enhanced apoptosis or modulation of signal transduction pathways by altered expression of key enzymes such as cyclooxygenases and protein kinases induced by phenolic compounds found in wine [47]. Quercetin is a wine flavone which has shown a wide spectrum of anticancer properties in different experimental models [30,34,48-50]. Other studies have demonstrated that (-)-catechin is able to inhibit cell growth in human cell lines from prostate cancer [51] as well cells from breast cancer [52]. One of the wine components that has been more widely studied for its numerous biological effects is the phytoalexin resveratrol. There are two isomeric forms of resveratrol: biologically inactive *cis*-resveratrol and active *trans*-resveratrol [53]. Several *in vitro* and *in vivo* studies indicate that *trans*-resveratrol appears to target more than one step in the neoplastic process. This polyphenolic compound can influence various signal pathways regulating the cell cycle, including those implicated in apoptosis [54-56], or in the modulation of tumor suppressor genes. *trans*-Resveratrol also appears to be an aryl hydrocarbon receptor antagonist therefore contributing to cancer prevention by inhibiting the uptake and activation of several dangerous carcinogens [57].

Cardioprotective Activity

The most common cause of death in industrialized countries are cardiovascular diseases followed by cancer, Alzheimer's Disease and accidents [58]. Flavonoids interfere at several points in the pathogenesis of cardiovascular diseases because of their cardioprotective activities. Although the precise mechanisms underlying these cardioprotective effects are not well understood, attenuation of platelet aggregation [59] and inhibition of smooth muscle proliferation, antiatherogenic effects [60,61], release of nitric oxide (NO), ability to regulate cyclooxygenase and lipoxygenase [62] activity and decreased LDL oxidation may play a role. Flavonoids show an antithrombotic activity owing to their ability to inhibit platelet aggregation and are able to increase blood vessel dilatation by inducing smooth muscle cells to relax. These characteristics account for their wide use in the treatment of venous insufficiency [4,63,64].

Cardiovascular diseases are frequently caused by atherosclerosis for which oxidative modification of the low density lipoproteins (LDL) has been proposed as an important initiating event. With their *in vitro* studies Kerry N. L. et al. confirmed that red wine inhibits the oxidation of human LDL collected from healthy volunteers by copper and azo-initiated systems. Therefore red wine's antioxidant components, e.g. phenolic compounds, appear to inhibit LDL oxidation in both a metal-dependent and a radical-dependent system [65]. Atherosclerosis is strongly correlated with hypercholesterolemia. Many researchers have reported that flavonoids are capable of reducing total cholesterol and LDL fraction in rats whose diet was supplemented with polyphenols extract [66]. Flavonoids are also able to influence hypercholesterolemia, for example by inhibiting HMG-CoA reductase, a key enzyme of cholesterol biosynthesis.

The high and complex content of polyphenols in wine most probably accounts for the benefic effects on the cardiovascular system that are associated with a regular intake of this beverage. It has been suggested that resveratrol could be responsible for the cardioprotective actions of red wine because of its antiarrhythmic effects [67]. According to the studies carried out by Shigematsu et al., resveratrol exerts powerful anti-inflammatory effects in the setting of Ischemia/Reperfusion (I/R) injury, that could also explain the cardioprotective effects of this compound. Furthermore they point out that resveratrol's ability to detoxify superoxide accounts for its antiadhesive and microvascular barrier preserving effects by detoxifycation of superoxide [68]. Interestingly a study regarding Italian red wine showed that anthocyanin fractions was the most effective both in scavenging reactive oxygen species and in inhibiting lipoprotein oxidation and platelet aggregation [69], suggesting that anthocyanins could be the key component in red wine that protects against cardiovascular disease.

Neuroprotective Activity

Numerous epidemiological studies indicate that antioxidants from diet can influence the incidence of many neurodegenerative disorders such as Alzheimer's and Parkinson's disease. The pathogenesis of these neurodegenerative diseases is characterized by a complex combination of genetic and non-genetic components. This multifactorial etiology suggests that polyphenols, which seem to have multiple targets, could find applications both in their prevention and therapeutic treatment [70].

According to nutritional studies green tea extracts or EGCG alone reduce risk of Parkinson's disease [71]. The neuroprotective effect of EGCG may depend partly from its free radical scavenging and metal chelator properties, as oxidative stress is implicated in the neurotoxic mechanisms correlated with this disease [70]. Although there are no relevant epidemiological studies regarding Alzheimer's disease (AD), there are several *in vitro* studies showing that green tea extracts are able to protect neurons from the amyloid β-induced damages [72,73]. EGCG can regulate the proteolytic processing of the Amyloid Precursor Protein (APP) both *in vitro* and *in vivo*. In neuronal cell cultures EGCG could promote the non-amyloidogenic α-secretase pathway [74], therefore restoring a normal cellular metabolic condition. Although EGCG has shown such promising activities it is still unclear weather the doses used in *in vitro* and *in vivo* assays would be safe and effective in humans [75].

According to some epidemiological studies indicate that a moderate consumption of wine is associated with a lower incidence of Alzheimer's disease [76,77]. Researchers have shown that resveratrol reduces the accumulation of reactive oxygen species induced by the amyloid β peptide in PC12 cells [78]. Recently, in two different APP695-transfected cell lines (HEK293 and N2A), Marambaud and coworkers demonstrated that resveratrol could decrease the secretion of the amyloid β peptide (1–40), this effect occurred without directly affecting β and γ-secretases [79]. Researchers speculate that resveratrol could activate the proteasome that degradates the amyloid β peptide. Other mechanisms involving intracellular signaling could also be implicated in the neuroprotective effect of resveratrol against the amyloid β peptide as the modulation of the nuclear factor-kappa B (NF-κB) activity or NF-κB/SIRT1 pathways [70].

Other polyphenols have shown neuroprotective effects. The flavonoid amentoflavone has shown strong neuroprotective affects probably mediated by the blockade of multiple cellular events leading to cell death following perinatal Hypoxic-ischemia (H-I) injury [80]. Different epidemiological studies revealed that Alzheimer's disease has a much lower prevalence in India where the yellow curry spice curcumin is widely in used. Curcumin is a pigment isolated from the plant *Curcuma longa* that inhibits the formation of reactive-oxygen species and has anti-inflammatory properties as a result of its ability to inhibit cyclooxygenases (COX) and other enzymes involved in inflammation [81]. Since Alzheimer's disease is characterized by chronic inflammation and oxidative damages in the brain, the relationship between a wide consumption of curcumin and a low incidence of AD has been investigated by many researchers. Experimental results show that when transgenic APPsw mice receive low doses of curcumin in their diet for 6 months, indices of inflammation and oxidative damages are reduced [82]. The EGb 761 ginkgo biloba extract, which contains 24% of flavonoids (quercetin, kaempferol and isorhamnetin, combined with a sugar) and 6% of terpenes, has been studied by two different research groups for its ability to protect primary hippocampal neurons and PC12 cells against the toxicity of the amyloid β peptide [72,83]. The observed protective effects originate from EGb 761 antioxidant activity but are also correlated to its capability of modulating the α-secretase pathway. In fact using hippocampal slices researchers demonstrated that EGb 761 positively influences the α-secretase pathway. This result was further assessed *in vivo*, using a transgenic animal model of Alzheimer's disease, which showed an enhancement of spatial learning and memory [84]. EGb 761 could also modulate the production of brain APP and the amyloid β peptide by lowering the levels of circulating free cholesterol [85] thus protecting cells against the amyloid β peptide toxicity [86]. EGb 761 is currently the focus of two phase III clinical trials, GEM study (Ginkgo Evaluation of Memory Study) in the United States and GuidAge study in France both with more than 3,000 individuals/study older than 70 years old [70].

Anti-Inflammatory and Antiallergic Activities

Polyphenols are able to inhibit some initial inflammatory processes, such as mastocyte, neutrophil and basophil degranulation, the formation of prostaglandines [87], lipid peroxidation [88] and the complex cascade of effects that follows the above mentioned processes.

Anthocyanin aglycones in particular have shown a strong inhibitory activity on COX-I and COX-II enzymes [4,63]. Flavonoids can prevent the synthesis and release of molecules which trigger inflammatory and allergic reactions such as histamine, cytokines [89], prostaglandines and leucotriens [90]. Apigenin and quercetin for example inhibit human basophils release of histamine.

Modulation of Enzymatic Activity

The ability of flavonoids to modulate different enzymatic activities involves various metabolic pathways contributing to their many biological activities such as antythrombotic, vessel protective [91], anti-inflammatory and anticarcinogenic properties.

The enzymes inhibited by flavonoids include hydrolases, oxidoreductases, DNA synthetases, RNA polymerases, phosphatases, protein phosphokinases, oxygenase, amino acid oxidases and so forth. Experimental results show that in some cases the type of inhibition is competitive, but more often it is allosteric. The ability of flavonoids to inhibit the activity of hyaluronidase enzymes is important in order to maintain the integrity of connective tissue which are a barrier against the spread of bacterial cells, metastases, and viruses. The best known example of an isomerase that is inhibited by flavonoids is the luteolin and quercetin inhibition of the DNA topoisomerase II [92]. Flavonoids are able to increase rhodopsin (photosensible retinic pigment) regeneration by acting on rhetinic enzymes, in particular on laccato dehydrogenase. This effect reduces the time of adaptation to darkness [93]. Quercetin for example is able to inhibit the activity of P450, cyclooxygenase, lipoxygenases and xantinoxydase [94].

Antimicrobial Activity

Several studies have indicated the antimicrobial activity of polyphenolic compounds, for example against *Staphylococcus aureous* e *S. epidermidis* [63]. Flavonoids from blueberries have an anti-adhesive activity that reduces the capacity of bacteria to stick to the walls of the urinary bladder, thus neutralizing one of the major bacterial pathogenicity mechanisms. Many of the bacterial strains usually encountered by humans are killed by flavonoids, however, the mechanisms by which this is accomplished are not known yet. Some flavonoids inhibit the activity of enzymes that are necessary for viral replication within the cells. This is the case of HIV *[95]*, *Herpes simplex*, influenza virus [96,97] and Rhinovirus [98].

It is important to note that all infectants, including viruses, may be eliminated through the immunostimulatory effect of flavonoid treatment. Flavonoids induce the production of Interferons (IFNs) [99] which have several antiviral effects, including fortification of the cellular membrane and induction of nucleases that attack viral genome. A study by Yao-Lan Li showed that orientin and vitexin, flavonoids isolated from *Trollius chinensis* Bunge (Ranunculaceae), possess strong antiviral activities against Parainfluenza type 3 (Para 3) virus [100].

Hormonal Activity

Phytoestrogens are produced by a wide variety of plants and include flavonoids, isoflavonoids, coumestans (coumestrol), and lignans. These compounds have estrogenic activity and are most abundant in leguminous plants, in particular soybean which contains high concentrations of daidzein and genistein [101]. Other isoflavones which are found in legumens are biochanin A and formononetin. Also kaempferol and quercetin can exhibit antiestrogenic activity [102].

Phytoestrogens act both through estrogen receptor-(ER) dependent and ER-independent mechanisms. Many legume extracts contain phytoestrogens with the ability to bind preferentially to Erβ and modulate the expression if of genes regulated by ER [103]. Of the seven legume extracts tested by Boue Stephen M et al, kudzu root extract showed the highest levels of estrogenic activity in both cell proliferation and transcriptional activation of ERβ and also displayed the highest binding affinity for ERβ. Kudzu fractions isolated by HPLC indicated several isoflavones, in particular puerarin, are responsible for the observed high estrogenic activity [104].

Phytoestrogens could be used to reduce fertility and/or to protect menopausal women against symptoms of menopause [105] and they have also been suggested to protect against hormone-related cancers such as those of breast or prostate [106,107]. Nevertheless recent studies indicate that these compounds could also be implicated in the development of breast cancer [108].

1.3. Chemical Characterization

Phenolic compounds analysis in plants and food is of great importance. In fact, phenols total amount and their identification can provide important information regarding the potential benefit of these plant secondary metabolites for human health. Moreover, the characterization of phenolic patterns can give significant indications to trace the origin of some natural products. For instance, flavonoids and caffeoylquinic acids can be used as fingerprints of plants [109]. Since homogentisic acid (2,5-dihydroxyphenylacetic acid), which was isolated from strawberry-tree (*Arbutus unedo* L.) honey, has been found in the nectar and has not been detected in any other type of honey originating from a diverse botanical source, it could well be used as a marker of this unifloral honey [110]. Also coumaric and gallic acids can be used for the authentication of Australian sunflower honey [111].

Usually phenolic compounds analysis involves both qualitative and quantitative aspects. During the years, traditional methods used to evaluate total phenolic amount have been integrated by increasingly sophisticated analytical techniques able to give complete information about each phenol structure. Nevertheless, at present many phenols remain unidentified and classes like tannins are poorly investigated.

Several spectrophotometric methods are still used to estimate phenolic content: the Folin Ciocalteu assay is based on an oxidation reaction and the results (usually expressed as gallic acid equivalents) allow to determine the total phenolic amount of samples; anthocyanins can be measured evaluating their color variation according to pH or after bleaching by means of sulphur dioxide [1]. Such methods are rather easy to use, but they are also relatively approximate because of different responses of the various phenol structures and the interference of other compounds (like sugars or ascorbic acid) [112]. This explains why literature data on phenols content are sometimes difficult to compare and often contradictory.

Powerful analytical techniques are represented by UV-Vis analysis coupled with chromatographic separation. Due to the extreme variability of these molecules, phenolic compounds show typical UV-Vis spectra that can be useful to determine their classification into a phenolic class rather than into another (table 1.3.1). The first practical use of such properties was the separation of phenols using the thin layer chromatography (TLC) method and the identification of phenolic compounds classes by specific reaction under UV light at different wavelengths or chromatic reaction with inorganic or organic compounds [113].

The natural evolution of such UV-Vis analysis and chromatographic separation was the development of high-performance liquid chromatography (HPLC) methods using UV-VIS detectors or diode array detectors (DAD). Such methods allow to easily characterize phenolic fractions in various samples, from raw vegetable material to processed food. The majority of the methods described in scientific papers use non-polar columns like C_{18} and polar eluent mixtures usually made of acidified water, and methanol or acetonitrile [114]. Sakakibara et al. developed a method for the determination of all the polyphenols in vegetables, fruits, and teas at once using an HPLC system and a photodiode array detector. This method allows to quantitatively determine individual classes of polyphenols, simple polyphenols, flavones, flavonols, flavanones, catechins, isoflavones, anthocyanidins, chalcones, and anthraquinones, including their glycosides, after a simple pretreatment involving homogenization in liquid nitrogen, lyophilization, and extraction with 90% methanol (recovery ranges from 68 to 92%, depending on the chemicals used) [115]. Recently, a standard analytical method was developed in order to analyze glycosylated flavonoids and other phenolic compounds in plant food materials [116]. This method uses an aqueous methanol extraction, followed by reverse phase liquid chromatographic separation, diode array and mass spectrometric detection.

Coupling mass spectrometry (MS) to HPLC apparatus is nowadays one of the most promising analytical procedures in phenolic compounds investigation. MS detector is extremely useful for the identification of phenolic compounds being able to elucidate the numerous and complex structures, even at low concentrations. The most widely used ionization methods for phenols analysis are the ion-spray techniques such as electrospray ionization (ESI), and atmospheric pressure chemical ionization (APCI). Today commercial HPLC–MS instruments can accommodate both of these techniques. APCI and ESI can be operated under both positive and negative ion modes and sensitivity and selectivity of detection can be increased using SIM (selected ion monitoring) instead of full scan acquisition mode. Tandem mass spectrometry, that is two (MS/MS) or more (MS^n) mass

Table 1.3.1. Typical phenolics UV-VIS spectra

	□	UV-Vis spectra
simple phenols	210-280	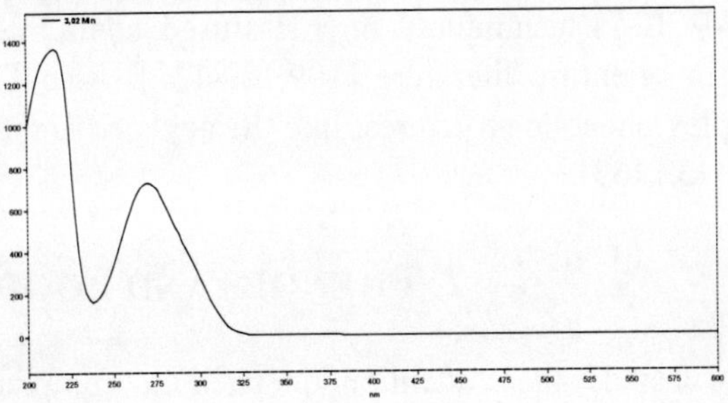 gallic acid
Hydroxycinnamic acids	310-330	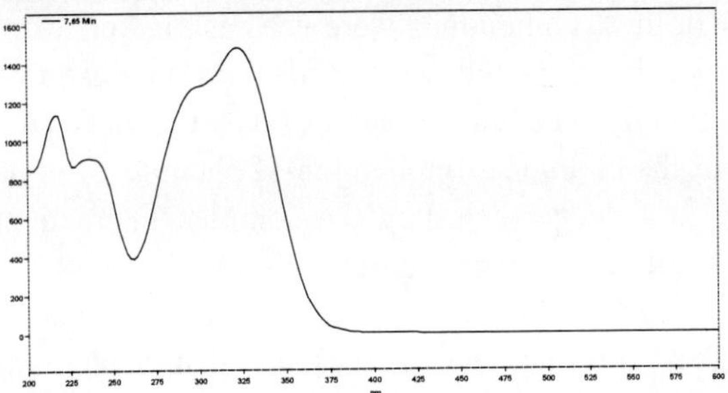 caffeic acid
Flavones / Flavonols	330-380	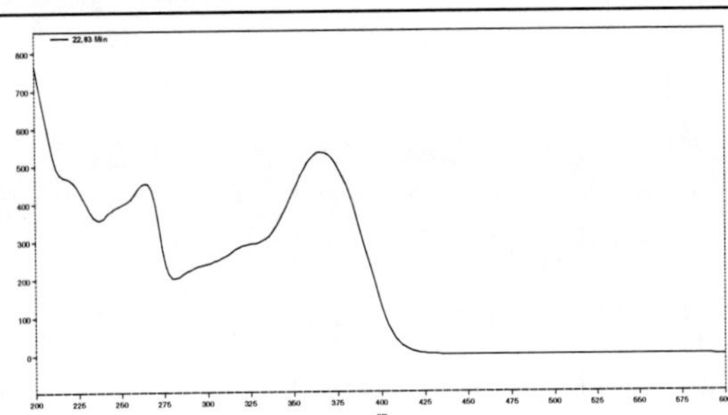 quercetin
Anthocyanins	520-540	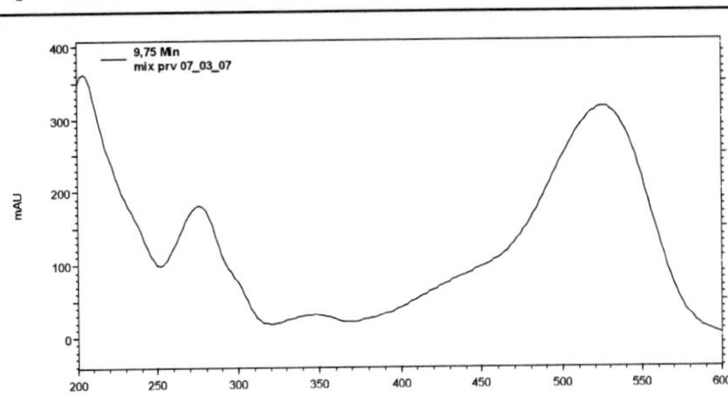 malvidin-3-*O*-glucoside

analyzers coupled in series, produce specific fragmentations of the precursor and daughter ions, and thus provide selective information on molecular structures. From the second half of the 90' publications on HPLC-DAD-ESI/MS methods for phenolic compounds in fruits, food and beverages have flourished [117-122]. More recently HPLC-DAD-ESI/MS/MS has been used to study anthocyanins [123,124], C-glycosyl flavones [125], acylated flavonoid-*O*-glycosides and methoxylated flavonoids [126], isoflavonoids [127] and lignins [128]. Even if HPLC-DAD-APCI/MS technique is now less used, some interesting applications on phenols can be found in scientific literature [109,129-131]. Also NMR (^{1}H and ^{13}C) is useful to elucidate complex phenolic structures, like the acylated anthocyanin-vinyl-flavanol pigments of aged wines [132,133].

2. Phenols and Food

During the last decades, attention on phenolic compounds has changed, focusing on diverse aspects according to the emerging interests in basic research or in everyday life aspects. At first, these compounds were used as markers of plant families, but gradually their biological properties attracted a great deal of interest from almost every branch of the scientific community. The huge amount of data that have since been obtained, have helped to clarify some of the biological implication of phenols, even in an everyday matter like human nutrition. The knowledge regarding the complex interactions between phenolic compounds and other inorganic and organic compounds and within phenols themselves, which take place from plants to foods, is increasingly getting clearer. This is particularly important for food producers as these information can be used to manufacture products that maintain most of the original phenolic content and to improve phenols stability during the phases of processing, storage and aging. Moreover, at present, it is possible to use by-products and agri-industrial wastes deriving from the processing of plant foods (citrus, olive, wine and fruit juices industries) to extract phenolic residues that can be reutilized [134-137].

2.1. Phenols in Food

Phenolic compounds can be found in a wide array of edible products such as fruit (apples, blackberries, cherries, citrus, cranberries, grapes, pears, plums, raspberries, and strawberries), vegetables (broccoli, cabbage, celery, onion and parsley), honey, wine, chocolate, tea, oils from olive and seeds, and so forth. table 2.1.1. reports some examples of phenolic compounds in food.

Foods from vegetable sources differ in phenols content both from a qualitative and a quantitative point of view. Many studies have been carried out in order to evaluate both the total amount of phenols and the relative amount of each class of these compounds or even of a single compound in food. Often literature data are difficult to compare due to both the diversity of measuring methods and the intrinsic variability of phenols content in vegetables (see paragraph 1.3). In addition, although raw material is the source of phenolic compounds, the exact nature of the substances that are introduced by humans depends on the processing and storage conditions of food. Phenols are highly reactive compounds that can react with oxygen, inorganic and organic molecules and are good substrates for enzymes such as oxidases, glycosidases and esterases [138]. The reduction of phenolic compounds content during food processing from raw vegetables to edible products can be related to the removal of parts of the plant which are rich in phenolic compounds, to the leakage of phenols into water or to their degradation through various processes. Food technology specialists are well aware of most of the major changes that occur during food processing. For instance, wine is a typical product for which technology can greatly influence phenolic composition throughout its modifications from grape into must and finally into wine. In grapes peel is rich in flavonols and, as for the red variety, also in anthocyanins; flesh is rich in hydroxycinnamic acids and seeds in galloylated proanthocyanidins. Consequently, white wine can be obtained from red grapes if skins are immediately removed after pressing; alternatively red wine is obtained if maceration with skins lasts long enough to extract anthocyanins.

Vegetables and fruit are the first and most important source of phenolics, many scientific papers have deled with both the total phenolic quantity in them and their chromatographic characterization. Furthermore, government structures, such as the United States Department of Agriculture (USDA), started to create databases on flavonoids [139] that are constantly updated by the scientific community [140]. Scientist are now mainly concentrated on elucidating the chemical structures and the various changes during processing, of phenolic compounds. Phenols like carnosol and rosmarinic acid, are found in many spices like rosemary, thyme, sage and oregano [141]. Interestingly rosemary showed the presence of several flavonoids (eriocitrin, luteolin 3'-*O*-β-D-glucuronide, hesperidin, diosmin, isoscutellarein 7-*O*-glucoside, hispidulin 7-*O*-glucoside, and genkwanin) with a diverse distribution in leaves, flowers, stems, and roots during plant growth [142]. Red cabbage extract contains a high fraction of anthocyanins (137.5 ± 2.9 mg/100 g, mainly cyanidin-3-diglucoside-5-glucoside derivatives) and when pickled, the product shows an extremely similar profile with only small variations in the relative abundances of the peaks [143].

Some of the most important world's fruit crops like apples, citrus and grapes, have been extensively studied. Apples and ciders are known sources of polyphenols, mainly flavan-3-ols ((-)-epicatechin, procyanidin B2) and hydroxycinnamic acids (chlorogenic acid) [144], but also protocatechuic acid [145], and chalcones [146]. Quercetin glucosides have been almost exclusively found in peel, while cyanidin 3-galactoside was found only in red apple peel [147]. Citrus fruits are usually eaten both as fresh products and juices, owing to their nutritional value and enjoyable flavor. Citrus fruits are rich in flavanones and show a distinct flavanone profile [148]. Sour oranges (*Citrus aurantium*) mainly contain naringin and neohesperidin (and have the highest quantity of total flavanones, 48 mg/100 g); sweet oranges (*C. sinensis*), tangerines (*C. reticulate*), and tangors are characterized by the presence of hesperidin and narirutin (and total flavanones are similar, about 20 mg/100 g); tangelos are halfway between sour and sweet oranges and their flavanone profile exhibits characteristics of both species (total flavanones 30 mg/100) [149]. Flavone-di-*C*-glycosides showed to have a different pattern of distribution in citrus fruits: 6,8-di-*C*-glucopyranosylapigenin is characteristic of orange juice, while 6,8-di-*C*-glucopyranosyldiosmetin is the most important *C*-glycoside in lemon and citron juice; in bergamot juice the concentrations of 6,8-di-*C*-glucopyranosylapigenin and 6,8-di-*C*-glucopyranosyldiosmetin are similar; clementine juice is distinctive as the amount of both *C*-glycosides is insignificant [150]. Anthocyanins are also found in citrus fruits and cyanidin-3-glucoside and its derivatives acylated with malonic acid have been detected [151]. Tropical fruits like guava, star fruit and langsat have a total amount of phenols which is higher than that of orange (75 ± 10 mg/100 g), while mangosteen, banana, water apple, kedondong, and papaia have a lower content of phenols compared to oranges [152].

Beverages obtained from fruits such as fruit juices, wines and liquers, show a typical phenolic pattern that correlates with the one of fruit of origin. Wines from fruits can be classified according to their total phenols content: high in total phenolics, 1500-2000 mg of gallic acid equivalent (GAE)/L (red wine, elderberry wine, blueberry wine, black currant wine); moderately high in total phenolics, 500-1000 mg GAE/L (icewine, cherry wine, raspberry wine, cranberry wine, plum wine); and low in total phenolics, 250-400 mg GAE/L (white wine, apple wine, peach wine, pear wine) [153]. A similar situation can be found in liquors obtained from berries and fruits, in particular total phenolic compounds are higher than 1000 mg GAE/L in cherry and red raspberry-black currant liquors [154].

Grape wine is a product for which a huge amount of work on phenols has been done and many reviews have been published. Almost all the classes of phenolics have been identified and several specific phenolic compounds have been characterized [1,155,156]. Obviously, grape variety and the kind of processing of the must till the wine is bottled, deeply affect the final phenolic compounds profile of wine [157]. Total phenolics content is higher in red wines and Cabernet Sauvignon; Merlot and Pinot noir usually show a 1000-3000 mg/L of GAE value [158,159]. Rosè and white wines show lower amount [1,160]. Studies on phenols allowed to distinguish significant differences between several varieties of wine. For instance, Tannat wines, show a high amount of delphinidin, petunidin and non-acylated glucosides, while malvidin and acetates are significantly higher in Cabernet-Sauvignon wines and peonidin and coumarates proportions are superior in Merlot [161]. Discriminant analysis revealed that flavanols, especially procyanidin B1 and B2, exert a profound influence on both cultivar and geographical origin-based differentiation. On the contrary, flavonols have a rather minor impact, assigned only to the geographical origin-based differentiation [162]. Several hydroxycinnamic acids (caffeic, ferulic, *p*-coumaric acids and their tartaric esters) have been identified [157], and some unusual ones, like 2-S-glutahtionylcaftaric acid, have been characterized [163]. Main flavonols are myricetin, quercetin, kaempferol and isorhamnetin and their 3-glucosides and 3-glucuronides. In addition, the methoxylated trisubstituted flavonols, laricitrin and syringetin, have been predominantly found as 3-glucosides. 3-galactosides of kaempferol and laricitrin, the 3-glucuronide of kaempferol, and the 3-(6''-acetyl)glucosides of quercetin and syringetin are minority flavonols [164]. Total anthocyanins are approximately 400 mg/L, while monomeric anthocyanins, mainly represented by malvidin-3-*O*-glucoside, range between 20-100 mg/L [1,158,159]. Peculiar ethyl-bridged flavanols are produced by the reaction of (+)-catechin with acetaldehyde under the typical acid condition of wines [165]. Anthocyanin-derived pigments composed of a pyranoanthocyanin moiety linked to substituted cinnamyl group have been recently characterized [166]. *trans*-Resveratrol has been found both in red and white wines, although production of this phytoalexin is higher red grapes [167,168]. Other stilbenes like the glucosidated forms *cis*-piceid and *trans*-piceid can be twice or three times the *trans*-resveratrol amount in grape-vines like Merlot [169].

Herbal teas obtained by infusions of fruits or herbs in hot water, are an everyday phenolic source. Tea is the most studied of these herb extracts. HPLC analysis of green tea shows that (-)-epigallocathechin-3-gallate is its main polyphenolic constituent (over 60% of the total catechins), followed by (−)-epigallocatechin, (−)-epicatechin and (−)-epicatechin-3-gallate [170]. Other compounds in green tea are the flavonols (quercetin, kaempferol and rutin) and phenolic acids [171]. As previously mentioned (see paragraph 1.2), the manufacturing process to obtain black tea modifies its original phenolic pool leading to the formation of dimers of catechins. Both green and black tea total polyphenols roughly amount to 1000 mg/L [172, while mate polyphenols are around 75 mg/100mL.

Edible oils from olives or seeds have been intensely studied because phenols, which are part of the so called unsaponifiable fraction, contribute to their protection from oxidation [173]. Usually, before the oils extraction from fruits or seeds, the amount phenolic compounds is higher, however during processing compounds with high polarity, especially glycosides, are lost. Moreover, during oil processing biotransformation occurs leading to the formation of new phenolic compounds [174]. Olive oil is characterized by: tyrosol and hydroxytyrosol and their derivatives, like oleuropein and ligstroside and their aldehydic forms [175-179]; *p*-coumaric, ferulic and caffeic acids [180]; luteolin and apigenin and lignans like pinoresinol [175,181]. The antioxidant activity of oils is directly connected with their phenolic content. In addition it is important to note that such activity is also influenced by the quality of phenolic compounds. Lignans, mainly pinoresinol derivatives, seem to have a low antioxidant activity, while secoridoids (oleuropein derivatives) have a higher antioxidant activity [182]. Oilseeds show typical differences according to their origin: grape-seed oils are rich in proanthocyanidins, sesame oil contains sesaminol and sesamol; rapeseed oil in rich in sinapic acid and other phenolic acids [183,184]; pumpkin oils contain hydroxycinnamic acids [185]; and soybean is very rich in isoflavones and some of them can be found in the oil [186].

Honey contains many phenolic compounds which vary according to the floral sources used by bees. Phenolic compounds like phenylacetic, caffeic, and protocatechuic acids [187], methyl siringate [188], gallic, ellagic and coumaric acids [111], tricetin, quercetin and its methyl derivatives [189,190], myricetin, kaempferol, pinobanksin pinocembrin [191], pinostrobin [192], acacetin, chrysin [193], and apigenin [194] have been found. Besides the important nutritional aspects connected with the presence of various phenolic compounds in honeys [192-195], for some of these substances it has been possible to correlate their presence in honey with their specific floral source. Thus phenolic compound act as markers and can be very useful when the information from pollen analysis is not sufficient [110,111,196]. Beverages obtained with honey, like mead, also show a polyphenolic profile correlated with that of the honeys that have been used.

Coffee (*Coffea arabica*) contains flavan-3-ols (catechins and proanthocyanidins), hydroxycinnamic acids (caffeoylquinic acid, caffeoylquinic acid derivatives, and *p*-coumaroylquinic acid), flavonols (quercetin, isoquercitrin, quercetin-3-O-arabinose, hyperoside, naringenin, luteolin, apigenin and some O-glucosides and C-glucosides of these compounds), and anthocyanidins [197,198]. Cocoa contains catechin, epicatechin, cyanidin-3-galactoside and cyanidin-3-arabinoside [199] and total phenolics (611 mg of gallic acid equivalents, GAE) and flavonoids (564 mg of epicatechin equivalents, ECE) amount per serving are much higher than black tea (124 mg of GAE and 34 mg of ECE, respectively), green tea (165 mg of GAE and 47 mg of ECE), and red wine (340 mg of GAE and 163 mg of ECE) [200].

Table 2.1.1. Phenolic compounds in food

Class		main constituents	dietary sources
Non flavonoid	Benzoic acids	gallic acid ellagic acid *p*-hydroxybenzoic tyrosol	honey grape passion fruit, strawberry olive, table olives
	Hydroxycinnamic acids	caffeic acid *p*-coumaric acid ferulic acid esters	asparagus, coffee, grape, olive asparagus, grape, spinach cabbage, grain, spinach, tomato, apricot, grape, wine, herbs
	Stilbenes	resveratrol (trans e cis)	grape, wine, peanuts
Flavonoid	Flavan-3-ols	catechin / epicatechina epigallocatechin epigallocatachin gallate	apple, black grape, red wine, tea green and black tea green and black tea
	Flavonols	quercetin kaempferol myricetin (and their glycosides)	grape, honey, hop, onion, tea, broccoli, endive, grapefruit, tea cranberry, grape, maize, wine
	Flavanones	hesperetin naringenin taxifolin (and their glycosides)	citrus fruits, cumin, peppermint citrus fruits, coffee citrus fruits
	Flavones	apigenin chrysin luteolin rutin	celery, cereals, honey, parsley honey, fruit skin cereals, herbs, olive broccoli, onion, tea
	Isoflavonoids	genistein daidzein	legumes, soybeans
	Anthocyanins	delphinidin cyanidin peonidin petunidin malvidin pelargonidin (and their glycosides)	black currant, blueberry cherry, raspberry, red cabbage blueberry, cranberry blueberry, black bean blueberry, myrtle, black grape, red wine red radish, strawberry

2.2. Bioavailability of Phenols

As illustrated in the previous paragraphs, over the past years many researchers have focused their attention on the potential benefic effects of polyphenols. Nevertheless, despite the enormous amount of data, the intriguing question weather these compounds have a real protective effect in humans remains unanswered. In fact, polyphenols are introduced through the food chain and undergo several complex metabolic reactions before they reach their potential site of action. During these biochemical and enzymatic processes phenolic compounds are extensively modified, thus becoming more or less bioavailable.

Usually polyphenols are present in food in the form of esters, glycosides, or polymers that cannot be absorbed in their native form but must be hydrolyzed by intestinal enzymes or by the colonic microflora, before they can be absorbed. During the course of absorption, polyphenols are then conjugated in the small intestine and later in the liver, owing to a physiologic metabolic detoxification process that mainly involves methylation, sulfation, and glucuronidation [201]. These polyphenols conjugates are chemically distinct from their parent compounds, differing in size, polarity and ionic form, thus their chemical behavior is likely to be different form that of their native compounds [202]. In order to understand the biological activities of polyphenols it is therefore essential to investigate their several mechanisms of action, not only considering the specific environment of their site of action, but also in view of the chemical form which they acquire going through metabolic processes.

Unfortunately, the biological activities of polyphenols have often been evaluated *in vitro* on pure enzymes, cultured cells, or isolated tissues by using polyphenol aglycones or some glycosides that are present in food. Therefore very little is known about the biological properties of the conjugated derivatives present in plasma or tissues [201]. Morover, much of the evidence on the prevention of diseases by polyphenols is derived from *in vitro* or animal experiments, which are often performed with doses much higher than those to which humans are exposed through the diet [203]. All of these aspects must be taken into account in the design of future experimental studies in the field of polyphenols; there is a need to try to model the human situation more closely.

The absorption and thus the bioavailability of polyphenols, could be affected by the direct interaction between these compounds and some components of food, such as proteins and polysaccharides, or by the indirect effects of the diet on various parameters of gut physiology (pH, intestinal fermentations, etc). Dietary fiber, for example, stimulating intestinal fermentation could influence the production of particular microbial metabolites. However existing data do not suggest a marked effect of the various diet components on polyphenol bioavailability [201].

In the small intestine conjugated polyphenols can penetrate the gut wall by passive diffusion [204], by means of specific carriers [205] or using both mechanisms depending on compounds concentration [206]. Polyphenols that are not absorbed in the small intestine reach the colon where the microflora can extensively metabolize them. It has been estimated that about 48% of dietary polyphenols are bioaccessible in the small intestine, while 42% become bioaccessible in the large intestine [207]. The identification and quantification of microbial metabolites represents an important field of research. Some microbial metabolites may have a physiologic effect; as in the case of hydroxyphenylacetic acids which have been suggested to inhibit platelet aggregation [208].

After intestinal absorption polyphenol metabolites are not free in the blood but are bond to albumin. The effect of albumin binding on the biological activity of polyphenols is unclear. Studies on the antioxidant activity of albumin-bound quercetin metabolites indicate that it should not influence its biological effects but possibly delay its clearance from plasma thus allowing an efficient distribution to target organs [209].

Many researchers have indicated the existence of an interindividual variability in the metabolization of some polyphenols. This could depend on several factors, including metabolic enzymes polymorphisms and the variability in intestinal microflora composition.

Colonic microflora composition, which has also been implicated in the protection from carcinogens, inflammation and oxidative stress [32]. is able to allow the metabolization of certain polyphenols. This is the case for example of the metabolite equol, produced from soya daidzein [210]. In fact there is a great interindividual variability in the capacity to produce equol. Only 30-40% of the occidental people ("equol producers") excrete significant quantities of equol after consumption of isoflavones. The corresponding percentage among the Asian populations is unknown, but a recent study suggested that the percentage in Japanese men could be as high as 60% [201].

Plasma concentrations reached after polyphenols consumption vary highly according to the nature of the polyphenol and the food source. Several studies indicate that isoflavones and quercetin have the longest permanence in the blood stream: on the order of 4–8 [211,212] and 17–18 [213] h, respectively. Some ellagitannins metabolites from pomegranate juice are detectable in human plasma and can persist in urine up to 48h [214].

One of the main objectives of bioavailability studies is to individuate the polyphenolic compound which is better absorbed and might lead to the formation of active metabolites. Manach et al have reviewed 97 studies of various classes of polyphenols in order to compare their bioavailability. They pointed out that bioavailability varies widely among polyphenols also depending on their dietary sources. Plasma concentrations of total metabolites range from 0 to 4 μmol/L, with an intake of 50 mg aglycone equivalents. The polyphenols that are most well absorbed in humans are isoflavones and gallic acid, followed by catechins, flavanones, and quercetin glucosides, with different kinetics. The least well-absorbed polyphenols are the proanthocyanidins, the galloylated tea catechins, and the anthocyanins [201].

Some researchers underline the fact that polyphenols may also have anti-nutritional effects. For example nonheme iron absorption is inhibited by green tea and rosemary extracts [215]. Furthermore, polyphenols may affect drug bioavailability and pharmacokinetics. For example Shirou Itagaki et al. have shown that ferulic acid is able to affect the transport of Nateglinide [216]. Many drugs have shown an increased bioavailability when taken after grapefruit juice ingestion, because of inhibition of Cytochrome P450 3A4 (CYP3A4) [217,218].

2.3. Phenolic Compounds and Sensory Properties

Nutritional characteristics of phenols usually regard their numerous biological activities (see paragraph 1.2) or their influence on the digestibility of nutrients. Negative effects due to the capacity of some phenolic compounds to bind organic molecules, like proteins and carbohydrates, or to chelate minerals, thus reducing food digestibility and nutrients bioavailability are often reported. Many phenolic compounds can also affect sensory characteristics of food and beverages. As the appearance of food, its color, smell, taste and consistence, have a great influence in inducing consumers to eat it, polyphenols play a major role in contributing to its attractiveness.

Phenolic compounds can determine the color of vegetables and their derived products, providing hues from yellow to orange, red, purple and even blue. Anthocyanins are primarily responsible for the often colorful aspect of vegetables, but they can also be added in food and beverages as natural colorants (e.g. food additive E126). The *in vivo* color of anthocyanins is affected by various factors such as the pH value of cell medium. Moreover, intramolecular copigmentation in acylated anthocyanins, and intermolecular copigmentation with flavones can stabilize the colors. Intramolecular copigmentation is due to interaction between the planar pyrylium ring and the aromatic acylating chains that protect the molecule from hydration in environmental conditions with pH values that range from acid to neutral. Free malonyl groups attached to the glucose at the C-3 position also stabilize the color by increasing the medium acidity in the cell vacuole [63]. The intermolecular copigmentation, generally with flavones and flavonols, determines the proper color of plant tissues. Studies demonstrated that usually the levels of copigments and anthocyanins are negatively correlated because flavones and anthocyanins share common precursors. In wine this correlation affects colors intensity [219]. Studies on red wines obtained from single cultivar grapes showed different behaviors connected with the evolution of the hue from purple-red to yellow-red. Therefore it is hard to predict colors evolution until stability is reached, owing to the formation of polymeric pigments [220,221]. Enzymatic oxidation is one of the major processes involving phenolic compounds. It starts as soon as the cell is damaged and contents of vacuoles mix together. This way various enzymes catalyze the transformation of phenols causing the browning of vegetables. One of the most active classes of enzymes involved in these reactions are polyphenol oxidases. These enzymes produce *o*-quinones followed by brown colored products known as melanins. Sometimes browning is desiderable, as in the case of cocoa, tea and coffee; but usually this modification is a problem for juices or puree obtained from fruit. The color of aged alcoholic products like wines, brandy etc is highly influenced by co-pigmentation due to the complex reactions that take place between phenolic compounds that lead to the formation of oligomeric and polymeric structures. Several experimental data indicate that incubation of (+)-catechin with glyoxylic acid caused the initial colorless solution to turn into brown after some time. The reactions implicated in the browning phenomenon start with the formation of bridged colorless derivatives, then xanthene and finally yellowish oxidation derivatives [222]. Acetaldehyde, furfural and HMF are also known to induce the polymerization of flavanols and anthocyanins [223,224] and the formation of dark derivatives.

The contribution of phenolic compounds to smell perceptions is less important, due to the low volatility of these molecules. Some volatile phenols like vanillin, eugenol, thymol and carvacrol are potent odorants responsible for the smell of spices and herbs. Phenols like guaiacol, 4-methylguaiacol, acetovanillone and vanillyl alcohol are found at much lower concentrations in vanilla beans than vanillin, but proved to have a smell as intense as vanillin [225]. Moreover, recently volatile phenols like ethyl and vinyl phenol and guaiacol have gained more interest due to their importance for smell in wine [226]. Interestingly, barrels used for wine, vinegar and other alcoholic spirits, can transfer the phenolic compounds produced from breakdown of lignins to their content which then acquires a smoky-burnt smell. Smoke flavorings are considered as additives of natural origin obtained from wood and contain several phenols like phenol, o-cresol, p-cresol, guaiacol, 4-methyloguaiacol and syringol derivatives [227].

Another sensory aspect of phenols is connected with taste. This perception is particularly complicated because it includes an initial sensation when food or beverages are introduced in the mouth and a sensation after deglutition (aftertaste). Additionally, tactile sensations such as texture, dryness and surface roughness, can be perceived in the mouth. Some phenolic compounds, especially those having a small molecular weight, are responsible for the bitter and sour taste of food, while tannins are related to astringency. Astringency is considered a tactile sensation and is caused by a reaction between tannins and salivary proteins which leads to a loss of mouth lubrication [132]. Anthocyanidins monoglucosides and monoglucosides coumarates do no contribute to astringency nor bitterness of wine, while they can contribute to increase the fullness sensation of these extracts. In wine, astringency usually increases with both the degree of polymerization and the extent of galloylation [219,228], while there are evidences that the reduction of astringency during ageing can be due both to polymerization and hydrolysis reactions [1,228,229]. The introduction of an ethyl-bond between each catechin unit can contribute to bitterness [230,231]. It is important to note that in wines, when ethanol level and pH values increase, the astringency perception is reduced: while pH affects only astringency, ethanol also contributes to the perception of tannin oligomers bitterness, especially at usual wine ethanol levels (11–15%) [232]. Phenols are important for olive oil taste and a good linear correlation between the bitter sensory notes and the oleuropein and ligstroside derivatives such as p-HPEA-EDA and 3,4-DHPEA-EDA has been found [233]. Moreover, fractions containing p-HPEA-EDA produce a strong burning pungent sensation. In contrast, the fraction containing 3,4-DHPEA-EDA only causes a slight burning sensation mainly perceived on the tongue [234]. A study on sorghum grain showed that bitterness and astringency of sorghum with and without tannins are perceived as similar [235]. Heiniö et al. found that phenolic acids, alkylresorcinols and lignans have a similar pattern of distribution in the rye grain as the flavor attributes: the phenolic compounds are located in the outer bran fractions being intense in flavor, but not in the mild-tasting inner layers of the grain [236]. Bitterness in carrots is highly related to falcarindiol and to a di-caffeic acid derivative present in peel [237]. Mate from reforested plants was considered more bitter than the beverage from the native plants, and had significantly higher caffeic acid and lower catechin, chlorogenic acid, caffeine, and gallic acid content than native plants [238].

3. CONCLUSION

The constant exposure to a variety of risk factors for cancer or cardiovascular diseases, such as daily stress, diets with a high cholesterol content and environmental pollution, have encouraged the elaboration of potentially preventive strategies for these diseases. Since ancient times polyphenolic compounds have been part of human beings diet and they have recently gained much attention because several epidemiological data indicate that a regular intake of polyphenols through the diet reduces the risk of developing progressive pathologies such as Alzheimer's or cardiovascular diseases.

Furthermore, *in vitro* experimental data have often been encouraging, but occasionally failed to be confirmed *in vivo*. A major part of these data were obtained using simplified experimental models or polyphenols concentrations which are seldom reached within the body. Therefore, information regarding polyphenols and their biological effects is often contradictory and difficult to compare. Experiments should be carried out taking into account critical aspects of polyphenols metabolization such as their real concentration within the body, the chemical nature of their derivatives and the final site of action of these modified molecules.

A better understanding of the biological effects and food distribution of polyphenols is desirable in order to individuate the best source of these substances, both in terms of nutritional value and appetizing characteristics. Nevertheless, in the case of an unbalanced diet or in pathological conditions, the use of polyphenols supplements may be advisable. Along with their biological effects polyphenols have also other interesting applications, for example as food addictives or as markers to track down the vegetable origin of natural products.

Concluding, while researchers struggle to investigate the benefic effects of polyphenolic compounds, a simple and rather old fashion consideration can easily be made by the authors: a moderate and varied intake of polyphenols should characterize our lifestyle and at present seems the best preventive strategy against degenerative diseases.

4. REFERENCES

[1] Ribéreau-Gayon, P; Glories, Y; Maujean, A; Dubourdieu, D (2000). *Handbook of enology, Vols 1 and 2*. Chichester, UK: Wiley.

[2] Rice-Evans, C A; Miller, N J; Paganga, G. Structure-Antioxidant activity relationships of flavonoids and phenolic acids. *Free Radical Biology and Medicine*. 1996, *20*, 933-956.

[3] Rice-Evans, C A; Miller, N J; Paganga, G. Antioxidant properties of phenolic compounds. *Trends in Plant science*. 1997, *2*, 152-159.

[4] Di Carlo, G; Mascolo, N; Izzo, A A; Capasso, F. Flavonoids: old and new aspects of a class of natural therapeutic drugs. *Life Sciences*, 1999, *65*, 337-353.

[5] Bravo, L. Polyphenols: Chemistry, dietary sources, metabolism, and nutritional significance. *Nutrition Reviews*, 1998, *56*, 317-333.

[6] Viitanen, P V; Devine, A L; Khan, M S; Deuel, D L; Van Dyk, D E; Daniell, H. Metabolic engineering of the chloroplast genome using the Echerichia coli ubiC gene reveals that chorismate is a readily abundant plant precursor for p-hydroxybenzoic acid biosynthesis. *Plant Physiology*, 2004, *136*, 4048-60.

[7] Yamauchi, K; Yasuda, S; Fukushima, K. Evidence for the biosynthetic pathway from sinapic acid to syringyl lignin using labeled sinapic acid with stable isotope at both methoxy groups in *Robinia pseudoacacia* and *Nerium indicum*. *Journal of Agricultural and Food Chemistry*, 2002, *50*, 3222-3227.

[8] Heim, K E; Tagliaferro, A R; Bobila, D J. Flavonoid antioxidants: chemistry, metabolism and structure-activity relationships. *Journal of Nutritional Biochemistry*, 2002, *13*, 572-584.

[9] Havsteen, B H. The biochemistry and medical significance of the flavonoids. *Pharmacology and Therapeutics*, 2002, *96*, 67– 202.

[10] Martens, S; Mithöfer, A. Flavones and Flavone Synthases. *Phytochemistry*, 2005, *66*, 2399-2407.

[11] Peterson, J J; Dwyer, J T; Beecher, G R; Bhagwat, S A; Gebhardt, S E; Haytowitz, D B; Holden J M. Flavanones in oranges, tangerines (mandarins), tangors, and tangelos: a compilation and review of the data from the analytical literature. *Journal of Food Composition and Analysis*, 2006, *19*, S66–S73.

[12] Wu, X; Beecher, G R; Holden, J M; Haytowitz, D B; Gebhardt, S E; Prior, R L. Concentrations of anthocyanins in common foods in the United States and estimation of normal consumption. *Journal of Agricultural and Food Chemistry*, 2006, *54*, 4069-4075.

[13] Kong, J-M; Chia, L-S; Goh, N-K; Chia, T-F; Brouillard, R. Analysis and biological activities of anthocyanins. *Phytochemistry*. 2003, *64*, 923–933.

[14] Steele, V E; Kelloff, G J.; Balentine, D; Boone, C W.; Mehta, R; Bagheri, D; Sigman, C C.; Zhu, S; Sharma, S. Comparative chemopreventive mechanisms of green tea, black tea and selected polyphenols extracts measured by *in vitro* bioassays. *Carcinogenes*, 2000, *21*, 63-67.

[15] Iqbal, M; Sharma, S D; Okazaki, Y; Fujisawa, M; Okada, S. Dietary supplementation of curcumin enhances antioxidant and phase II metabolizing enzymes in ddY male mice: possible role in protection against chemical carcinogenesis and toxicity. *Pharmacology and Toxicology*, 2003, 92, 33–38.

[16] Chang, T K H; Chen, J; Yeung, E Y H. Effect of Ginkgo biloba extract on procarcinogen-bioactivating human CYP1 enzymes: Identification of isorhamnetin, kaempferol, and quercetin as potent inhibitors of CYP1B1. *Toxicology and Applied Pharmacology,* 2006, *213*, 18–26.

[17] Pohl, C; Will, F; Dietrich, H; Schrenk, D. Cytochrome P450 1A1 expression and activity in Caco-2 Cells: modulation by apple juice extract and certain apple polyphenol. *Journal of Agricultural and Food Chemistry*, 2006, *54*, 10262-10268.

[18] Peng, G; Dixon, D A; Muga, S J; Smith, T J; Wargovich, M J. Green tea polyphenol epigallocatechin-3-gallate inhibits cyclooxygenase-2 expression in colon carcinogenesis. *Molecular Carcinogenesis*, 2006, *45*, 309-319.

[19] Fujii, H; Yokozawa, T; Kim, Y A; Tohda, C; Nonaka, G I. Protective effect of grape seed Polyphenols against high glucose-induced stress. *Bioscience, Biotechnology and Biochemistry*, 2006, *70*, 2104-2111.

[20] Hong, J; Bose, M; Ju, J; Ryu, J H; Chen, X; Sang, S; Lee, M J; Yang, C S. Modulation of arachidonic acid metabolism by curcumin and related b-diketone derivatives: effects on cytosolic phospholipase A2, cyclooxygenases and5-lipoxygenase. *Carcinogenesis*, 2004, *25*, 1671-1679.

[21] Serraino, I; Dugo L; Dugo, P; Mondello, L; Mazzon, E; Dugo, G; Caputi, A P; Cuzzocrea, S. Protective effects of cyanidin-3-*O*-glucoside from blackberry extract against peroxynitrite-induced endothelial dysfunction and vascular failure. *Life Sciences*, 2003, *73*, 1097–1114.

[22] Jiao, H L; Ye, P; Zhao, B L. Protective effects of green tea polyphenols on human Hepg2 cells against oxidative damage of fenofibrate. *Free Radical Biology and Medicine*, 2003, *35*, 1121–1128.

[23] Guo, Q; Zhao, B; Li, M; Shen, S; Xin, W. Studies on protective mechanisms of four components of green tea polyphenols against lipid peroxidation in synaptosomes. *Biochimica et Biophysica Acta,*1996, *13*, 210-22.

[24] Osawa, T. Protective role of dietary polyphenols in oxidative stress. *Mechanisms of ageing and development*, 1999, *111*, 133–139.

[25] Kagan, V E; Tyurina, Y Y. Recycling and redox cycling of phenolic antioxidants. *Annals of the N.Y. Academy of Sciences,* 1998, *854*, 425–434.

[26] Ohshima, H; Yoshie, Y; Auriol, S; Gilibert, I. Antioxidant and pro-oxidant actions of flavonoids: effects on DNA damage induced by nitric oxide, peroxynitrite and nitroxyl anion. *Free Radical Biology and Medicine,* 1998, *25*, 1057–1065.

[27] Sahu, S C; Gray, G C. Lipid peroxidation and DNA damage induced by morin and naringenin in isolated rat liver nuclei. Food and Chemical Toxicology, 1997, *35*, 443–447.

[28] Almaraz-Abarca, N; Campos, M G; Alvila-Reyes, J A; Naranjo-Jimeneza, N; Corral, J H; Gonzalez-Valdez, L S. Antioxidant activity of polyphenolic extract of monofloral honeybeecollected pollen from mesquite (*Prosopis juliflora*, Leguminosae). *Journal of Food Composition and Analysis*, 2007, *20*, 119–124.

[29] Meiers, S; Kemeny, M; Weyand, U; Gastpar, R; von Angerer, E; Marko, D. The anthocyanidins cyanidin and delphinidin are potent inhibitors of the epidermal growth-factor receptor. *Journal of Agricultural and Food Chemistry*, 2001, *49*, 958–962.

[30] Rosner, K; Röpke, C; Pless, V; Skovgaard, G L. Late type apoptosis free lethal effect of quercetin in human melanoma. *Bioscience, Biotechnology and Biochemistry*, 2006, *70*, 2169-2177.

[31] Jiang, H; Zhang, L; Kuo, J; Kuo, K; Gautam, S C; Groc, L; Rodriguez, A I; Koubi, D; Hunter, T J; Corcoran, G B; Seidman, M D; Levine, R A. Resveratrol-induced apoptotic death in human U251 glioma cells. *Molecular Cancer Therapeutics*, 2005, *4*, 554–561.

[32] Dolara, P; Luceri, C; De Filippo, C; Femia, A P; Giovannelli, L; Caderni, G; Cecchini, C; Silvi, S; Orpianesi, C; Cresci, A. Red wine polyphenols influence carcinogenesis, intestinal microflora, oxidative damage and gene expression profiles of colonic mucosa in F344 rats. *Mutation Research*, 2005, *591*, 237–246.

[33] Cao, H; Hininger-favier, I; Kelly, M A; Benaraba, R; Dawson,H D; Coves, S; Roussel, A M; Anderson, R A. Green tea polyphenol extract regulates the expression of genes involved in glucose uptake and insulin signaling in rats fed a high fructose diet. *Journal of Agricultural and Food Chemistry*, 2007, *55*, 6372-6378.

[34] Xing, N; Chen, Y; Mitchell, S H; Young C Y F. Quercetin inhibits the expression and function of the androgen receptor in LNCaP prostate cancer cells. *Carcinogenesis*, 2001, *22*, 409-414.

[35] Luceri, C; Caderni, G; Sanna, A; Dolara, P. Red wine and black tea polyphenols modulate the expression of cycloxygenase-2, inducible nitric oxide synthase and glutathione-related enzymes in azoxymethane-induced F344 rat colon tumors. *The Journal of Nutrition*, 2002, *132*, 1376–1379.

[36] Shoji, T; Masumoto, S; Moriichi,N; Kobori, M; Kanda, T; Shinmoto,H; Tsushida, T. Procyanidin trimers to pentamers fractionated from apple inhibit melanogenesis in B16 Mouse Melanoma Cells. *Journal of Agricultural and Food Chemistry*, 2005, *53*, 6105-6111.

[37] Roy, G.; Lombardía, M.; Palacios, C.; Serrano, A.; Cespón C.; Ortega, E.; Eiras, P.; Lujan, S.; Revilla, Y.; Gonzalez-Porqué, P. Mechanistic aspects of the induction of apoptosis by lauryl gallate in the murine B-cell lymphoma line Wehi 231. *Archives of Biochemistry and Biophysics*, 2000, *383*, 206-214.

[38] Calcabrini, A; Garcıa-Martınez, M J; Gonzalez, L; Tendero, M J; Ortuno, M T A; Crateri, P; Lopez-Rivas, A; Arancia, G; Gonzalez-Porque´,P; Martın-Perez, J.

Inhibition of proliferation and induction of apoptosis in human breast cancer cells by lauryl gallate. *Carcinogenesis,* 2006, *27*, 1699–1712.

[39] Seerama, N P; Adams, L S; Henning, S M; Niu, Y; Zhang, Y; Nair, M G; Hebera, D. In vitro antiproliferative, apoptotic and antioxidant activities of punicalagin, ellagic acid and a total pomegranate tannin extract are enhanced in combination with other polyphenols as found in pomegranate juice. *Journal of Nutritional Biochemistry*, 2005, *16*, 360– 367.

[40] Nagle, D G; Ferreira, D; Zhou, Y D. Epigallocatechin-3-gallate (EGCG): chemical and biomedical perspectives. *Phytochemistry*, 2006, *67*, 1849–1855.

[41] Lazzé, M.C.; Pizzala, R; Savioa, M; Stivala, L A; Prosperi, E; Bianchi, L. Anthocyanins protect against DNA damage induced by *tert*-butyl-hydroperoxide in rat smooth muscle and hepatoma cells. *Mutation Research*, 2003, *535*, 103–115.

[42] Feng, Q; Torii, Y; Uchida, K; Nakamura, Y; Hara, Y; Osawa, T. Black tea polyphenols, theflavins, prevent cellular DNA damage by inhibiting oxidative stress and suppressing cytocrome P450 1A1 in cell cultures. *Journal of Agricultural and Food Chemistry,* 2002, *50*, 213-220.

[43] Murata, M; Midorikawa, K; Koh, M; Umezawa, K; Kawanishi, S. Genistein and daidzein induce cell proliferation and their metabolites cause oxidative dna damage in relation to isoflavone-induced cancer of estrogen-sensitive organs. *Biochemistry,* 2004, *43,* 2569-2577.

[44] Ross, J. A. Maternal diet and infant leukemia: a role for DNA topoisomerase II inhibitors? *International Journal of Cancer, Supplement,* 1998, *11*, 26-28.

[45] Strick, R; Strissel, P L; Borgers, S; Smith, S L; Rowley, J. D. Dietary bioflavonoids induce cleavage in the *MLL* gene and may contribute to infant leukemia. *Proc. Natl. Acad. Sci,* 2000, *97*, 4790-4795.

[46] Bandele, O J; Osheroff, N. Bioflavonoids as Poisons of Human Topoisomerase IIα and Iiβ *Biochemistry*, 2007, *46*, 6097-6108.

[47] Soleas, G J; Grass, L P; Josephy, D; Goldberg D M; Diamandis, E P. A comparison of the anticarcinogenic properties of four red wine Polyphenols. *Clinical Biochemistry*, 2002, *35*, 119–124.

[48] Choi, J,A; Kim, J Y; Lee, J Y; Kang, C M; Kwon, H J; Yoo, Y D; Kim, T W; Lee Y S; Lee, S J. Induction of cell cycle arrest and apoptosis in human breast cancer cells by quercetin. *International Journal of Oncology,* 2001, *19*, 837-44.

[49] Ranelletti, F O; Maggiano, N; . Serra, F G; Ricci, R; Larocca, L M; Lanza, P; Scambia, G; Fattorossi, A; Capelli, A; Piantelli, M; Quercetin inhibits p21-RAS expression in human colon cancer cell lines and in primary colorectal tumors. *International Journal of Cancer*, 2000, *85*, 438-445

[50] Chakraborty, R N D S; Ghosh, S; Sengupta, A; Das S. Comparative evaluation of cancer chemopreventive efficacy of alpha-tocopherol and quercetin in a murine model. *Journal of experimental and clinical cancer research,* 2004, *23*, 251-258.

[51] Chung, L Y; Cheung, T C, Kong, S K; Fung, K P; Choy, Y M; Chan, Z Y; Kwok, T,T. Induction of apoptosis by green tea catechins in human prostate cancer DU145 cells. *Life Sciences,* 2001, *68*, 1207–1214.

[52] Damianaki, A; Bakogeorgou, E; Kampa, M; Notas, G; Hatzoglou, A; Panagiotou, S; Gemetzi, C; Kouroumalis, E; Martin, P M; Castanas, E. Potent inhibitory action of red

wine polyphonols on human breast cancer cells. *Journal of Cellular Biochemistry*, 2000, *78*, 429–441.

[53] Anekonda, T S. Resveratrol-A boon for treating Alzheimer's Disease. *Brain Research Reviews,* 2006, *52*, 316-326.

[54] Jiang, H; Zhang, L; Kuo, J; Kuo, K; Gautam, S C; Groc, L; Rodriguez, A I; Koubi, D; Hunter, T J; Corcoran, G B; Seidman, M D; Levine, R A. Resveratrol-induced apoptotic death in human U251 glioma cells. *Molecular Cancer Therapeutics*, 2005, *4*, 554–561.

[55] Benitez, D A; Pozo-Guisado, E; Clementi, M; Castellón, E; Fernandez-Salguero, M. Non-genomic action of resveratrol on androgen and oestrogen receptors in prostate cancer: modulation of the phosphoinositide 3-kinase pathway. *British Journal of Cancer*, 2007, *96*, 1595-1604.

[56] Park, J W; Woo, K J; Lee, J T; Lim, J H; Lee, T J; Kim, S H; Choi, Y H, Kwon, T K. Resveratrol induces pro-apoptotic endoplasmic reticulum stress in human colon cancer cells. *OncologyReports*, 2007, 18, 1269-1273.

[57] Casper, R; Quesne, M; Rogers, I M; Shirota, T; Jolivet, A E; Milgrom, E; Savouret, J F. Resveratrol has antagonist activity on the aryl hydrocarbon receptor: implications for prevention of dioxin toxicity, *Molecular Pharmacology*, 1999, *56*, 784–790.

[58] National Vital Statistics Report, *53*, Number 5 (October 2004); http://www.cdc.gov/nchs/products/pubs/pubd/nvsr/nvsr.htm

[59] Freedman, J E; Parker, C; Li, L; Perlman, J A; Frei, B; Ivanov, V; Deak, L R; Iafrati, M D; Folts, J D. Select flavonoids and whole juice from purple grapes inhibit platelet function and enhance nitric oxide release. *Circulation,* 2001, *103*, 2792-2798.

[60] Aviram, M; Dornfeld, L; Kaplan, M; Coleman, R; Gaitini, D; Nitecki, S; Hofman, A; Rosenblat, M; Volkova, N; Presser, D; Attias, J; Hayek, T; Fuhrman. B. Pomegranate juice flavonoids inhibit low-density lipoprotein oxidation and cardiovascular diseases: studies in atherosclerotic mice and in humans. *Drugs under experimental and clinical research,* 2002; *28*, 49-62.

[61] Nikitina, N A; Sobenin, I A; Myasoedova, V A; Korennaya, V V; Mel'nichenko, A,A; Khalilov, E M; Orekhov, A,N. Antiatherogenic effect of grape flavonoids in an ex vivo model. *Bulletin of experimental biology and medicine,* 2006, *141*, 712-715.

[62] Burnett, B P; Jia, Q; Zhao, Y; Levy, R M. A Medicinal extract of *Scutellaria baicalensis* and *Acacia catechu* acts as a dual inhibitor of cyclooxygenase and 5-lipoxygenase to reduce inflammation. *Journal of Medicinal Food,* 2007, *10*, 442–451.

[63] Harborne, J B; Williams, C A; Advances in flavonoid research since 1992. *Phytochemistry,* 2000, *55*, 481-504.

[64] Christie, S; Walker, A F; Lewith, G T. Flavonoids - A new direction for the treatment of fluid retention? *Phytotherapy Research*, 2001, *15*, 467-475.

[65] Kerry, N L; Abbey, M. Red wine and fractionated phenolic compounds prepared from red wine inhibit low density lipoprotein oxidation *in vitro. Atherosclerosis,* 1997, *135*, 93-102.

[66] Zdunczyk, Z; Frejnagel, S; Wròblewska, M; Juskiewicz, J; Oszmianski, J; Estrella, I. Biological activity of polyphenol extracts from different plant sources. *Food Research International*, 2002, *35*, 183–186.

[67] Zhang, Yan; Liu, Y; Wang, T; Li, B; Li, H; Wang, Z; Yang, B. Resveratrol, a natural ingredient of grape skin: antiarrhythmic efficacy and ionic mechanisms. *Biochemical and Biophysical Research Communications,* 2006, *340*, 1192–1199.

[68] Shigematsu, S; Ishida, S; Hara, M; Takahashi, N; Yoshimatsu, H; Sakata. T; Korthuis, R J.. Resveratrol, a red wine constituent polyphenol, prevents superoxide-dependent inflammatory responses induced by ischemia/reperfusion, platelet-activating factor, or oxidants free radical. *Biology and Medicine*, 2003, *34*, 810–817.

[69] Ghiselli, A; Cardini, M; Baldi, A; Scaccini, C. Antioxidant activity of different phenolic fractions separated from an italian red wine. *Journal of Agricultural and Food Chemistry,* 1998, *46*, 361-367.

[70] Ramassamy, C. Emerging role of polyphenolic compounds in the treatment of neurodegenerative diseases: A review of their intracellular targets. *European Journal of Pharmacology,* 2006, *545*, 51–64.

[71] Checkoway, H; Powers, K; Smith-Weller, T; Franklin, G M; Longstreth Jr., W T; Swanson, P D. Parkinson's disease risks associated with cigarette smoking, alcohol consumption, and caffeine intake. *American Journal of Epidemiology,* 2002, *155*, 732–738.

[72] Bastianetto, S; Yao, Z X; Papadopoulos, V; Quirion, R. Neuroprotective effects of green and black teas and their catechin gallate esters against betaamyloid- induced toxicity. *European Journal of Neuroscience*, 2006, 23, 55–64.

[73] Choi, Y.T; Jung, C H; Lee, S R; Bae, J H; Baek, W K; Suh, M H; Park, J; Park, C W; Suh, S,I. The green tea polyphenol (−)-epigallocatechin gallate attenuates beta-amyloid-induced neurotoxicity in cultured hippocampal neurons. *Life Sciences*. 2001, *70*, 603–614.

[74] Levites, Y; Amit, T; Mandel, S; Youdim, M B. Neuroprotection and neurorescue against Abeta toxicity and PKC-dependent release of nonamyloidogenic soluble precursor protein by green tea polyphenol (−)-epigallocatechin-3-gallate. FASEB Journal, 2003, *17*, 952–954.

[75] Rezai-Zadeh, K; Shytle, D; Sun, N; Mori, T; Hou, H; Jeanniton, D; Ehrhart, J; Townsend, K; Zeng, J; Morgan, D; Hardy, J; Town, T; Tan, J. Green tea epigallocatechin-3-gallate (EGCG) modulates amyloid precursor protein cleavage and reduces cerebral amyloidosis in Alzheimer transgenic mice. *The Journal of Neuroscience*, 2005, *25*, 8807-8814.

[76] Lindsay, J, Laurin, D; Verreault, R; Hebert, R; Helliwell, B; Hill, G B; McDowell, I. Risk factors for Alzheimer's disease: a prospective analysis from the Canadian Study of Health and Aging. *American Journal of Epidemiology*, 2002, *156*, 445–453.

[77] Truelsen, T; Thudium, D; Gronbaek, M. Amount and type of alcohol and risk of dementia: the Copenhagen City Heart Study. *Neurology*, 2002, *59*, 1313–1319.

[78] Jang, J H; Surh, Y J. Protective effect of resveratrol on beta-amyloidinduced oxidative PC12 cell death. *Free Radical Biology and Medicine*, 2003, *34*, 1100–1110.

[79] Marambaud, P; Zhao, H; Davies, P. Resveratrol promotes clearance of Alzheimer's disease amyloid-beta peptides. *Journal of Biological Chemistry,* 2005, *280*, 37377–37382.

[80] Shin, D H; Bae, Y C; Kim-Han, J S; Lee, J H; Choi, I Y; Son, K H; Kang, S S; Kim, W K; Hee Han, B. Polyphenol amentoflavone affords neuroprotection against neonatal

hypoxic-ischemic brain damage via multiple mechanisms. *Journal of Neurochemistry*, 2006, 96, 561–572.

[81] Zhang, H,Y; Zhang, H Y. Can food-derived multipotent agents reduce the risk of Alzheimer's disease. *Trends in Food Science and Technology,* 2007, *18*, 492-495.

[82] Lim, G P; Chu, T; Yang, F; Beech, W; Frautschy, S A; Cole, G M. The curry spice curcumin reduces oxidative damage and amyloid pathology in an Alzheimer transgenic mouse. *Journal of Neuroscience*, 2001, *21*, 8370–8377.

[83] Yao, Z; Drieu, K; Papadopoulos, V. The Ginkgo biloba extract EGb 761 rescues the PC12 neuronal cells from beta-amyloid-induced cell death by inhibiting the formation of beta-amyloid-derived diffusible neurotoxic ligands. *Brain Research*, 2001, *889*, 181–190.

[84] Colciaghi, F; Borroni, B; Zimmermann, M; Bellone, C; Longhi, A, Padovani, A; Cattabeni, F; Christen, Y; Di Luca, M. Amyloid precursor protein metabolism is regulated toward alpha-secretase pathway by Ginkgo biloba extracts. *Neurobiology of Disease*, 2004, *16*, 454–460.

[85] Yao, Z X; Han, Z; Drieu, K; Papadopoulos, V. Ginkgo biloba extract (Egb 761) inhibits beta-amyloid production by lowering free cholesterol levels. The *Journal of Nutritional Biochemistry*, 2004, *15*, 749–756.

[86] Bodovitz, S; Klein, W L. Cholesterol modulates alpha-secretase cleavage of amyloid precursor protein. *Journal of Biological Chemistry*, 1996, *271*, 4436–4440.

[87] Djoko, B; Chiou, R Y Y; Shee, J J; Liu, Y W. Characterization of Immunological Activities of Peanut Stilbenoids, Arachidin-1, Piceatannol, and Resveratrol on Lipopolysaccharide-Induced Inflammation of RAW 264.7 Macrophages. *Journal of Agricultural and Food Chemistry*, 2007, *55*, 2376-2383.

[88] Rivero-Peärez, M D; Muniz, P; Lez-Sanjoseä, M G; Antioxidant profile of red wines evaluated by total antioxidant capacity, scavenger activity, and biomarkers of oxidative stress methodologies. *Journal .of Agricultural and Food Chemistry,* 2007, *55*, 5476-5483.

[89] Sharma, V; Mishra, M; Ghosh, S; Tewari, R; Basu, A; Seth, P; Sen, E. Modulation of interleukin-12 mediated inflammatory response in human astrocytes by flavonoids: Implications in neuroprotection. *Brain Research Bulletin,* 2007, *73*, 55–63.

[90] Yamada, K; Shoji, K; Mori, M; Ueyama, T; Matzuo, N; Oka, S; Nishiyama, K; Sugano, M. Structure-activity relationship of polyphenols on inibition of chemical mediator release fro rat peritoneal exudates cells. *In Vitro Cellular and Developmental Biology,* 1999, *35*, 169-174.

[91] Jiménez. R; López-Sepúlveda, R; Kadmiri, M; Romero, M; Vera, R; Sánchez, M; Vargas, F; O'Valle, F; Zarzuelo, A; Dueñas, M; Santos-Buelga, C; Duarte, J. Polyphenols restore endothelial function in DOCA-salt hypertension: Role of endothelin-1 and NADPH oxidase. *Free Radical Biology and Medicine*, 2007, *43*, 462–473.

[92] Cantero, G; Campanella, C; Mateos, S; Cortes, F. Topoisomerase II inhibition and high yield of endoreduplication induced by flavonoids luteolin and quercetin. *Mutagenesis*, 2006, *21*, 321-325.

[93] Matsumoto, H; Nakamura, Y; Tachibanaki, S; Kawamura, S; Hirayama, M. Stimulatory effect of cyanidin 3-glycosides on the regeneration of rhodopsin. *Journal of Agricultural and Food Chemistry*, 2003, *51*, 3560-3563.

[94] Peterson, J; Dwyer, J. Flavonoids: dietary occurrence and biochemical activity. *Nutrition Research*, 1998, *18*, 1995-2018.

[95] Wang, L X; Heredia, A, Song, H J. Resveratrol glucuronides as the metabolites of resveratrol in humans: characterization, synthesis, and anti-HIV activity. *Journal of Pharmaceutical Sciences,* 2004, *93*, 2448-2457.

[96] Li, Y L; Ma, S C; Yang, Y T. Antiviral activities of flavonoids and organic acid from *Trollius chinensis* Bunge. *Journal of Ethnopharmacology*, 2002, *79*, 365-368.

[97] Song, J M; Lee, K H; Seong, B L, Antiviral effect of catechins in green tea on influenza virus. *Antiviral Research*, 2005, *68*, 66–74.

[98] Esquenazi, D; Wigg, M D; Miranda, M M F S; Rodrigues, H M; Tostes J B F; Rozental, S; da Silva, A J R; Alviano, C S. Antimicrobial and antiviral activities of polyphenolics from *Cocos nucifera* Linn. (Palmae) husk fiber extract. *Research in Microbiology*, 2002, *153*, 647-652.

[99] Chang, S L; Chiang, Y M; Chang, C L T; Yeh, H H; Shyur, L F; Kuo, Y H; Wu, T K; Yang, W C. Flavonoids, centaurein and centaureidin, from *Bidens pilosa*, stimulate IFN-gamma expression. *Journal of Ethnopharmacology,* 2007, *112*, 232–236.

[100] Li, Yao-Lan; Ma, S C; Yang, Y T; Ye, S M; But, P P H. Antiviral activities of flavonoids and organic acid from *Trollius chinensis* Bunge. *Journal of Ethnopharmacology*, 2002, *79*, 365–368.

[101] Mazur, W M; Duke, J A; Wahala, K; Rasku, S; Adlercreutz, H. Isoflavonoids and lignans in legumes: Nutritional and health aspects in humans. *Journal of Nutritional Biochemistry,* 1998, *6*, 193-200.

[102] Harris, D M; Besselink, S M; Henning, Go,V L; Heber, D.. Phytoestrogens induce differential estrogen receptor alpha- or beta-mediated responses in transfected breast cancer cells. *Experimental Biology and Medicine*, 2005, *230*, 558–568.

[103] Katzenellenbogen, B S; Choi, I; Delage-Mourroux, R T; Ediger, R; Martini, P G V; Montano, M; Sun, J; Weis, K; Katzenellenbogen, J A. Molecular mechanisms of estrogen action: selective ligands and receptor pharmacology. *Journal of Steroid Biochemistry and Molecular Biology*, 2000, *74*, 279–285.

[104] Boue, S; Wiese, T E; Nehls, S; Burow, M; Elliott, S; Carter-Wientjes, C H; Shih, B Y; Mclachlan, J A; Cleveland, T E. Evaluation of the estrogenic effects of legume extracts containing phytoestrogens. *Journal of Agricultural and Food Chemistry*, 2003, *51*, 2193-2199.

[105] Prouillet, C; Maziére, J C; Maziére, C; Wattela, A; Braziera, M; Kamela, S D. Stimulatory effect of naturally occurring flavonols quercetin and kaempferol on alkaline phosphatase activity in MG-63 human osteoblasts through ERK and estrogen receptor pathway. *Biochemical Pharmacology,* 2004, *67*, 1307–1313.

[106] Bianco, N R; Chaplin,L J; Montano, M M; Differential induction of quinone reductase by phytoestrogens and protection against oestrogen-induced DNA damage. *Biochemical Journal,* 2005, *385*, 279–287.

[107] Vij, U; Kumar, A. Phyto-oestrogens and prostatic growth *National Medical Journal of India,* 2004,*17*, 22-26.

[108] Rice, S; Whitehead, S A. Phytoestrogens and breast cancer – promoters or protectors? *Endocrine-Related Cancer*, 2006, *13*, 995–1015.

[109] Lai, J-P; Lim, Y H; Su, J; Shen, H-M; Ong, C N. Identification and characterization of major flavonoids and caffeoylquinic acids in three Compositae plants by LC/DAD-APCI/MS. *Journal of Chromatography B*, 2007, *848*, 215-225.

[110] Cabras, P; Angioni, A; Tuberoso, C; Floris, I; Reniero, F; Guillou, C; Ghelli, S. Homogentisic acid: a phenolic acid as a marker of Strawberry-Tree (*Arbutus unedo*) honey. *Journal of Agricultural and Food Chemistry*, 1999, *47*, 4064-4067.

[111] Yaoa, L; Jiang, Y; Singanusong, R; Datta, N; Raymont, K. Phenolic acids in Australian Melaleuca, Guioa, Lophostemon, Banksia and Helianthus honeys and their potential for floral authentication. *Food Research International*, 2005, *38*, 651-658.

[112] Stratil, P; Klejdus, B; Kubáň V. Determination of phenolic compounds and their antioxidant activity in fruits and cereals *Talanta*, 2007, *71,* 1741-1751.

[113] Wagner, H. and Bladt, S. (1996). *Plant Drug Analysis. A Thin Layer Chromatography Atlas* (2nd ed.). New York, NY: Springer.

[114] Merken, H M; Beecher, G R. Measurement of food flavonoids by High-Performance Liquid Chromatography: A Review. *Journal of Agricultural and Food Chemistry*, 2000, *48*, 577-599.

[115] Sakakibara, H; Honda, Y; Nakagawa, S; Ashida, H; Kanazawa, K. Simultaneous determination of all polyphenols in vegetables, fruits, and teas. *Journal of Agricultural and Food Chemistry*. 2003, *51*, 571-581.

[116] Lin, L.-Z.; Harnly, J. M. A screening method for the identification of glycosylated flavonoids and other phenolic compounds using a standard analytical approach for all plant materials. *Journal of Agricultural and Food Chemistry*. 2007, *55*, 1084-1096.

[117] Dugo, P; Mondello, L; Errante, G; Zappia, G; Dugo, G. Identification of anthocyanins in berries by narrow-bore high-performance liquid chromatography with electrospray ionization detection. *Journal of Agricultural and Food Chemistry*, 2001, *49*, 3987-3992.

[118] Tomas-Barberan, F A; Gil, M I; Cremin, P; Waterhouse, A L; Hess-Pierce, B; Kader, A A. HPLC-DAD-ESIMS analysis of phenolic compounds in nectarines, peaches, and plums. *Journal of Agricultural and Food Chemistry*, 2001, *49*, 4748-4760.

[119] Mattivi, F; Guzzon, R; Vrhovsek, U; Stefanini, M; Velasco, R. Metabolite profiling of grape: flavonols and anthocyanins. *Journal of Agricultural and Food Chemistry*, 2006, *54*, 7692-7702.

[120] Romani, A; Ieri, F; Turchetti, B; Mulinacci, N; Vincieri, F F; Buzzini, P. Analysis of condensed and hydrolysable tannins from commercial plant extracts. *Journal of Pharmaceutical and Biomedical Analysis*, 2006, *41*, 415-420.

[121] Murkovic, M; Lechner, S; Pietzka, A; Bratacos, M; Katzogiannos, E. Analysis of minor components in olive oil. *Journal of Biochemical and Biophysical Methods*, 2004, *61*, 155-160.

[122] Es-Safi, N-E; Cheynier, V; Moutounet, M. Implication of phenolic reactions in food organoleptic properties. *Journal of Food Composition and Analysis*. 2003, *16*, 535–553.

[123] Heier, A; Blaas, W; Dross, A; Wittkowski, R. Anthocyanin analysis by HPLC/ESI-MS. *American Journal of Enology and Viticulture*, 2002, *53*, 78-86.

[124] Montoro, P; Tuberoso, C I G; Piacente, S; Perrone, A; Cabras, P; Pizza, C. Characterisation by liquid chromatography-electrospray tandem mass spectrometry of anthocyanins in extracts of *Myrtus* communis L. berries used for the preparation of myrtle liqueur. *Journal of Chromatography A*, 2006, *1112*; 232-240.

[125] Ferreres, F; Silva, B M; Andrade, P B; Seabra, R M; Ferreira, M A. Approach to the study of C-glycosyl flavones by Ion Trap HPLC-PAD-ESI/MS/MS: Application to seeds of Quince (*Cydonia oblonga*). *Phytochemical Analysis*. 2003, *14*, 352–359.

[126] Parejo, I; Jáuregui, O; Viladomat F; Bastida, J; Codina, C. Characterization of acylated flavonoid-O-glycosides and meth,oxylated flavonoids from *Tagetes maxima* by liquid chromatography coupled to electrospray ionization tandem mass spectrometry. *Rapid Communications in Mass Spectrometry*, 2004, *18*, 2801–2810.

[127] Farag, M A; Huhman, D V; Lei, Z; Sumner, L W. Metabolic profiling and systematic identification of flavonoids and isoflavonoids in roots and cell suspension cultures of *Medicago truncatula* using HPLC–UV–ESI–MS and GC–MS. *Phytochemistry*, 2007, *68*, 342-354.

[128] Willför, S M; Smeds, A I; Holmbom, B R. Chromatographic analysis of lignins. *Journal of Chromatography A*, 2006, *1112,* 64-77.

[129] Jean-Denis, J B; Pezet, R; Tabacchi, R. Rapid analysis of stilbenes and derivatives from downy mildew-infected grapevine leaves by liquid chromatography–atmospheric pressure photoionisation mass spectrometry. *Journal of Chromatography A*, 2006, *1112,* 263-268.

[130] Counet, C; Callemien, D; Collin, S. Chocolate and cocoa: New sources of *trans*-resveratrol and *trans*-piceid. *Food Chemistry*, 2006, *98,* 649-657.

[131] Alonso-Salces, R M; Ndjoko, K; Queiroz, E F; Ioset, J R; Hostettmann, K; Berrueta, L A; Gallo, B; Vicente F. On-line characterisation of apple polyphenols by liquid chromatography coupled with mass spectrometry and ultraviolet absorbance detection. *Journal of Chromatography A*, 2004, *1046,* 89-100.

[132] Mateus, N; Carvalho, E; Carvalho, A R F; Melo, A; Gonzalez-Paramas, A M; Santos-Buelga, C; Silva, A M S; de Freitas, V. Isolation and structural characterization of new acylated anthocyanin-vinyl-flavanol pigments occurring in aging red wines. *Journal of Agricultural and Food Chemistry*, 2003, *51*, 277-282.

[133] Mateus, N; Silva, A M S; Rivas-Gonzalo, J C; Santos-Buelga, C; de Freitas, V. A new class of blue anthocyanin-derived pigments isolated from red wines. *Journal of Agricultural and Food Chemistry*, 2003, *51*, 1919-1923.

[134] Baydar, N G; Ozkan, G; Cetin, E S. Characterization of grape seed and pomace oil extracts. *Grasas y Aceites*, 2007, *58*, 29-33.

[135] Jing, P; Giusti, M M. Effects of extraction conditions on improving the yield and quality of an anthocyanin-rich purple corn (*Zea mays* L.) color extract. *Journal of Food Science*, 2007, *72*, C363-C368.

[136] Makris, D P; Boskou, G; Andrikopoulos, N K. Recovery of antioxidant phenolics from white vinification solid by-products employing water/ethanol mixtures. *Bioresource Technology*, 2007, *98*, 2963-2967.

[137] Makris, D P; Boskou, G; Andrikopoulos, N K. Polyphenolic content and in vitro antioxidant characteristics of wine industry and other agri-food solid waste extracts. *Journal of Food Composition and Analysis*, 2007, *20*, 125-132.

[138] Cheynier, V. Polyphenols in foods are more complex than often thought. *American Journal of Clinical Nutrition*, 2005, *81*, 223S–229S.

[139] USDA Database for the Flavonoid Content of Selected Foods – 2003, http://www.nal.usda.gov/fnic/foodcomp/Data/Flav/flav.html

[140] Chun, O K; Chung, S J; Song, W O. Estimated dietary flavonoid intake and major food sources of US adults. *Journal of Nutrition*, 2007, *137*, 1244-1252

[141] Kulišič, T; Kriško, A; Dragovič-Uzelac, V; Miloš, M; Pifat G. The effects of essential oils and aqueous tea infusions of oregano (*Origanum vulgare* L. spp. hirtum), thyme (*Thymus vulgaris* L.) and wild thyme (*Thymus serpyllum* L.) on the copper-induced oxidation of human low-density lipoproteins. *International Journal of Food Sciences and Nutrition*, 2007, *58*, 87-93.

[142] Del Baño, M J; Lorente, J; Castillo, J; Benavente-García, O; Marín, M P; Del Río, J A; Ortuño, A; Ibarra I. Flavonoid distribution during the development of leaves, flowers, stems, and roots of Rosmarinus officinalis. Postulation of a biosynthetic. *Journal of Agricultural and Food Chemistry*, 2004, *52*; 4987-4992.

[143] McDougall, G J; Fyffe, S; Dobson, P; Stewart, D. Anthocyanins from red cabbage – stability to simulated gastrointestinal digestion. *Phytochemistry*, 2007, *68*, 1285–1294.

[144] Alonso-Salces, R M; Korta, E; Barranco, A; Berrueta, L A; Gallo, B; Vicente, F. Determination of polyphenolic profiles of Basque Cider apple varieties using accelerated solvent extraction. *Journal of Agricultural and Food Chemistry*, 2001, *49*, 3761-3767.

[145] Wu, J H; Gao, H Y; Zhao, L; Liao, X; Chen, F; Wang, Z; Hu X. Chemical compositional characterization of some apple cultivars *Food Chemistry*, 2007, *103*, 88-93.

[146] D'Abrosca, B; Pacifico, S; Cefarelli, G; Mastellone, C; Fiorentino, A. 'Limoncella' apple, an Italian apple cultivar: Phenolic and flavonoid contents and antioxidant activity. *Food Chemistry*, 2007, *104*, 1333-1337.

[147] Khanizadeh, S; Tsao, R; Rekika, D; Yang, R; DeEll, J. Phenolic composition and antioxidant activity of selected apple genotypes. *Journal of Food Agriculture and Environment*, 2007, *5*, 61-66.

[148] Abeysinghe, D C; Li, X; Sun, C D; Zhang, W S; Zhou, C H; Chen, K S. Bioactive compounds and antioxidant capacities in different edible tissues of citrus fruit of four species. *Food Chemistry*, 2007, *104*, 1338-1344.

[149] Peterson, J; Dwyer, J. Flavonoids: dietary occurrence and biochemical activity. *Nutrition Research*, 1998, *18*, 1995-2018.

[150] Caristi, C; Bellocco, E; Gargiulli, C; Toscano, G; Leuzzi, U. Flavone-di-C-glycosides in citrus juices from southern Italy. *Food Chemistry*, 2006, *95*, 431-437.

[151] Lee, H S. Characterization of major anthocyanins and the color of Red-Fleshed Budd Blood Orange (*Citrus sinensis*). *Journal of Agricultural and Food Chemistry*, 2002, *50*, 1243-1246.

[152] Lim, Y Y; Lim, T T; Tee, J J. Antioxidant properties of several tropical fruits: A comparative study. *Food Chemistry*, 2007, *103*, 1003-1008.

[153] Rupasinghe, H P V; Clegg, S. Total antioxidant capacity, total phenolic content, mineral elements, and histamine concentrations in wines of different fruit sources. *Journal of Food Composition and Analysis*, 2007, *20*, 133-137.

[154] Heinonen, I M; Lehtonen, P J; Hopia, A I. Antioxidant activity of berry and fruit wines and liquors *Journal of Agricultural and Food Chemistry*, 1998, *46*, 25-31.

[155] Pour Nikfardjam, M S; Márk, L; Avar, P; Figler, M; Ohmacht, R. Polyphenols, anthocyanins, and trans-resveratrol in red wines from the Hungarian Villány region. *Food Chemistry*, 2006, *98*, 453-462.

[156] Gomez-Alonso, S; Garcia-Romero, E; Hermosin-Gutierrez, I. HPLC analysis of diverse grape and wine phenolics using direct injection and multidetection by DAD and fluorescence. *Journal of Food Composition and Analysis*, 2007, *20*, 618-626.

[157] Bautista-Ortin, A B; Fernandez-Fernandez, J I; Lopez-Roca, J M; Gómez-Plaza, E. The effects of enological practices in anthocyanins, phenolic compounds and wine colour and their dependence on grape characteristics. *Journal of Food Composition and Analysis*, 2007, *20*, 546-552.

[158] Cliff, M A; King, M C; Schlosser, J. Anthocyanin, phenolic composition, colour measurement and sensory analysis of BC commercial red wines. *Food Research International*, 2007, *40,* 92-100.

[159] Katalinić, V; Milos, M; Modun, D; Musić, I; Boban, M. Antioxidant effectiveness of selected wines in comparison with (+)-catechin. *Food Chemistry*, 2004, *86,* 593-600.

[160] Paixao, N; Perestrelo, R; Marques, J C; Câmara J S. Relationship between antioxidant capacity and total phenolic content of red, rose and white wines. *Food Chemistry*, 2007, *105*, 204-214.

[161] Gonzalez-Neves, G; Franco, J; Barreiro, L; Gil, G; Moutounet, M; Carbonneau A. Varietal differentiation of Tannat, Cabernet-Sauvignon and Merlot grapes and wines according to their anthocyanic composition. *European Food Research and Technology*, 2007, *225*, 111-117.

[162] Makris, D P; Kallithraka, S; Mamalos, A. Differentiation of young red wines based on cultivar and geographical origin with application of chemometrics of principal polyphenolic constituents. *Talanta*, 2006, *70*, 1143-1152.

[163] Boselli, E; Minardi, M; Giomo, A; Frega, N G. Phenolic composition and quality of white d.o.c. wines from Marche (Italy). *Analytica Chimica Acta*, 2006, *563*, 93–100.

[164] Castillo-Munoz, N; Gomez-Alonso, S; Garcia-Romero, E; Hermosín-Gutiérrez, I. Flavonol profiles of Vitis vinifera red grapes and their single-cultivar wines. *Journal of Agricultural and Food Chemistry*, 2007, *55*, 992-1002

[165] Drinkine, J; Lopes, P; Kennedy, J A; Teissedre, P-L; Saucier, C. Ethylidene-bridged flavan-3-ols in red wine and correlation with wine age. *Journal of Agricultural and Food Chemistry*, 2007, *55*, 6292-6299.

[166] Oliveira, J; de Freitas, V; Silva, A M S; Mateus, N. Reaction between hydroxycinnamic acids and anthocyanin-pyruvic acid adducts yielding new portisins. *Journal of Agricultural and Food Chemistry*, 2007, *55*, 6349-6356.

[167] Gerogiannaki-Christopoulou, M; Athanasopoulos, P; Kyriakidis, N; Gerogiannaki, I A; Spanostrans, M.. Resveratrol in wines from the major Greek red and white grape varieties. *Food Control*, 2006, *17*, 700–706.

[168] Kolouchová-Hanzlíková, I; Melzoch, K; Filip, V; Šmidrkal, J. Rapid method for resveratrol determination by HPLC with electrochemical and UV detections in wines. *Food Chemistry*, 2004, *87*, 151–158.

[169] Lee, J; Rennaker, C. Antioxidant capacity and stilbene contents of wines produced in the Snake River Valley of Idaho. Food Chemistry, 2007, 105, 195-203.

[170] Moyers, S B; Kumar, N B. Green tea polyphenols and cancer chemoprevention: Multiple mechanisms and endpoints for phase II trias. *Nutrition Reviews*, 2004, *62*, 204-211.

[171] Graham, H N. Green tea composition, consumption, and polyphenol chemistry. *Preventive Medicine, 1992, 21*, 334-350.

[172] Bravo, L; Goya, L; Lecumberri, E. LC/MS characterization of phenolic constituents of mate (Ilex paraguariensis, St. Hil.) and its antioxidant activity compared to commonly consumed beverages. *Food Research International*, 2007, *40,* 393-405.

[173] Caballero, B; Trugo, L C; Finglas, P M. (2003). Encyclopedia of food sciences and nutrition (2nd ed.). Oxford, UK: Academic Press, Elsevier Science Ltd.

[174] Artajo, L S; Romero, M P; Motilva, M J. Transfer of phenolic compounds during olive oil extraction in relation to ripening stage of the fruit. *Journal of the Science of Food and Agriculture*, 2006, *86*, 518-527.

[175] Mateos, R; Espartero, J L; Trujillo, M; Ríos, J J; León-Camacho, M; Alcudia, F; Cert A. Determination of phenols, flavones, and lignans in Virgin Olive Oils by Solid-Phase Extraction and High-Performance Liquid Chromatography with Diode Array Ultraviolet Detection. *Journal of Agricultural and Food Chemistry*, 2001, *49*, 2185-2192.

[176] Paiva-Martins, F; Gordon, M H; Gameiro P. Activity and location of olive oil phenolic antioxidants in liposomes. *Chemistry and Physics of Lipids*, 2003, *124*, 23–36.

[177] Owen, RW, Haubner, R, Wurtele, G; Hull, W E; Spiegelhalder, B; Bartsch, H. Olives and olive oil in cancer prevention. *European Journal Of Cancer Prevention*, 2004, 13, 319-326.

[178] Krichene, D; Taamalli, W; Daoud, D; Salvador, M D; Fregapane, G; Zarrouk, M. Phenolic compounds, tocopherols and other minor components in virgin olive oils of some Tunisian varieties. *Journal of Food Biochemistry*, 2007, *31*, 179-194.

[179] Sotiroudis, T G; Kyrtopoulos, S A; Xenakis, A; Sotiroudis, G T. Chemopreventive potential of minor components of olive oil against cancer. Italian Journal of Food Science, 2003, *15*, 169-185.

[180] Keceli, T; Gordon, M H. Ferric ions reduce the antioxidant activity of the phenolic fraction of virgin olive oil. *Journal of Food Science*, 2002, *67*, 943-947.

[181] Brenes, M; Hidalgo, F J; Garcia, A; Rios, J J; Garcia, P; Zamora, R; Garrido, A. Pinoresinol and 1-acetoxypinoresinol, two new phenolic compounds identified in olive oil. *Journal of the American Oil Chemists Society*, 2000, *77*, 715-720.

[182] Franconi, F; Coinu, R; Carta, S; Urgeghe, P P; Ieri, F; Mulinacci, N; Romani, A. Antioxidant effect of two Virgin Olive Oils depends on the concentration and composition of minor polar compounds *Journal of Agricultural and Food Chemistry*, 2006, *54*, 3121-3125.

[183] Thiyam, U; Stöckmann, H; Zum Felde, T; Schwarz, K. Antioxidative effect of the main sinapic acid derivatives from rapeseed and mustard oil by-products. *European Journal of Lipid Science and Technology*, 2006, *108*, 239-248.

[184] Vuorela, S; Meyer, A S; Heinonen, M. Impact of isolation method on the antioxidant activity of rapeseed meal phenolics *Journal of Agricultural and Food Chemistry*, 2004, *52*, 8202-8207.

[185] Tuberoso, C I G; Kowalczyk, A; Sarritzu, E; Cabras, P. Determination of antioxidant compounds and antioxidant activity in commercial oilseeds for food use. *Food Chemistry*, 2007, *103*, 1494-1501.

[186] Shahidi, F. (2002). Phytochemicals in oilseeds. In Phytochemicals in nutrition and health (pp. 139–156). Boca Raton, FL, USA: CRC Press.

[187] Dimitrova, B; Gevrenova, R; Anklam, E. Analysis of phenolic acids in honeys of different floral Origin by solid-phase extraction and high-performance liquid chromatography. *Phytochemical Analysis*, 2007, *18*, 24–32.

[188] Inoue, K; Murayama, S; Seshimo, F; Takeba, K; Yoshimura, Y; Nakazawa, H. Identification of phenolic compound in manuka honey as specific superoxide anion radical scavenger using electron spin resonance (ESR) and liquid chromatography with coulometric array detection. *Journal of the Science of Food and Agriculture*, 2005, *85*, 872-878.

[189] Yao, L; Jiang, Y; Singanusong, R; Datta, N; Raymont, K. Phenolic acids and abscisic acid in Australian Eucalyptus honeys and their potential for floral authentication. *Food Chemistry*, 2004, *86*, 169–177.

[190] Yao, L; Jiang, Y; D'Arcy, B; Singanusong, R; Datta, N; Caffin, N; Raymont, K. Quantitative High-Performance Liquid Chromatography analyses of flavonoids in Australian eucalyptus honeys. *Journal of Agricultural and Food Chemistry*, 2004, *52*, 210-214.

[191] Arráez-Román, D; Gómez-Caravaca, A M; Gómez-Romero, M; Segura-Carretero, A; Fernández-Gutiérrez, A. Identification of phenolic compounds in rosemary honey using solid-phase extraction by capillary electrophoresis–electrospray ionization-mass spectrometry. *Journal of Pharmaceutical and Biomedical Analysis*, 2006, *41*, 1648–1656.

[192] Fahey, J W; Stephenson, K K. Pinostrobin from honey and Thai Ginger (*Boesenbergia pandurata*): a potent flavonoid inducer of mammalian Phase 2 chemoprotective and antioxidant enzymes. *Journal of Agricultural and Food Chemistry*, 2002, *50*, 7472-7476.

[193] Fiorani, M; Accorsi, A; Blasa, M; Diamantini, G; Piatti, E. Flavonoids from Italian multifloral honeys reduce the extracellular ferricyanide in human red blood cells. *Journal of Agricultural and Food Chemistry*, 2006, *54*, 8328-8334.

[194] Baltrušaitytė, V; Venskutonis, P R; Čeksterytė, V. Radical scavenging activity of different floral origin honey and beebread phenolic extracts. *Food Chemistry*, 2007, *101*, 502–514.

[195] Gheldof, N; Engeseth, N J. Antioxidant capacity of honeys from various floral sources based on the determination of oxygen radical absorbance capacity and inhibition of in vitro lipoprotein oxidation in human serum samples. *Journal of Agricultural and Food Chemistry*, 2002, *50*, 3050-3055.

[196] Tomás-Barberán, F A; Martos, I; Ferreres, F; Radovic, B S; Anklam, E. HPLC flavonoid profiles as markers for the botanical origin of European unifloral honeys. *Journal of the Science of Food and Agriculture*, 2001, *81*, 485-496.

[197] Sanchez-Rabaneda, F; Jauregui, O; Casals, I; Andrés-Lacueva, C; Izquierdo-Pulido, M; Lamuela-Raventós R M. Liquid chromatographic/electrospray ionization tandem mass spectrometric study of the phenolic composition of cocoa (*Theobroma cacao*). *Journal of Mass Spectrometry*, 2003, *38*, 35-42.

[198] Ramirez-Coronel, M A; Marnet, N; Kolli, V S K; Roussos, S; Guyot, S; Augur, C. Characterization and estimation of proanthocyanidins and other phenolics in coffee Pulp (*Coffea arabica*) by Thiolysis-High-Performance Liquid Chromatography. *Journal of Agricultural and Food Chemistry*, 2004, *52*, 1344-1349

[199] Niemenak, N; Rohsius, C; Elwers, S; Ndoumou, D O; Lieberei R. Comparative study of different cocoa (Theobroma cacao L.) clones in terms of their phenolics and anthocyanins contents. *Journal of Food Composition and Analysis*, 2006, *19*, 612-619.

[200] Lee, K W; Kim, Y J; Lee, H J; Lee, C Y. Cocoa has more phenolic phytochemicals and a higher antioxidant capacity than teas and red wine. *Journal of Agricultural and Food Chemistry*, 2003, *51*, 7292-7295.

[201] Manach, C; Scalbert, A; Morand, C; Rémésy, C; Jiménez, L. Polyphenols: food sources and bioavailability. *The America Journal of Clinical Nutrition*, 2004, *79*, 727-47.

[202] Kroon, P A; Clifford, M N; Crozier, A; Day, A J; Donovan, J; Manach, C; Williamson, G. How should we asses the effects of exposure to dietary polyphenols in vitro? *The America Journal of Clinical Nutrition,* 2004, *80*, 15-21.

[203] Scalbert, A; Johnson, I T; Saltmarsh, M. Polyphenols: antioxidants and beyond. The American *Journal of Clinical Nutrition*, 2005, *81*, 215S–7S.

[204] Zhang. Li; Lin, G; Kovacs, B; Jani, M; Krajcsi, P; Zuo, Z; Mechanistic study on the intestinal absorption and disposition of baicalein. *European Journal of Pharmaceutical Sciences,* 2007, *31*, 221–231.

[205] Wolffram, S; Block, M; Ader, P. Quercetin-3-Glucoside is transported by the glucose garrier SGLT1 across the brush border membrane of rat small intestine. *The Journal of Nutrition*, 2002, *132*, 630–635.

[206] Starp, C; Alteheld, B; Stehle, P. Characteristics of (+)-catechin and (-)-epicatechin transport across pig intestinal brush border membranes. *Annals of Nutrition and Metabolism,* 2006, *50*, 59-65.

[207] Saura-Calixto, F; Serrano, J; Goni, I. Intake and bioaccessibility of total polyphenols in a whole diet. *Food Chemistry*, 2007, *101*, 492–501.

[208] Kim, D H; Jung, E A; Sohng, Han, M,J. Intestinal bacteria metabolism of flavonoids and its relation to some biological activities. *Archives of Pharmacal Research*, 1998, *21*, 17-23.

[209] Murota, K; Hotta, A; Ido, H; Kawai, Y; Moon, J H; Sekido, K; Hayashi, H; Inakuma, T; Junji, T. Antioxidant capacity of albumin-bound quercetin metaboites after onion consumption in humans. *The Journal Medical. Investigation*, 2007, *54*, 370-374.

[210] Atkinson, C; Berman, S; Humbert, O; Lampe, J W. In vitro incubation of human feces with daidzein and antibiotics suggests interindividual differences in the bacteria responsible for equol production. *The Journal of Nutrition,* 2004, *134*, 596–599.

[211] King, R A; Bursill, D B. Plasma and urinary kinetics of the isoflavones daidzein and genistein after a single soy meal in humans. *American Journal of Clinical Nutrition*, 1998, 67, 867–72.

[212] Moon, Y J; Sagawa, K; Frederick, K; Zhang, S; Morris, M E. Pharmacokinetics and bioavailability of the isofl avone biochanin A in rats. *The AAPS* American Association of Pharmaceutical Scientists *Journal,* 2006, *8*, 433-442.

[213] Olthof, M R; Hollman P C H; Vree, T B; Katan, M B. Bioavailabilities of quercetin-3-glucoside and quercetin-4'- glucoside do not differ in humans. *The Journal of Nutrition*, 2000, *130*, 1200–1203.

[214] Seeram, N P; Henning, S M; Zhang, Y; Suchard, M; Li, Z; Heberm D. Pomegranate juice ellagitannin metabolites are present in human plasma and some persist in urine for up to 48 hours. *The Journal of Nutrition*, 2006, *136*, 2481–2485.

[215] Samman, S; Sandström, B; Toft, M B; Bukhave, K; Jensen, M; Sørensen, S S; Hansen, M. Green tea or rosemary extract added to foods reduces nonheme-iron absorption. *American Journal of Clinical Nutrition,* 2001, *73*, 607–12.

[216] Itagaki, S; Kobayashi, Y; Otsuka, Y; Kubo, S; Kobayashi, M; Hirano, T; Iseki, K. Food-drug interaction between ferulic acid and nateglinide involving the fluorescein/h+ cotransport system. *Journal of Agricultural and Food Chemistry*, 2005, *53*, 2499-2502.

[217] Lilja, J J; Neuvonen, M; Neuvonen, P J. Effects of regular consumption of grapefruit juice on the pharmacokinetics of simvastatin. *British Journal of Clinical Pharmacology,* 2004, *58*, 56–60.

[218] Jetter, A; Kinzig-Schippers, M; Walchner-Bonjean, M; Hering, U; Bulitta, J; Schreiner, P; Sörgel, F; Fuhr, U. Effects of grapefruit juice on the pharmacokinetics of sildenafil. *Clinical Pharmacology and Therapeutics*, 2002, *71*, 21-9.

[219] Preys, S; Mazerolles, G; Courcoux, P; Samson, A; Fischer, U; Hanafi, M; Bertrand, D; Cheynier, V. Relationship between polyphenolic composition and some sensory properties in red wines using multiway analyses. *Analytica Chimica Acta*, 2006, *563*, 126-136.

[220] Gutiérrez, I H; Sánchez-Palomo E L; Espinosa, A V. Phenolic composition and magnitude of copigmentation in young and shortly aged red wines made from the cultivars, Cabernet Sauvignon, Cencibel, and Syrah. *Food Chemistry*, 2005, *92*, 269-283.

[221] García-Falcón, M S; Pérez-Lamela, C; Martínez-Carballo, E; Simal-Gándara J. Determination of phenolic compounds in wines: Influence of bottle storage of young red wines on their evolution. *Food Chemistry*, 2007, *105*, 248-259.

[222] Es-Safi, N-E; Cheynier, V; Moutounet, M. Implication of phenolic reactions in food organoleptic properties. *Journal of Food Composition and Analysis*, 2003, *16*, 535–553.

[223] Es-Safi, N; Fulcrand, H; Cheynier, V; Moutounet, M. Studies on the acetaldehyde-induced condensation of (-)-epicatechin and malvidin 3-*O*-glucoside in a model solution system. *Journal of Agricultural and Food Chemistry*, 1999, *47*, 2096–2102.

[224] Es-Safi, N, Cheynier, V, Moutounet, M. Study of the reaction between (+)-catechin and furfural derivatives in the presence of anthocyanins and their implication in food color change. *Journal of Agricultural and Food Chemistry*, 2000, *48*, 5946–5954.

[225] Pérez-Silva, A; Odoux, E; Brat, P; Ribeyre, F; Rodriguez-Jimenes, G; Robles-Olvera, V; García-Alvarado, M A; Günata, Z. GC–MS and GC–olfactometry analysis of aroma compounds in a representative organic aroma extract from cured vanilla (*Vanilla planifolia* G. Jackson) beans. *Food Chemistry*, 2006, *99*, 728-735

[226] Caboni, P; Sarais, G; Cabras, M; Angioni, A. Determination of 4-ethylphenol and 4-ethylguaiacol in wines by LC-MS-MS and HPLC-DAD-fluorescence. *Journal of Agricultural and Food Chemistry*, 2007, *55*, 7288-7293.

[227] Kostyra, E; Baryłko-Pikielna, N. Volatiles composition and flavour profile identity of smoke flavourings. *Food Quality and Preference*, 2006, *17*, 85-95.

[228] Vidal, S; Francis, L; Guyot, S; Marnet, N; Kwiatkowski, M; Gawel, R; Cheynier, V; Waters, E J. The mouth-feel properties of grape and apple proanthocyanidins in a wine-like medium. *Journal of The Science of Food and Agriculture*, 2003, *83*, 564-573.

[229] Cheynier, V; Duenas-Paton, M; Salas, E; Maury, C; Souquet, J M; Sarni-Manchado, P; Fulcrand, H. Structure and properties of wine pigments and tannins. *American Journal of Enology and Viticulture*, 2006, *57*, 298-305.

[230] Vidal, S; Francis, L; Williams, P; Kwiatkowski, M; Gawel, R; Cheynier, V; Waters E. The mouth-feel properties of polysaccharides and anthocyanins in a wine like medium. *Food Chemistry*, 2004, *85*, 519-525.

[231] Vidal, S; Francis, L; Noble, A; Kwiatkowski, M; Cheynier, V; Waters E. Taste and mouth-feel properties of different types of tannin-like polyphenolic compounds and anthocyanins in wine. *Analytica Chimica Acta*, 2004, *513*, 57-65

[232] Fontoin, H; Saucier, C; Teissedre, P-L; Glories Y. Effect of pH, ethanol and acidity on astringency and bitterness of grape seed tannin oligomers in model wine solution. *Food Quality and Preference*, 2007 (In Press, Corrected Proof).

[233] Gutiérrez-Rosales, F; Rios, J J; Gomez-Rey, M L. Main polyphenols in the bitter taste of Virgin Olive Oil. Structural confirmation by On-Line High-Performance Liquid Chromatography Electrospray Ionization Mass Spectrometry. *Journal of Agricultural and Food Chemistry*, 2003, *51*, 6021-6025.

[234] Andrewes, P; Busch, J L H C; de Joode, T; Groenewegen, A; Alexandre, H. Sensory properties of Virgin Olive Oil polyphenols: Identification of deacetoxy-ligstroside aglycon as a key contributor to pungency. *Journal of Agricultural and Food Chemistry*, 2003, *51*, 1415-1420.

[235] Kobue-Lekalake, R I; Taylor, J R N; de Kock H L. Effects of phenolics in sorghum grain its bitterness, astringency and other sensory properties. *Journal of the Science of Food and Agriculture*, 2007, *87*, 1940-1948.

[236] Heiniö, R-L; Liukkonen, K-H; Myllymäki, O; Pihlava, J-M; Adlercreutz, H; Heinonen, S-M; Poutanen, K. Quantities of phenolic compounds and their impacts on the perceived flavour attributes of rye grain. *Journal of Cereal Science*, 2007, (In Press, Corrected Proof).

[237] Kreutzmann, S; Christensen, L P; Edelenbos M. Investigation of bitterness in carrots (*Daucus carota* L.) based on quantitative chemical and sensory analyses. *LWT - Food Science and Technology*, 2007, (In Press, Corrected Proof).

[238] Streit, N M; Rychecki Hecktheuer, L H; Weber do Canto, M; Mallmann, C A; Streck, L; Vey Parodi T; Pedrolo Canterle L. Relation among taste-related compounds (phenolics and caffeine) and sensory profile of erva-mate (*Ilex paraguariensis*). *Food Chemistry*, 2007, *102*, 560-564.

In: Progress in Food Chemistry
Editor: E. N. Koeffer, pp. 47-72

ISBN: 978-1-60456-303-0

Chapter 2

METHOD VALIDATION AND UNCERTAINTY ESTIMATE IN THE QUANTIFICATION OF TOXIC METALS IN FOODS OF ANIMAL ORIGIN

Giovanni Forte **[*]** ***and Beatrice Bocca***

Department of Environment and Primary Prevention,
Istituto Superiore di Sanità, Viale Regina Elena 299, 00161 Rome, Italy

ABSTRACT

Foods of animal origin, such as honey, milk and offal, are able to accumulate toxic metals posing a risk to health of general consumers and more vulnerable groups. For this reason, the European Commission Regulation No. 1881/2006 recommended maximum levels for metals as contaminants in food matrices. On this basis, the development of quantification methods supported by validation figures and uncertainty associated with each quantity become the central point to assure the quality and comparability of the final data. In this work, procedures based on microwave digestion with oxidizing agents followed by detection with sector field inductively coupled plasma mass spectrometry were developed and validated to measure arsenic, cadmium and lead in honey, cow milk, infant formulas and offal. Limits of detection and quantification, sensitivity, specificity, linearity range, trueness/recovery, repeatability, within-laboratory reproducibility and robustness were the main issues of the validation process. The analytical information obtained from the validation study was then used to calculate the method uncertainty without no extra work to be done. The benefit of this approach lies in its conceptual simplicity, low cost and application to routine analysis. The methods were applied to a number of marketed samples so as to contribute to the knowledge of the daily human exposure to metals from stable and special foods.

Keywords: Arsenic, cadmium, lead, honey, cow milk, infant formulas, offal, method validation, measurement uncertainty

---

[*] Author for correspondence: E-mail:giovanni.forte@iss.it

INTRODUCTION

Except for occupationally exposed individuals, ingestion of contaminated food represents the major route of exposure to metals such as arsenic (As), cadmium (Cd) and lead (Pb). Honey, milk and offal of animals are kinds of foodstuffs exposed to metals as a consequence of both the intentional contamination from agricultural practices and packaging materials, and unintentional contamination through environmental pollution of air, soil and water. Honeybees are indeed continuously exposed to potential pollutants present in the widespread foraging area and carry metals from the nectar flowers to honey. Large amounts of heavy metals were found in honey from hives located near extra-urban crossroads and steelworks [1-3]. Similarly, offal of animals grazing in polluted areas accumulated toxic metals more than offal of animals living in rural areas and kidney of animals accumulated Cd more than any other foods [4-6]. Milk is prone to contaminants not only via animal feedings but also by industrial treatments and leaching from metallic materials with which milk comes into contact [7]. Also, additives or mineral supplements added to infant formulas to better simulate the composition of breast milk and to impart health benefits can determine the levels of metals in the final products [8].

High concentrations of As, Cd and Pb in foodstuffs are undesirable for their known toxicity. The most toxic forms of As in food are the inorganic As(3) and As(5), classified by the International Agency for Research on Cancer (IARC) as human carcinogens [9]. Skin lesion, peripheral neuropathy, anaemia and development of diabetes, are all hallmarks of chronic As ingestion [10]. Cadmium binding metallothioneins accumulated mainly in kidney and liver, but also in muscle, bones and skin. It causes renal and kidney dysfunction, and negative effects on hemopoietic, cardiovascular and skeletric systems [11]; it is also considered as carcinogenic and genotoxic agent [12]. Lead by binding thiolic groups of proteins and making enzymes inactive, and by replacing other ions in various metabolic functions, is able to adversely affects the heme-biosynthesis, and gastrointestinal, nervous and cardiovascular systems [13].

In particular, milk and honey represent priority foods to be investigated because they are mainly consumed by children and infants, which are especially vulnerable to the effects of ingestion of contaminants. In consideration of the gastrointestinal assimilation of infants higher than that of adults and that developing organs and tissues are more susceptible to toxic effects of chemicals, metals in food can be more harmful to children than adults [14]. For example, exposure of Pb in the early age increases the risk for mild mental retardation, attention deficit hyperactivity disorder and other developmental disabilities [15, 16]. Moreover, absorption of metals in infants was found higher when they were on a milk diet, probably due to binding to readily absorbed milk proteins [17].

To reduce the risk of disease and disability arising from the exposure to heavy metals, both EU and US policies define and update standards, guidelines and recommendations to be adopted in the member states with regards to food control and food safety. In fact, the Commission Regulation no. 1881/2006 of 19 December 2006 established the maximum level (ML) for certain metals in foodstuffs. In particular, it was established in cow milk, infant and follow-up formulas a ML of 0.020 mg/kg for Pb; in offal of animals a ML of 0.5 mg/kg for Pb and a ML of 0.5 mg/kg in liver and 1.0 mg/kg in kidney for Cd [18]. For honey, a ML has not been settled so far, even if the Codex Alimentarius reported that "honey shall be free from heavy metals in amounts which may represent a hazard to human health" [19]. The Joint FAO/WHO Expert Committee on Food Additives (JECFA) has established the Provisional Tolerable Weekly Intakes (PTWIs) for chemicals, i.e., the amount of a contaminant that can be ingested over a lifetime without an appreciable risk. In particular, cumulative exposure from different sources should not exceed the PTWIs of 15, 7 and 25 μg/kg/body weight/week for As, Cd and Pb, respectively [11, 13, 20]. The US Environmental Protection Agency (EPA) established the oral Reference Dose (RfD) for substances that are not likely to be a risk [21]. The RfD were settled at 0.3 μg/kg per day and 1 μg/kg per day in food for As and Cd, respectively. The US Agency for Toxic Substances and Disease Registry (ATSDR) chose to adopt a practice similar to that of the EPA's RfD for deriving substance specific health guidance levels for non-neoplastic endpoints. It derived a Minimal Residue Level (MRL) for As of 0.3 μg/kg per day and for Cd of 0.2 μg/kg per day [22]. No MRL and RfD have been derived for Pb till now. Finally, based on the available data on feed-to-food transfer, the European Food Safety Authority (EFSA) Panel for contaminants emanated updated opinions on As, Cd and Pb as undesirable substances in animal feed [23-25].

As a consequence of these strict imposed regulations, national authorities have the responsibility to monitor that metals in food are at levels below the toxicological reference intakes. In several cases, data on contamination and exposure to metals through food are not collected or are incomplete in a way that any inter-country comparisons are difficult. This happens because, first of all, metals are present at very low concentrations in food so as to require that laboratories have very sensitive and specific instrumentation for accurate quantifications. Secondly, laboratories produced results that are not associated with a statement of their uncertainty so they are not traceable to common primary references. In the official control of food, several legislations prescribed that the analytical methods developed have to be fully validated and results must be expressed with their expanded uncertainty, so that the measurement data encompass two essential criteria, i.e., the utility and the reliability [26-29]. The validation process is the procedure used to demonstrate that a specific analytical method measures what it is intended to measure, making the adopted approach suitable for the intended purpose. The objective of the validation is to measure the different effects, throughout the whole analytical system, that can influence the final result, and to ensure that there are no other effects that have to be taken into account [30]. Internationally accepted protocols have been established for the validation of a method and they are based on the evaluation of a number of method–performance parameters, namely, limits of detection and quantification, sensitivity, specificity, linearity, repeatability, reproducibility, trueness and robustness [31-34]. The measurement uncertainty is described by the International Vocabulary of Basic and General Terms in Metrology as "a parameter associated with the result of a measurement, that characterises the dispersion of the values that could reasonably be attributed to the measurand" [35]. It allows the comparison of results among different laboratories at both national and international level, and is crucial for the traceability of the procedure and is strictly required for laboratories that need the accreditation to the International Organization for Standardization (ISO) rules reported in the ISO/IEC 17025:1999 [36, 37]. Some texts provides examples on how identify, quantify and combine all individual uncertainty sources that contribute to the overall uncertainty of the method [38, 39]. Recently, the use of experimental data from precision and trueness studies is also suggested in the estimation of uncertainty [40]. This last approach has the advantage of using all the information generated during validation and its benefit appears to lie in the conceptual simplicity as well as in the minimization of costs. The step next to the validation, is the demonstration that the validated method is also characterized by practicability and applicability. To this end, the method should be applied to a number of real samples to give evidence that it can be easily used in the lab for a certain amount of time without losing the adequate analytical performances.

In this context, three methods based on microwave (MW)-assisted acid digestion and sector field inductively coupled plasma mass spectrometry (SF-ICP-MS) for the quantification of Cd and Pb in honey and offal of animals and of As, Cd and Pb in milk were developed and validated. The method validation consisted of a specificity test to ensure that the method responded to the specific analyte, a linearity check to study the relationship between signal and concentration unit, a bias study using Certified Reference Materials (CRMs) or spiked samples to demonstrate that the method was not significantly biased, and a precision study to cover the effects of variability in operators and equipments. More, the robustness of the method when subjected to different operative changes and its stability in time by the use of control charts were also assessed. In addition, from the validation data obtained, expanded uncertainties were calculated following the recommendations given by international standard guides. The methods were then applied to different kinds of honey, cow milk, infant formulas and edible bovine, ovine and porcine offal in order to contribute to the assessment of metal contamination in foodstuffs available on the Italian market.

In-House Validation Parameters and Performance Criteria

Validation has been performed by conducting an in-house validation study. In fact, the analytical study involved a single laboratory and different methods were used to analyse different matrices under various conditions over a reasonable time interval [41]. The approach consisted in the assessment of a set of performance characteristics (linearity, limit of detection, limit of quantification, sensitivity, specificity, trueness/recovery, repeatability, within-laboratory reproducibility and robustness) and their conformity to well defined criteria of acceptability. For each validation parameter, the definition, the way of calculation and expression of results, and the acceptability criteria are reported below.

Linearity

Linearity defines the ability of the method to obtain test results proportional to the analyte concentration [33]. It represents the range of analyte concentrations over which the method may be applied and it can be different for different matrices. In this study, it was determined by the measurement of real samples spiked with 10 different concentrations of the analyte of interest. The measurement response was plotted against the analyte concentration and a correlation coefficient is calculated. A correlation coefficient of > 0.990 was considered as evidence of acceptable fit of the data to the regression line.

Limit of Detection (LoD)

For this analytical parameter there is a great variety of terminology and formulations. The Association of Official Analytical Chemists (AOAC) refers to limit of detection (LoD) as "the lowest content that can be measured with reasonable statistical certainty" [42] , while the ISO prefers the general term "minimum detectable net concentration' [43] and International Union of Pure and Applied Chemistry (IUPAC) uses "minimum detectable (true) value" [44]. Another definition for LoD is "the lowest concentration of analyte in a sample that can be detected, but not necessarily quantified under the stated conditions of the test" [45]. The EURACHEM Guide reported that for validation purposes it is sufficient to provide an indication of the level at which detection becomes problematic and the "mean sample value + 3 standard deviation (SD)" approach can be used [33]. Following this approach, LoD was determined by repeating the analysis of 10 independent test samples measured once each and was expressed as the analyte concentration the response of which is equivalent to the mean sample response + 3 SD. The LoD value is different for different types of sample [33]. For this reason, when the determination were made using reagent blanks the term instrumental LoD (ILoD) was used and results were expressed in ng of element per ml of blank solution; when the test sample was represented by the sample matrix or a matrix that matched the sample matrix the terminology method LoD (MLoD) was used and this value was reported in ng of element per g of sample weight.

As regards the acceptability criteria to be used for LoD, Regulation 333/2007 about the methods of analysis for the official control of Cd and Pb in food specifies that the LoD must be no more than one tenth of the ML values reported in Regulation 1881/2006. If the ML for Pb is less than 0.1 mg/kg, the LoD should be no more than one fifth of that value [18, 27].

Limit of Quantification (LoQ)

Limit of quantification (LoQ) is the lowest concentration of analyte that can be determined with an acceptable level of precision and accuracy and it is expressed as the analyte concentration corresponding to the sample test value + 10 SD [33]. Practically, it was calculated on 10 independent test samples measured once each and was dependent on the types of test sample. The ILoQ was used when the test sample was represented by reagent blanks and reported in ng of element per ml of blank solution; the MLoQ was used when the test sample is the real matrix and reported in ng of element per g of sample weight. The LoQ value recommended by the Regulation 333/2007 should be no more than one fifth of the ML values given in the Regulation 1881/2006, and no more than two fifth if the ML for Pb is less than 0.1 mg/kg [18, 27].

Sensitivity

Sensitivity is defined as the gradient of the calibration curve, which corresponds to a change in analyte concentration [35, 46]. A method is called sensitive if a small change in concentration causes a large change in the measured signal and it depends on the instrument settings [32]. Experimentally, it was calculated using samples containing a low concentration of the analytes of interest, and, in ICP-MS, expressed as instrumental counts per second (cps) relative to a defined concentration in the selected matrix.

Specificity

Specificity ensures that the method responds to the specific analyte of interest only, and not to other interferents or contaminants [33]. This characteristic is predominantly a function of the measuring technique used, but can vary according to class of compound or matrix. In ICP-MS measurements, specificity involves the process of selection of analytical mass and instrumental resolution and confirmation that at those conditions interferences are not significant. To this end, samples were spiked with various suspected interferences in the presence of the analytes of interest. After the analysis, if the presence of the interfering ion led to a false identification of the analyte and if the quantification was influenced notably, adequate correction factors (CF) were mathematically calculated. The order of correction was arranged so that only the "true", i.e. interference-free, values were quantified. In this study, two different correction formulas were used, one for the interference of molybdenum oxide ($^{98}Mo^{16}O$) on ^{114}Cd and the other for the isobaric interference of tin (^{114}Sn) on ^{114}Cd. In the first case, the correction equation used was: $I(^{114}Cd) = I(^{114}\text{ mass}) - [CF \times I(^{98}Mo)]$. The CF was daily calculated because it varied with the instrumental conditions. In the second case, the equation was: $I(^{114}Cd) = I(^{114}\text{ mass}) - [0.0268 \times I(^{118}Sn)]$, where the value 0.0268 was the ratio of the relative abundances of ^{114}Sn and ^{118}Sn.

Accuracy

Accuracy is defined as the closeness of agreement between a quantity value obtained by measurement and the true value of the measurand [35]. It is determined by determining trueness and precision [34].

Trueness

Trueness is the closeness of agreement between the average value obtained from a large series of test results and an accepted reference value [34, 47]. Two basic techniques for practical assessment of trueness are available: checking against certified values given by CRMs or against typical materials spiked with known concentration of pure certified reference standards (recovery test) [33].

A CRM means a material that has a specified analyte content assigned to it [41]. The ideal CRM is a natural matrix reference material, closely similar to the samples of interest. To check trueness using a CRM, the mean and the SD of 10 replicate tests were determined and compared with the certified value. The trueness was then calculated by dividing the estimated mean concentration by the certified value and multiply by 100, to express the result as a percentage. The deviation of the experimentally estimated mean content from the certified value (i.e., bias) shall not lie outside the limit ± 10% as recommended by the Commission Decision 2002/657/EC [41]. When a suitable CRM is not available, recovery can be determined and it represents the percentage of the true concentration of a substance recovered during the analytical procedure [33]. Recovery (%) was calculated by fortifying 20 aliquots of real matrix with relevant concentrations of the analytes and expressed as (Concentration found – Concentration originally present) x 100/(Concentration theoretical). The fortification was added before the digestion, i.e., prior to the addition of chemical reagents. Recovery data were only acceptable when they are within ± 10% of the target value [41]. In this work, the trueness was evaluated through the use of the CRM 151 skim milk powder, and of the CRM 185R bovine liver (both purchased from the Institute for Reference Materials and Measurements, IRMM, Geel, Belgium) certified for the elements Cd and Pb. The certified values were 101 ± 8 ng/g for Cd and 2002 ± 26 ng/g for Pb in milk, and 544 ± 17 ng/g for Cd and 172 ± 9 ng/g for Pb in bovine liver. In addition, recovery tests were performed for Cd and Pb in honey and for As in milk by spiking the raw material with known amount of the analytes. In particular, 0.80 ng/g and 8.00 ng/g of Cd and Pb, respectively, were added in the case of honey, and the concentration of 90.0 ng/g of As was selected for milk.

Precision

Precision is the closeness of agreement between independent test results obtained under stipulate conditions [34, 47]. Precision is expressed as repeatability and within-laboratory reproducibility and computed as the RSD % of the test result. Less precision is determined by a larger RSD.

Repeatability (r)

Repeatability requires that mutually independent test results are obtained with the same method on a test material in the same laboratory with the same equipment by the same operator within a short interval of time [47]. Experimentally, it was determined by calculated the RSD_r % on 30 independent samples analysed in the same operative conditions. The RSD_r equal or better than 10% for analyte concentration from 10 to 100 ng/g and as better as possible for concentrations lower than 10 ng/g was used as the criteria of acceptability applied to repeatability results.

Within-Laboratory Reproducibility (R)

Within-laboratory reproducibility requires that test results are carried out within the same laboratory, over a longer period of time, by different analysts, using different reagent lots, in different environmental conditions and even using different instrumentation [47]. In this study, it was measured by analyzing 30 independent samples in different days by changing analyst, instrumentation model (two different version of the SF-ICP-MS, i.e., Element 1 and Element 2), reagent lots, pipettes and expressed as RSD_R %. The Commission Decision 2002/657/EC recommends the RSD for the within-laboratory reproducibility be equal to or less than 20% when the analyte concentration ranges 10-100 ng/g and as better as possible for concentrations lower than 10 ng/g [41].

Robustness

Robustness testing deals with the critical operational parameters and the tolerances for their control. Robustness is the capacity of a method to remain unaffected by deliberate variations in the analytical protocol [33]. It is necessary to identify the variables in the method which have the most significant effect and ensure that, when using the method, they are closely controlled. In the case of trace analysis using MW digestion and ICP-MS quantification, parameters such as concentration of reagents, MW irradiation power and time, radiofrequency (RF) power, flow gas rates, spray chamber temperature can be varied. Practically, the first set of data was acquired under standard operative conditions, while the second one was obtained under dissimilar instrumental working conditions. Then, concentration values obtained from the two sets of results (10 independent samples for each set and for each matrix) were statistically compared through the t-test. If the test gave a p value less than 0.05 the two sets of data were significantly different and the method was not robust to the selected changes.

Calculation of Measurement Uncertainty

Uncertainty can be obtained either by calculating all the sources of uncertainty individually or by grouping different sources of uncertainty when possible. The first method is known as the "bottom–up" approach as proposed by the ISO [38]. However, identifying and quantifying all the sources of uncertainty individually is not simple, so other, more holistic, approaches based on calculating uncertainty using information from the in-house validation process have been proposed [39, 40, 48, 49]. These documents planned to include the estimates of reproducibility SD and of the bias coming from CRM/recovery study as the main components of the overall uncertainty. Then, uncertainty includes any other sources of uncertainty that are not covered by the validation study data.

Following this approach, in this study the relative combined uncertainty (u_{comb}) was calculated by this formula $u_{comb} = \sqrt{u_R^{\,2} + u_{tru/rec}^{\,2} + u_{other}^{\,2}}$. The first term of uncertainty, u_R, accounted for the contribution from long-term random variability estimated from reproducibility experiments. The second term, $u_{tru/rec}$, accounted for the systematic variability typically associated to the analysis of CRMs or spiked samples. The last term, u_{other}, included uncertainties sources coming from any other components associated to effects un-completely accounted for in the validation study. It should be mentioned that contributions to the uncertainty coming from operator effects, calibration uncertainty, reagent batches, ancillary equipment (i.e., pipettes) and laboratory effects were all included in the reproducibility SD. For this reason, u_{other} was judged unnecessary at this stage.

In this work, the relative contributions actually calculated were as follows:

1) u_R was the RSD_R obtained during the reproducibility test;

2) u_{tru} was calculated with the following formula

$$\sqrt{\left(\frac{u_{CRM}}{Conc_{CRM}}\right)^2+\left(\frac{SD_{estimated}}{Conc_{estimated}\sqrt{n}}\right)^2}$$; the first term was the uncertainty of the CRM given by the formula $\frac{SD_{CRM}}{\sqrt{6}}$ (the SD_{CRM} was available in the manufacture certificate and $\sqrt{6}$ represented triangular distribution), and the second term was the uncertainty of the estimated value of the CRM expressed as the RSD on replicated measurements. The u_{rec} was calculated in the same way, but the uncertainty on the CRM was replaced by the uncertainty on the standard solution purity (u_{STD}) used for spiking samples that follows a rectangular distribution (i.e., $\frac{SD_{STD}}{\sqrt{3}}$). The n was the number of replicates on each CRM or on fortified samples.

Finally, the relative expanded uncertainty (U) was calculated by multiplying the relative combined uncertainty by a coverage factor of 2, that accounts for an appropriate level of confidence of 95%.

SHEWHART CONTROL CHARTS

Control charts are constructed to decide whether a process is under statistical control and to monitor any departures from this state. They are based on monitoring events, which are very unlikely when the controlled process is stable. Any incidence of such an event is taken as an alarm signal suggesting that stability of the process was broken and the process changed. Upon receiving such signal, possible causes of the change should be investigated and some correcting steps taken.

The Shewhart control chart consists of the following [50]:

- Points representing mean of measurements of a quantity in samples versus time,
- A central line (CL), drawn at the mean,
- Upper (UL) and lower (LL) control limits that indicate the threshold at which the process output is considered out of control.

Generally, the UL and LL in the chart represented the ± 3SD of the CL, where the CL is the mean value of all the observations, and SD is the associated standard deviation. The ± 3SD limits means that the ca. 99.7% of all the point in the chart fall in the normal area. The UL and LL are also called “action limits” because when a point is placed outside that values actions should be undertaken to solve the occurred problem. Normally, in the chart are also reported two other lines, placed at the CL ± 2SD level and are called “warning limits”. In this regard, a point outside this limit and below the UC could indicate that the system should be monitored because something is changing. A light corrective action at this level could represent the best compromise in terms of efforts to maintain the system under control and the high costs involved in the worst case. In this study, Shewhart control charts, constructed following this rationale, were used to monitor the stability of each validated method over a long period of time.

Sample Selection and Treatment

Honey

The Lime Tree honey was selected for method development and calculation of validation parameters. The validated method was then applied to nine different types of honey, namely Acacia, Chestnut, Country Flowers, Lime Tree, Multiflora, Orange Tree, Rosemary, Strawberry and Honeydew originated from different regions of Italy. Samples were packaged in glass jars and bought in farms and stores. In order to reduce the heterogeneity of the raw honey mass and to have a sub-sampling as much representative as possible, containers with honey were heated in a water bath at 50°C and sonicated for 10 min. Sub-aliquots of approximately 1.5 g were weighed and transferred into Teflon vessels, added with 6 ml of nitric acid (HNO_3) (65%, Merck, Darmstadt, Germany) and 1 ml of hydrogen peroxide (H_2O_2) (30%, Merck) and further digested in a MW oven (MLS-1200, FKV, Sorisole, Italy). The MW irradiation programme consisted of two steps (2 min each) at a power of 250 W and 0 W, followed by four steps (5 min each) at 250 W, 500 W, 650 W and 250 W. After cooling at room temperature, the digested sample solutions were quantitatively transferred into disposable flasks, diluted to 15 g with high purity deionised water (Easy-pure, PBI, Milan, Italy) and stored at 4 °C until analysis. The reagent blanks were prepared following the same procedure.

Milk

Aliquots of powdered cow milk were used to validate the procedure and then the validated method was applied to three cow milk samples and to six milk-based infant formulas available on the Italian market. The formulas (six different brands) were bought at pharmacies and stored in Pb-free cans. The formula samples were all classified as starter formulas, i.e. for infants from the first day to 5-6 months of age, with the exception of one follow-up formula, used from 5 to 12 months of age. All formulas excepted one were enriched with Fe. Aliquots of approximately 0.5 g of powdered milk samples were transferred into Teflon vessels and 6 mL of HNO_3 (65%, Merck) and 1 mL of H_2O_2 (30%, Merck) were added. The MW irradiation programme was: 2 min at a power of 250 W, 2 min at 0 W, 5 min at 250 W, 5 min at 500 W, 5 min at 650 W, and 5 min at 250 W. The digested solutions were transferred into disposable flasks and diluted to 15 g with high purity deionized water (Easy-pure) and stored at 4 °C until analysis. Blanks, CRM 151 skim milk powder (IRMM) and all samples were digested by means of the same procedure.

Offal

The method was validated on calf liver and subsequently applied on eight different varieties of offal (spleen, lung and kidney of calf; liver, lung, kidney and heart of lamb; and kidney of pig). Offal were bought in supermarkets and come from animals farmed in Italy and not over 1 year of age. Visible fat and connective tissues were previously removed and samples were homogenized by a turbo homogenizer (HMHF, PBI, Milan, Italy). Sub-aliquots of approximately 2 g were transferred into Teflon vessels and added with 6 ml of a 5:1 (v/v) mixture of HNO_3 (67%, ROMIL, Cambridge, UK) and H_2O_2 (30%, Merck). Calf liver was MW digested under the following MW irradiation programme: 10 min at 250 W, 5 min at 400 W, 5 min at 500 W and 5 min at 600 W. After cooling at room temperature, the digested sample solutions were water diluted to ca. 17 g and stored at 4 °C. Reagent blanks, CRM 185R bovine liver (IRMM) and all kinds of offal were prepared following the same procedure.

SF-ICP-MS Method Development

SF-ICP-MS Description

A SF-ICP-MS instrumentation was used for the quantification of the analytes of interest, namely, As, Cd and Pb in food matrices. The SF-ICP-MS was characterised by a double focusing reverse Nier–Johnson geometry and sampler and skimmer cones in Ni alloy. The instrument was equipped with a Meinhard nebulizer, a water cooled spray chamber and a guard electrode device. It can operate at three different resolutions, i.e. Low Resolution (LR, $m/\Delta m = 300$), Medium Resolution (MR, $m/\Delta m = 4000$), and High Resolution (HR, $m/\Delta m = 10{,}000$).

The critical instrumental parameters, such as argon flow rates, torch position, lenses and RF power were daily optimized so as to reach a signal for 1 ng/ml of ^{115}In of > 900,000 cps in LR, > 90,000 cps in MR and > 20,000 in HR. These counts were chosen as acceptability limits before starting the analysis. Also the oxides formation was daily minimized on the BaO^+/Ba^+ ratio, and a value less than 0.002 was considered as appropriate.

The optimized instrumental settings for As, Cd and Pb quantification in all matrices were as follows: RF generator, 1.25 kW; plasma gas flow, 15 l/min; auxiliary and sample gas flows, 1.0 l/min; peristaltic pump flow rate, 1.0 ml/min; temperature of the spray chamber, 10 °C. A summary of the SF-ICP-MS characteristics and conditions, and of the isotopes and resolution settings chosen for metal quantification is reported in table 1.

Analysis and Control Checks

The standard addition calibration was used to determine the content of As, Cd and Pb in the samples. This procedure consisted in adding known amounts of the standard analyte to the test portions before analysis. This procedure is designed to minimise sample-specific matrix effects. Mixed calibration curve standards were daily prepared by diluting solutions of 1000 μg/l from certified standard stocks (Spex, Edison, USA) and analyzed at the beginning of the running sequence. Calibration curves were constructed on at least five levels (including zero) and a correlation coefficient $R^2 > 0.995$ was considered as the acceptability criteria [41]. The amount of the standard analyte added was between two and five times the estimated amount of the analyte in the sample [41]. In honey, R^2 (averaged on different days of analysis) of 0.9991 for Cd and 0.9992 for Pb were obtained; the R^2 in milk were 0.9997 for Pb, 0.9998 for Cd and 0.997 for As; the R^2 in offal were 0.9992 for Cd and 0.9995 for Pb. Only in the case of As, the correlation was slightly worse because of the low sensitivity typical when the HR setting was applied.

Table 1. SF-ICP-MS characteristics and conditions

Spectrometer	Element (Thermo-Fischer, Bremen, Germany)
Geometry	Double focusing reverse Nier-Johnson
Sample introduction device	Meinhard-type glass nebulizer; water-cooled Scott spray chamber; torch with guard electrode
Interface	Sampler and skimmer cones of Ni
RF generator (kW)	Power output, 1.25
Argon flows (l/min)	Plasma, 15; auxiliary, 1.0; sample, 1.0
Resolution used (m/Δm)	300, LR; 10,000, HR
Signal optimization on ^{115}In (cps)	> 900,000, LR; > 20,000, HR
Oxide ions optimization	$BaO^+/Ba^+ < 0.002$
Scanning conditions	Electric; number of scans, 20 in LR and in HR
Mass, search and integration windows (%)	100, 100, 100 in LR; 100, 90, 80 in HR
Analytical mass (amu)	^{75}As in HR, ^{114}Cd and ^{208}Pb in LR
Internal standard mass (amu)	^{69}Ga for ^{75}As; ^{115}In for ^{114}Cd and ^{208}Pb
Interferent mass (amu)	^{114}Sn, ^{98}Mo

The reagent blanks carried the entire preparation procedure and analysis scheme. The final solution contained the same acid concentration as sample solutions for analysis. Reagent blanks were analyzed after the calibration curve and before samples in the running sequence and subtracted to the sample analyte concentration when their values were greater than the method detection limit to correct for contributions to the signal not attributable to the sample (e.g. contributions from reagents and/or vessels). In this study, reagent blanks were always under the detection limit of the methods.

The internal standardisation was used to correct temporal variation of the signal drifts. It consisted in the normalisation of all data to a non-analyte isotope added in the same and known concentration in all samples and standards. In this work, the internal standardization with ^{115}In for Cd and Pb in honey, milk and offal, and ^{69}Ga for As in milk, both at the concentration of 1 ng/ml in calibrants and samples was applied. The selection of the internal standard was based on the best compromise among different isotopic properties: freedom from interferences, presence at very low concentration in the original matrix and physical-chemical properties as similar as possible to those of the analytes.

For the interference study, interference check samples were analyzed at the beginning and at the end of the run. The interferents (Mo and Sn in the present study) were added at concentrations up to five-times higher that the actual content of samples.

Random variation in performance of the analytical process was monitored by monitoring the value of a control sample (CS) digested and analyzed during the routine analysis of samples. The measured value for the CS was plotted on the control charts and as long as the CS value was acceptable it was likely that results from samples in the same batch as the CS could be taken as reliable.

RESULTS

Table 2 summarizes practical assessment, way of expression, and acceptance criteria in the validation of SF-ICP-MS-based methods for As, Cd and Pb quantification in food of animal origin. Table 3 reports the results for trueness, recovery, repeatability and reproducibility obtained in the SF-ICP-MS measurements of metals in the selected foodstuffs. The contribution of the single uncertainty sources, and the combined and the expanded uncertainty in the analysis of metal in foods are reported in table 4. Table 5 shows the Cd and Pb levels in different varieties of Italian honeys, while table 6 gives the As, Cd and Pb concentration found in cow milk and starter and follow-up infant formulas. Data on the levels of Cd and Pb in offal of calf, lamb and pig are reported in table 7. Figure 1 shows the Shewhart control charts obtained in one-year analysis of Cd (1a) and Pb (1b) in honey. Figure 2 shows the specificity in the SF-ICP-MS analysis of As in milk obtained by working in HR mode.

DISCUSSION

The results on the validation study, the uncertainty of the measurements, and the application to real samples were discussed for each matrix individually.

HONEY

The ILoD were 0.003 and 0.03 ng/ml and ILoQ were 0.008 and 0.09 ng/ml for Cd and Pb, respectively. The MLoD and MLoQ were 0.07 and 0.20 ng/g for Cd and 0.70 and 2.10 ng/g for Pb. The MLoDs were more than ten-times lower than the levels found in honey samples assuring that the analyte signal in samples is well distinguishable from that of the background. The linearity was tested using a concentration range of 0.05-5 ng/ml for Cd and 0.50-50 ng/ml for Pb and R^2 values of 0.9991 for Cd and 0.9992 for Pb were obtained. Correlation coefficients respected the established limit showing proportionality between intensity and increased metal content over two orders of magnitude of concentration. For the calculation of sensitivity, a concentration of 0.05 ng/ml and 0.5 ng/ml for Cd and for Pb respectively, and instrumental responses of 2300 and 186,000 cps were obtained. The

Table 2. Validation study for SF-ICP-MS analysis of As, Cd and Pb in food of animal origin

Characteristics evaluated	Practical assessment	Expression	Criteria of acceptability
Linearity	Analysis of 10 independent spiked samples	R^2	$R^2 \geq 0.990$
ILoD ILoQ	Analysis of 10 independent reagents blanks Analysis of 10 independent reagents blanks	$Conc_{blank} + 3SD_{blank}$ $Conc_{blank} + 10SD_{blank}$	
MLoD MLoQ	Analysis of 10 independent samples Analysis of 10 independent samples	$Conc_{sample} + 3SD_{sample}$ $Conc_{sample} + 10SD_{sample}$	MLoD should be < 1/10 (or < 1/5 when Pb is less than 0.1 mg/kg) of the ML reported in the Regulation 1881/2006 MLoQ should be < 1/5 (or < 2/5 when Pb is less than 0.1 mg/kg) of the ML reported in the Regulation 1881/2006
Specificity	Analysis of 5 samples spiked with possible interferences	cannot be expressed, must be demonstrated	
Repeatability (r)	Analysis of 30 independent samples under the same operative conditions	$RSD_r \% = (SD_r/Conc)\ 100$	< 10% for concentration between 10 and 100 μg/kg; as better as possible for concentration < 10 μg/kg
Within laboratory reproducibility (R)	Analysis of 30 independent samples by changing analyst, instrument, pipettes and reagent lot	$RSD_R \% = (SD_R/Conc)\ 100$	< 20% for concentration between 10 and 100 μg/kg; as better as possible for concentration < 10 μg/kg
Trueness	Analysis of 20 independent aliquots of skim milk powder CRM 151 and bovine liver CRM 185R	$(Conc_{estimated}/Conc_{theoretical})\ 100$ Or expressed as $Bias \% = [(Conc_{estimated} - Conc_{theoretical})/Conc_{theoretical}]\ 100$	Within ± 10%
Recovery	Analysis of 20 independent spiked samples	$(Conc_{estimated}/Conc_{theoretical})\ 100$ Where $Conc_{estimated} = Conc_{found} - Conc_{originally\ present}$	Within ± 10%
Robustness	Analysis of 20 independent samples, 10 with the original method and 10 by changing MW procedure, instrumental parameters and concentrations reagent	p value from t-test	$p > 0.05$

Table 3. Results for trueness/recovery and precision for As, Cd and Pb quantification in food of animal origin

Element	Parameter	Honey	Milk	Offal
As	Recovery (%)	-	102	-
	Repeatability (%)	-	3.54	-
	Reproducibility (%)	-	4.32	-
Cd	Trueness (bias, %)	-	1.00	1.34
	Recovery (%)	104	-	-
	Repeatability (%)	10.7	4.90	2.25
	Reproducibility (%)	15.2	4.96	1.99
Pb	Trueness (bias, %)	-	-2.40	5.65
	Recovery (%)	98.5	-	-
	Repeatability (%)	18.5	5.72	1.49
	Reproducibility (%)	21.4	5.06	6.55

Table 4. Relative standard uncertainty (in %) budget for As, Cd and Pb in the matrices under study

Element	Uncertainty	Honey	Milk	Offal
As	u_R	-	4.30	-
	$u_{tru/rec}$	-	0.64	-
	u_{comb}	-	4.30	-
	U	-	8.70	-
Cd	u_R	15.2	5.00	1.99
	$u_{tru/rec}$	2.90	3.20	1.27
	u_{comb}	15.5	6.00	2.37
	U	31.0	12.0	4.74
Pb	u_R	21.4	5.10	6.55
	$u_{tru/rec}$	3.50	1.30	2.14
	u_{comb}	21.7	5.10	6.90
	U	43.4	10.2	13.8

sensitivity for both elements resulted to be satisfactory for the purpose. As regards the specificity test, in the case of Cd, the signal at mass 114 (the most abundant isotope for Cd)was checked for the potential interference from the molecular specie $^{98}Mo^{16}O$ and the isobaric specie ^{114}Sn. The formation of $^{98}Mo^{16}O$ was found not to be negligible and because this interference could not be solved even in the HR setting, Cd signal was registered in LR mode and further corrected by the appropriate CF (see experimental section). In its turn, the contribution of ^{114}Sn on the mass 114 resulted to be negligible and corrections were not necessary. As regards Pb, its signal presented no significant interference on the most abundant mass so it was quantified in LR mode without corrections. Due to the lack of CRM for Cd and Pb based on a matrix of honey, recovery test were performed (see table 3). To this end, honey was fortified with 0.8 ng/ml of Cd and 8 ng/ml of Pb before digestion, and after that it was MW digested and SF-ICP-MS analyzed. Results gave a very high recovery efficiency, i.e., 104% for Cd and 98.5% for Pb, thus the deviations from the theoretical value laying well within the recommended ± 10% range [41]. This result made also confident that the matrix mineralization process avoided significant analyte loss or contamination. The method showed a rather high imprecision under repeatability conditions and, as expected, it worsened under reproducibility conditions (Cd, 15.2%; Pb, 21.4%). Anyway, the observed imprecision of ca. 20% was acceptable considering that the analytes were quantified at the level of few ng/g, or fractions [41]. The precision study suggested that some differences in metal concentration occur when testing more aliquots from the same raw mass. This outcome reflects the intrinsic heterogeneity of the raw honey and the fact that a honey-based multi-elemental CRM has not been produced till now. The method's robustness was assessed by comparing the mean concentration value obtained from two sets of results, one acquired under standard operative conditions (see experimental section), while the second one was obtained after changing the following instrumental settings: peristaltic pump flow rate, 1.3 ml/min, RF power at 1.35 kW, plasma flow rate at 16 l/min, temperature of the spray chamber set at 20 °C. These parameters are able to affect the ICP-MS results interfering both with the sample introduction speed (the first), and with nebulization and ionisation efficiency (the other three). Mean results from the two data sets were subjected to the t-test obtaining as result a $p > 0.1$ for Cd and Pb demonstrating that the selected changes did not influence the method performances. The results on the uncertainty contributions (see table 4) showed the u_R as the heaviest contribution to the combined uncertainty since this component derives from the day to day variability of the method. In fact, the u_R was 15.2% for Cd and 21.4% for Pb, while the u_{rec} was 2.90% for Cd and 3.50% for Pb. The uncertainty associated to the recovery was ca. 1/5 of u_R. The combined uncertainty u_{comb} was 15.5% for Cd and 21.7% for Pb. Applying the coverage factor of 2, the relative expanded uncertainties (U) were 31.0% and 43.4% for Cd and Pb, respectively.

Nine varieties of Italian honeys coming from different geographical regions were analyzed in triplicate using the described in-house validated procedure (see table 5).

Table 5. Levels (in ng/g) of Cd and Pb in honey

Type	Area of origin, place of sampling	Cd	Pb
Acacia	Northern, supermarket	0.61 ± 0.12	12.0 ± 3.2
Chestnut	Southern, supermarket	0.55 ± 0.17	21.5 ± 6.0
Chestnut	Northern, supermarket	0.93 ± 0.06	11.7 ± 1.2
Chestnut	Central, rural area, farm	0.90 ± 0.38	16.9 ± 0.8
Country Flowers	Central, rural area, farm	1.04 ± 0.23	11.1 ± 1.7
Lime	Central, supermarket	0.59 ± 0.15	13.7 ± 3.4
Multiflora	Island (Sicily), supermarket	< MLoQ	11.1 ± 2.3
Multiflora	Southern, rural area, farm	0.75 ± 0.13	4.56 ± 0.75
Orange tree	Southern, rural area, farm	0.55 ± 0.06	5.17 ± 0.64
Rosemary	Island (Sardinia), urban area, supermarket	0.74 ± 0.06	7.72 ± 0.87
Strawberry	Central, urban area, supermarket	1.37 ± 0.17	30.5 ± 4.5
Honeydew	Central, supermarket	4.96 ± 0.08	117 ± 4
Honeydew	Northern, cooperative	2.06 ± 0.17	30.8 ± 1.2

Cadmium content ranged from < 0.2 to 1.37 ng/g, whereas Pb levels were from 4.56 to 30.5 ng/g in flower honeys. The concentration of metals presented only slight variations depending on the variety of flower considered. Higher levels of Cd and Pb were found in Strawberry honey, while Orange tree honey and a sample of Multiflora honey showed the lowest concentration of Pb. Dark honeys, i.e. the Honeydew honeys, presented an higher concentration of metals in comparison with the light ones, with a mean of 3.51 ng/g for Cd and 74.1 ng/g for Pb. So far, it is difficult to extrapolate a link between geographical origin and type of production (e.g., intensive or limited productions) and environmental contamination. For example, no significant differences were observed between samples of the same variety but originating from different Italian regions, as in the case of Multiflora and Chestnut honey samples. Moreover, only light evidence related elemental concentration to environmental pollution. For instance, the Orange tree and the Multiflora honey samples coming from rural areas, that are characterized by a very low density of automotive traffic, presented low levels of Pb (ca. 5.00 ng/g); conversely, the higher Cd and Pb concentrations were found in the Strawberry honey produced in an industrialized area. On the other hand, two Chestnut honey samples from supermarkets gave a concentration of metals similar to that found in the same kind of honey purchased from country amateurs. Figure 1 shows the Shewhart control charts for Cd (1a) and Pb (1b) in honey. The CL was the mean value of independent measurements of Lime honey (CS), as obtained under reproducibility conditions. Warning and action limits were calculated as CL ± 2SD and CL ± 3SD, respectively. During the routine analysis of honey samples, three aliquots of CS was digested and analyzed along with samples, and the mean value plotted on the charts. This procedure was uninterruptedly used for more than one year. All the points were acceptable (i.e. always inside the ± 1SD) and placed randomly around the CL. This finding proved the method was stable with time and, in other words, that the results from real samples processed together with CS were reliable.

1a.

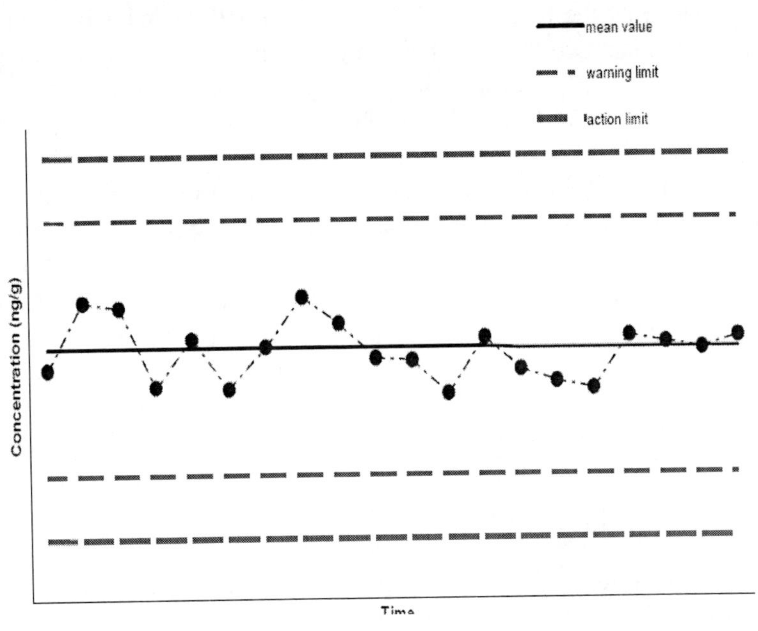

Figure 1. Continued on next page.

1b.

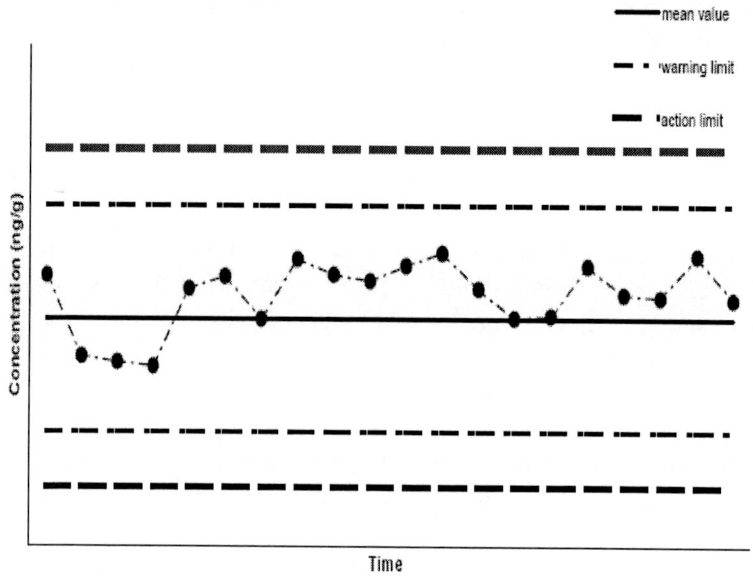

Figure 1. Shewhart control chart for Cd (1a) and Pb (1b) in honey.

MILK

The ILoDs (ng/ml) and ILoQs (ng/ml) were 0.04 and 0.13 for As, 0.007 and 0.02 for Cd, and 0.01 and 0.03 for Pb. The MLoDs (ng/g) and MLoQs (ng/g) were as follows: As, 3.04 and 9.12; Cd, 0.49 and 1.46; Pb, 0.62 and 1.85. Considering the maximum value of Pb of 20 ng/g in milk provided by the Regulation 1881/2006, the MLoD and MLoQ for Pb were less than one fifth and than two fifth of that value, respecting the requisites given by the Regulation 333/2007 [18, 27]. The linearity was tested using a concentration range of 0.5-50 ng/ml for As and Cd, and 10-1000 ng/ml for Pb. The R^2 values over the linearity range were 0.992 for As, 0.9993 for Cd, and 0.9996 for Pb. These values for Cd and Pb were above the critical limit. Spiked samples with a concentration of 1 ng/ml for As, Cd and Pb was used for the sensitivity calculation and counts of 900, 101,700 and 371,200, respectively, were obtained. Obviously, the sensitivity for As was lower than that of the other elements because acquired in HR mode which is characterized by scarce sensitivity and high specificity. In fact, as shown in figure 2, the HR mode was able to unequivocally separate ^{75}As from interfering masses, namely $^{59}Co^{16}O$, $^{35}Cl^{40}Ar$ and $^{39}K^{36}Ar$. These molecules were not negligible considering the high abundance of K and Cl ions in milk and of oxygen in the digested samples. Figure 2 shows the As spectra obtained at different resolutions: in the LR setting (figure 2a) only one peak was observed, indicating this resolution as inadequate to separate the As peak from the interfering species. When the MR mode (figure 2b) was used, the As peak was still not completely free from interferences. In the HR mode (figure 2c) the interferences were shifted well away from the As peak, thus enabling the specific quantification of As.

In the case of Cd, the signal at mass 114 was checked for the interferences from $^{98}Mo^{16}O$ and ^{114}Sn. The former specie was found of some concern and its contribution was corrected by a daily CF. Table 3 shows the trueness results for Cd and Pb calculated on the CRM 151. Expressing the results as bias (see table 2), values of + 1.00% for Cd and - 2.40% for Pb were obtained; the deviations from the theoretical value were very small and laid within the criteria reported in legislation [41]. In consideration of the fact that As was not certified in the CRM 151, the recovery test for this metal was performed adding a concentration of 90 ng/g. The estimated concentration (i.e. 91.8 ng/g) was very close to that added and the recovery of 102% agreed with the established criteria [41]. This result substantiated the absence of analyte losses, contaminations and interferences during sample treatment and analysis. The precision of the method was calculated on real samples in the case of Cd and Pb, while on spiked samples in the case of As because its concentration was below the MLoD in all samples. For all elements an RSD of about 5% was observed under both repeatability and reproducibility conditions and the criteria of acceptability were fulfilled [41]. Four relevant operative parameters were changed to estimate method's robustness. In particular, two parameters are known to affect the sample introduction in the plasma, i.e. the speed of the peristaltic pump (raised from 1.0 to 1.3 ml/min) and the temperature of the spray chamber (raised from 10 to 20°C). The remaining two parameters potentially affect the efficiency of MW digestion, i.e. the composition of the digestion acidic mixture (3 mL of HNO_3, 1 mL of H_2O_2) and the MW steps (2 min at 250 W, 2 min at 0 W, 5 min at 400 W, 5 min at 0 W, 5 min at 600 W). Results did not statistically differ when obtained under these new operative conditions ($p > 0.1$ for the three elements), and it was concluded therefore that the method was robust when subjected to the selected variations. In the estimation of uncertainty (table 4), the u_R, which included factors such as analyst, instrumentation, pipettes, standard solutions and calibration, represented the main contribution to the overall uncertainty. The contribution of recovery was low for As and Pb while more significant for Cd (3.20%). The u_{comb} was 4.30% for As, 6.00% for Cd and 5.10% for Pb. The u_{comb} values matched well with the method reproducibility (see table 3). The U were 8.70% for As, 12.0% for Cd and 10.2% for Pb.

The described method was applied to the analysis of cow milk and starter and follow-up infant formulas marketed in Italy. Results reported in table 6 are the mean values obtained from 3 independent aliquots for each brand. Results showed As levels below the MLoD (< 3.0 ng/g) in all the collected samples, whereas Cd ranged 2.30-4.55 ng/g in cow milk and 2.31-7.84 ng/g (mean value equal to 5.27 ng/g) in infant formulas. Lead ranged 8.89-15.9 ng/g in cow milk and < MLoQ (i.e. < 1.85 ng/g)-12.1 ng/g in infant formulas. No differences in Cd content was found between cow milk and formulas, and among the different brands. Lead showed detectable levels in cow milk, while it was under the limit for the majority of infant formulae, except for two cases. In particular, these two infant formulae showed also the highest Cd concentration (7.20 and 7.84 ng/g). Considering the ML admitted for Pb in milk (20 ng/g), Pb was found at acceptable levels in all samples.

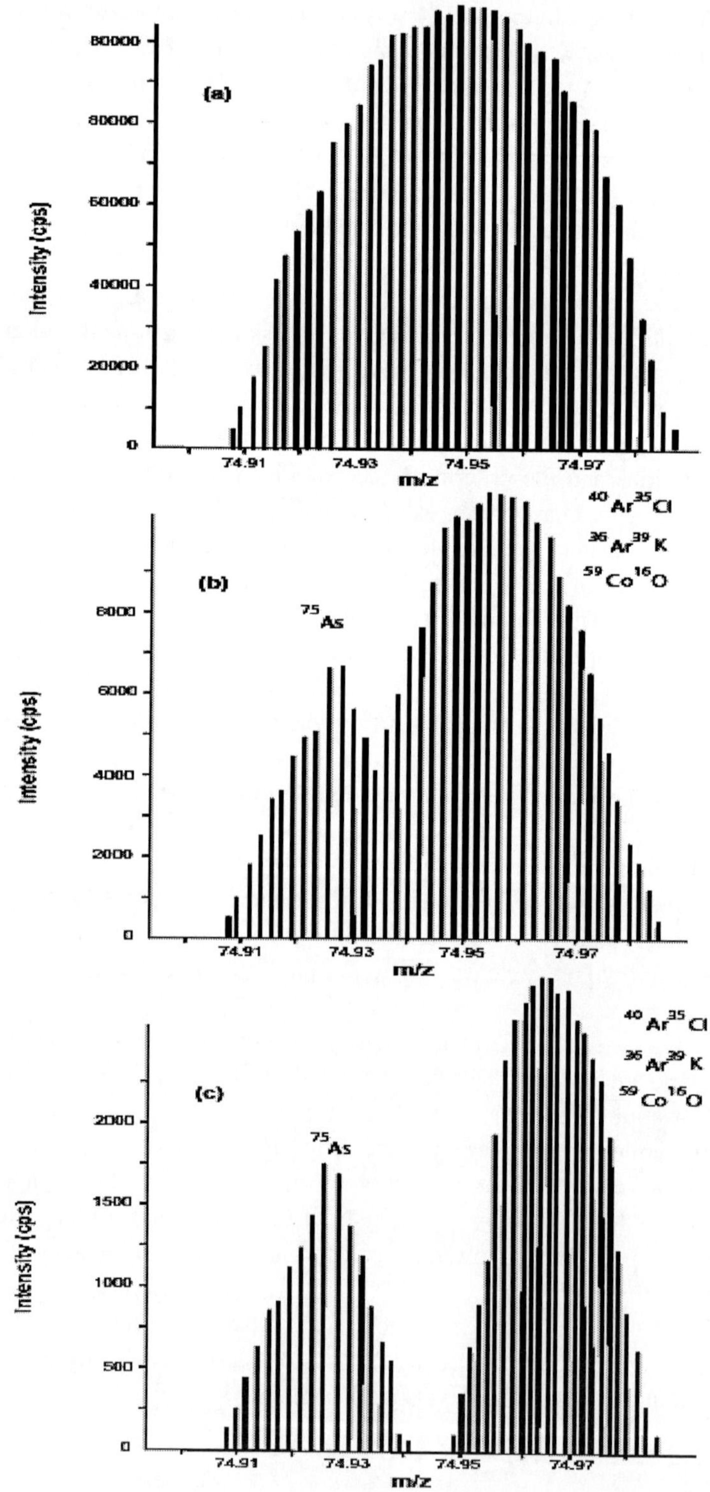

Figure 2. Typical SF-ICP-MS spectra of As in milk: (a) LR setting; (b) MR setting; (c) HR setting.

The control charts for As, Cd and Pb in milk were constructed as reported for honey (data not shown). Points were the mean of three independent aliquots of the cow milk (used as CS) digested and analyzed along with samples. As for honey, the process was controlled for more than year and points were within the ± 1SD, indicating that the method was stable for long time and that results on real samples were reliable.

Table 6. Levels (in ng/g) of As, Cd and Pb in milk

	Type	As	Cd	Pb
Cow milk	Whole	< MLoD	4.02 ± 0.69	8.89 ± 3.70
	Whole	< MLoD	2.30 ± 0.87	10.9 ± 4.6
	Partially skim	< MLoD	4.55 ± 2.53	15.9 ± 4.40
Starter infant formulas	-	< MLoD	2.31 ± 0.34	< MLoQ
	Fe enriched	< MLoD	5.88 ± 0.64	< MLoQ
	Fe enriched	< MLoD	7.20 ± 0.49	12.1 ± 1.2
	Fe enriched	< MLoD	4.65 ± 0.97	< MLoQ
	Fe enriched	< MLoD	7.84 ± 1.65	4.22 ± 1.14
Follow-up infant formulas	Fe enriched	< MLoD	3.77 ± 0.86	< MLoQ

OFFAL

The ILoDs and ILoQs were 0.005 and 0.015 ng/ml for Cd, and 0.06 and 0.18 ng/ml for Pb; the MLoDs and MLoQs were 3.5 and 10.8 ng/g for Cd, and 2.0 and 6.0 ng/g for Pb. The MLoD and MLoQ for Pb were ca. 20 times lower than the criteria established by the Regulation 333/2007 for a maximum permitted concentration of 500 ng/g in offal [18, 27]. The MLoD and MLoQ for Cd were ca. 15 and 10 times lower than the criteria established for a Cd ML of 500 ng/g in liver [18, 27]. The linearity was tested in the range 0.125-32 ng/ml for both elements. Linearity was of two orders of magnitude with R^2 equal to 0.9996 for Cd and to 0.9997 for Pb over the tested concentration range. A concentration of 0.25 ng/ml for Cd and Pb were added to samples for assessing the sensitivity in matrix and instrumental responses of 26,253 and 166,752 cps for Cd and Pb, respectively, were obtained. For Cd, the most abundant mass was selected and interferences from $^{98}Mo^{16}O$ and ^{114}Sn on that mass were carefully evaluated. The interference study did not indicate any considerable contribution from both species and analyte signals did not necessitate of mathematical corrections. The trueness was checked throughout the use of the CRM 185R bovine liver where Cd and Pb have certified values (table 3). The found values were very close to the certified ones with bias of + 1.34% for Cd and + 5.65% for Pb and, thus in fully agreement with the legislative recommendation (i.e. ± 10%) [41]. Comparing repeatability and reproducibility results (table 3), the RSD for Cd remained similar at ca. 2%, the RSD for Pb increased from 1.49% to 6.55%. The method was, thus, considered precise when subjected to run to run variations. To assess the robustness, the variations applied to the original protocol were: HNO_3 65% from Merck (this might affect the blank levels); peristaltic pump flow rate of ca. 1.3 ml/min and spray chamber kept at room temperature (these parameters might interfere with the sample introduction in the plasma); ^{103}Rh as the IS at the concentration of 1 ng/ml (it might influence the correction of instrumental drifts). Because the final data did not statistically differ from one to another operative condition ($p > 0.1$ for both elements), it can be concluded that the selected variations did not introduce any worsening of the method performances. The results on the uncertainty (table 4) showed that, for Cd, u_R and u_{tru} contributed for the 50% each to the combined uncertainty, while in the case of Pb the u_R had the largest part in the uncertainty being the 75% of the u_{comb}. The U were 4.74% for Cd and 13.8% for Pb at the mean concentrations found in real samples.

Offal (liver, kidney, spleen, lung and hearth) of different types of animals were analyzed for Cd and Pb content using the method here validated (table 7). As regards Cd, its content in calf decreased as follows: kidney > liver >> spleen and lung. In lamb it was not detected in all offal and in pig liver it was found at the highest level (114 ng/g). The results indicated that kidney and liver are the critical organs for accumulation of Cd. In fact, its elimination rate from these two organs is relatively low partly due to the link with metallothioneins in these tissues. With reference to Pb, in calf it was undetectable in spleen and lung, and at level of tens of ng/g in liver and kidney. In lamb, Pb accumulated in liver and kidney at levels of hundreds of ng/g, more than in lung (72.2 ng/g) and heart (below 6 ng/g). In pig liver it was found below 10 ng/g. The higher Pb concentration in lamb than in calf and pig can be ascribed to the fact that lambs were more prone to contamination due to their grazing outside, on the contrary, calves and pigs are fed indoors. Finally, Cd and Pb values here found were below the ML recommended for these contaminants in offal [18].

Table 7. Levels (in ng/g) of Cd and Pb in offal

	Type	Cd	Pb
Calf	Liver	58.2 ± 1.8	31.8 ± 1.2
	Kidney	96.4 ± 4.5	22.9 ± 1.3
	Spleen	< MLoD	< MLoQ
	Lung	< MLoD	< MLoQ
Lamb	Liver	< MLoD	279 ± 11
	Kidney	< MLoD	172 ± 10
	Lung	< MLoD	72.2 ± 2.7
	Heart	< MLoD	< MLoQ
Pig	Liver	114 ± 9	9.19 ± 0.43

CONCLUSION

The validation process and the calculation of the uncertainty associated to values are crucial points for laboratories who want to undertake preliminary actions towards food safety standards. Some international guidelines issued by AOAC, EURACHEM, ISO and IUPAC which define validation and standardization frameworks for analytical chemistry, are recommended to be followed. The efforts in approaching such quality system led benefits to laboratories in terms of quality of the produced analytical data, comparison of results among teams and minimization of costs. The validation process consists in the determination of a number of parameters, namely, limits of detection and quantification, sensitivity, specificity, linearity, repeatability, reproducibility, trueness and robustness and in the check of their full compliance with established acceptability criteria. These criteria are the basis for the final acceptability of the analytical data and of the validated method. At this point, laboratories can be sure that all the different effects that might led to variations in the final data have been taken into account. Among the various validation parameters, the measurements used to calculate method reproducibility and accuracy can be subsequently used to quantify the uncertainty of results; this means that each laboratory can easily perform an in-house calculation of the uncertainty associated to values and this approach has the advantage of limiting extra-work and costs. Also the robustness is an important parameter to be calculated because it indicates that the method does not change its performances when some alterations to the original protocol were applied; this serves to demonstrate that the validated method is suitable for the purpose also in the presence of sudden changes that can happen during the routine analysis. To monitor if the analytical procedure is able to maintain the performances over the time, the use of the Shewhart control charts is strictly recommended. The charts highlight the state-of-the-art of the method performances with time through the analysis of control samples. In case of deviation from the normality the adoption of a corrective action is required to lead again the method under control. The next and unavoidable step is the daily application of the validated method to the analysis of real samples for a certain amount of time.

Following this rationale, an in-house validation study was applied to the SF-ICP-MS determination of metals (As, Cd and Pb) that are considered contaminants to be monitored in food control national plans because toxic to animals and humans. The validation figures obtained in each method fully satisfied the criteria recommended by the international quality standards above mentioned. Among them, the trueness results ranged from 97.6% (Pb, milk) to 106% (Pb, offal). The precision of the methods were below 7% for all elements in milk and offal, whereas worsened in honey (up to ca. 20%). For all matrices, the uncertainty coming from the reproducibility measurements contributed most to the overall method uncertainty. In particular, the U for milk and offal were below the 15%, while raised to ca.40% in honey. The high uncertainty related to honey analysis can be ascribed to the high heterogeneity of the raw mass. All methods were robust versus operative changes both on the sample treatment phases and on ICP-MS settings and showed long-term stability with values never above the warning line of the control charts. Finally, the validated analytical procedures were applied to milk, honey and offal sampled on the Italian market to have a picture of their possible contamination by As, Cd and Pb. In this context, Cd and Pb were found at level of fractions or few ng/g in honey and milk. Arsenic was not detected in cow milk and in infant formulas. Whereas, the highest Cd and Pb values were found in liver and kidney of animals (i.e. at level of hundreds of ng/g). In conclusion, the metal contents in food of animal origin were below the ML reported by the Regulation 1881/2006, and thus, even if samples were not numerous, products seemed to be safe for Italian consumers, both adults and children. The analytical approach used can be adapted in the future to achieve a satisfactory quality level in the case of the routine analysis of a wider range of metals in other kinds of foods.

ACKNOWLEDGEMENTS

This work was carried out in the framework of the activity of the Community Reference Laboratory for Chemical Elements in Food of Animal Origin at the Istituto Superiore di Sanità of Rome (CRL-ISS).

REFERENCES

[1] Bromenshenk, J. J. and Carlson, S. R. (1985). Pollution monitoring of Pugget Sound with honey bees. *Science*, *227*, 632–634.

[2] Jones, K. B. (1987). Honey as an indicator of heavy metal contamination. *Water, Air, Soil Poll.*, *33*, 179-189.

[3] Leita, L., Muhlbachova, G., Cesco, S., Barbattini, R. and Mondini, C. (1996). Investigation on the use of honeybees and honeybee products to assess heavy metal contamination. *Environ. Monit. Assess.*, *43*, 1-9.

[4] Abou-Arab, A. A. K. (2001). Heavy metals contents in Egyptian meat and the role of detergent washing of their levels. *Food Chem. Toxicol.*, *39*, 593–599.

[5] Miranda, M., López-Alonso, M., Castillo, C., Hernández, J. and Benedito, J. L. (2005). Effects of moderate pollution on toxic and trace metal levels in calves from a polluted area of northern Spain. *Environ. Pollut.*, *31*, 543–548.

[6] Sedki, A., Lekouch, N., Gamon, S. and Pineau, A. (2003). Toxic and essential trace metals in muscle, liver and kidney of bovines from a polluted area of Morocco. *Sci. Total Environ.*, *317*, 201–205.

[7] Dabeka R. W. and McKenzie, A. D. (1987). Lead, cadmium, and fluoride levels in market milk and infant formulas in Canada, *J. AOAC*, *70*, 754-757.

[8] FAO/WHO Food Standards Programme, Codex Alimentarius, Codex Standard for infant formula. *CODEX STAN* 72-1981, 1-7.

[9] IARC. (2004). Monographs on the Evaluation of Carcinogenic Risks to Humans. Volume 84. Lyon, France.

[10] FAO/WHO. (1983). Arsenic. Safety evaluation of certain food additives and contaminants. *WHO food additive series*. Volume 18. Geneva, Switzerland.

[11] FAO/WHO. (2001). Cadmium. Safety evaluation of certain food additives and contaminants. *WHO food additive series*. Volume 46. Geneva, Switzerland.

[12] IARC. (1997). Monographs on the Evaluation of Carcinogenic Risks to Humans. Volume 58. Lyon, France.

[13] FAO/WHO. (2000). Lead. Safety evaluation of certain food additives and contaminants. *WHO food additive series*. Volume 44. Geneva, Switzerland.

[14] WHO/ENHIS. Exposure of children to chemical hazards in food. *Fact sheet* no. 4.4. May 2007.· Code: RPG4_Food_Ex1.

[15] Pocock S. J., Smith M. and Baghrst P. (1994). Environmental lead and children's intelligence: a systematic review of the epidemiological evidence, *Brit. Med. J.*, *309*, 1189-1197.

[16] Needleman H. L. and Gatsonis C. A. (1990). Low-level lead exposure and IQ of children. A meta-analysis of modern studies, *JAMA*, *263*, 673-678.

[17] Jensen, A. A. (1991). Levels and trends of environmental chemicals in human milk. In: A. A. Jensen, and S. A. Slorach (Eds.). *Chemical contaminants in human milk*. (pp. 45–198) Boston, USA: CRC Press Inc.

[18] Commission Regulation (EC) No. 1881/2006 of 19 December 2006 setting maximum levels for certain contaminants in foodstuffs. *OJ L364*, 5–24.

[19] FAO/WHO. Food Standards Programme, Codex Alimentarius, Revised Codex Standard for Honey, *CODEX STAN* 12-1981, Rev.1 (1987), Rev.2 (2001), 1-7.

[20] FAO/WHO. (1989). Arsenic. Safety evaluation of certain food additives and contaminants. *WHO food additive series*. Volume 24. Geneva, Switzerland.

[21] United States Environmental Protection Agency, IRIS Data Base, 2001.

[22] US Agency for Toxic Substances and Disease Registry. Minimal Risk Levels (MRLs) for Hazardous Substances (December 2006). Available from URL: http://www.atsdr.cdc.gov/mrls/.

[23] Opinion of the Scientific Panel on Contaminants in the Food Chain on a request from the Commission related to arsenic as undesirable substance in animal feed. (2005). *The EFSA Journal*, *180*, 1-35.

[24] Opinion of the Scientific Panel on Contaminants in the Food Chain on a request from the Commission related to cadmium as undesirable substance in animal feed. (2004). *The EFSA Journal*, *72*, 1-24.

[25] Opinion of the Scientific Panel on Contaminants in the Food Chain on a request from the Commission related to lead as undesirable substance in animal feed. (2004). *The EFSA Journal*, *71*, 1-20.

[26] Commission Regulation (EC) No 882/2004 of the European Parliament and of the Council of 29 April 2004 on official controls performed to ensure the verification of compliance with feed and food law, animal health and animal welfare rules. *OJ L165*, 1–141.

[27] Commission Regulation (EC) No 333/2007 of 28 March 2007 laying down the methods of sampling and analysis for the official control of the levels of lead, cadmium, mercury, inorganic tin, 3-MCPD and benzo(a)pyrene in foodstuffs. *OJ L88*, 29-38.

[28] FAO/WHO. (2001). Food Standards Programme, Codex Alimentarius Commission - Procedural Manual - Twelfth Edition (pp 1-175). FAO/WHO, Rome, Italy.

[29] A Report of a Joint FAO/IAEA Expert Consultation. (1998). Food and nutrition paper, volume 68. Validation of analytical methods for food control. (pp. 1-20). FAO, Rome, Italy.

[30] Taverniers, I., De Loose, M. and Van Bockstaele, E. (2004). Trends in quality in the analytical laboratory. II. Analytical method validation and quality assurance. *TrAC*, *23*, 535-552.

[31] Association of Official Analytical Chemists. (1989). Guidelines for collaborative study-procedures to validate characteristics of a method of analysis. *J. AOAC Int.*, *72*, 694–704.

[32] Thompson, M., S. L. R. Ellison, S. L. R. and Wood, R. (2002). Harmonized guidelines for single laboratory validation of methods of analysis (IUPAC Technical Report). *Pure Appl. Chem.*, *74*, 835–855.

[33] Eurachem. (1998). The fitness for purpose of analytical methods. A laboratory guide to method validation and related topics. Teddington, United Kingdom: Eurachem-*LGC.*

[34] ISO 5725-1:1994. Accuracy (trueness and precision) of measurement methods and results. *ISO*, Geneva, Switzerland.

[35] VIM. (1993). International Vocabulary of Basic and General Terms in Metrology, 2nd edition, *ISO*, Geneva, Switzerland.

[36] Taverniers, I., Van Bockstaele, E. and De Loose, M. (2004). Trends in quality in the analytical laboratory. I. Traceability and measurement uncertainty of analytical results. *TrAC*; *23*, 480-490.

[37] ISO 17025:1999. General requirement for the competence of calibration and testing laboratories. *ISO*, Geneva, Switzerland.

[38] ISO/IEC 98:1995. Guide to the expression of uncertainty in measurement (GUM*). ISO,* Geneva, Switzerland.

[39] Ellison, L. R., Rosslein M. and Williams, A. (2000). Eurahem/Citac Guide CG 4: Quantifying uncertainty in analytical measurement (QUAM) (2nd edition). Teddington, United Kingdom: Eurachem-LGC.

[40] ISO/TS 21748:2004. Guidance to the use of repeatability, reproducibility and trueness estimates in measurement uncertainty estimation. *ISO*, Geneva, Switzerland.

[41] Commission Decision 2002/657/EC of 12 August 2002 implementing Council Directive 96/23/EC concerning the performance of analytical methods and the interpretation of results. *OJ L221*, 8– 36.

[42] AOAC Peer Verified Methods Advisory Committee. AOAC Peer Verified Methods Program - Manual on policies and procedures. AOAC International, 1998, pp 1-35. Gaithersburg, MD, USA

[43] ISO 11843-1:1997. Capability of detection - Part 1 Terms and definitions. *ISO*, Geneva, Switzerland.

[44] Currie, L. A. (1995). Nomenclature in evaluation of analytical methods, including detection and quantification capabilities. (IUPAC Recommendations 1995). *Pure Appl. Chem.*, *67*, 1699 – 1723

[45] NATA Tech Note #17. (1997). Requirements for the Format and Content of Test Methods and Recommended Procedures for the Validation of Test Methods. NATA, Sidney, Australia.

[46] Freiser H. and Nancollas, G. H. (1987). IUPAC, Compendium of Analytical Nomenclature (2nd edition). Oxford, UK: *Blackwell Science*.

[47] ISO Standard 3534-1:2006. Statistics - Vocabulary and symbols - Part 1: General statistical terms and terms used in probability.

[48] Gluschke, M., Wellmitz, J. and Lepom, P. (2005). A case study in the practical estimation of measurement uncertainty. *Accred. Qual. Assur*., *10*, 107-111

[49] Feinberg, M., Boulanger, B., Dewé, W. and Hubert, P. (2004). New advances in method validation and measurement uncertainty aimed at improving the quality of chemical data. *Anal. Bional. Chem*., *380*, 502-514

[50] ISO 8250:2004. Shewhart control chart. *ISO*, Geneva, Switzerland.

In: Progress in Food Chemistry
Editor: E. N. Koeffer, pp. 73-103
ISBN: 978-1-60456-303-0

Chapter 3

STUDY OF THE ALCOHOLIC FERMENTATION OF MUST STABILIZED BY PULSED ELECTRIC FIELDS — EFFECT OF SO_2

Teresa Garde-Cerdán[1,2], Margaluz Arias-Gil[2], A. Robert Marsellés-Fontanet[3], M. Rosario Salinas[1], Carmen Ancín-Azpilicueta[2] and Olga Martín-Belloso[3*]

[1] Cátedra de Química Agrícola, E.T.S.I. Agrónomos, Universidad de Castilla-La Mancha, Campus Universitario, 02071 Albacete, Spain

[2] Departamento de Química Aplicada, Universidad Pública de Navarra, Campus de Arrosadía s/n, 31006 Pamplona, Spain

[3] CeRTA-UTPV, Food Technology Department, University of Lleida, Avda. Rovira Roure, 191, 25198 Lleida, Spain

ABSTRACT

Pulsed electric field (PEF) technology has been used to preserve fruit juice and to delay spoilage by microorganism. In vinification, sulphur dioxide (SO_2) is used as antimicrobial and as antioxidant. The aim of this study was to assess the effect of the sulphur dioxide content on the nitrogen metabolism (consumption of amino acids and formation of biogenic amines) and the production of volatile compounds throughout the alcoholic fermentation of must processed by PEF. Taking advantage of the fact that PEF treatments allow reducing the level of sulphur dioxide and, at the same time, guarantee the biochemical and microbiological stability of the must this study could be a starting point leading to an effective reduction of the sulphur dioxide content in wines. For this purpose, must of *Vitis vinífera* var. *Parellada* was stabilized by a PEF treatment and inoculated with *Saccharomyces cerevisiae* Na33 strain. The fermentations were carried out with and without SO_2.

From the results obtained, it was observed that the PEF treatment led to four logarithmic reductions of the microbial population of *Parellada* must without modifying the content of fatty acids and free amino acids of *Parellada* grape juice, which are

* e-mail: omartin@tecal.udl.es

essential for the development of the yeast during fermentation. As far as the development of the wine alcoholic fermentation is concerned, results showed that yeast consumed preferably the amino acids in the first half of fermentation in presence of SO_2. The final concentration of amino acids in the wines obtained using PEF was greater when the must fermented without SO_2 than when the latter compound was present. Therefore, it could be stated that the presence of SO_2 facilitated the consumption of amino acids and, hence, the wine may have higher microbiological stability than that obtained from fermentation without SO_2. Regarding the biogenic amines, they were mainly synthesized after the consumption of the first 25% of sugars and their formation was qualitative and quantitatively low. The SO_2 concentration did not affect the formation of biogenic amines during the alcoholic fermentation. On the other hand, the evolution of the volatile compounds profile throughout the fermentations with and without SO_2 was similar. The content of volatile acids in the wine obtained using SO_2 was not significantly different than that fermented without adding this compound. However, the final content of total alcohols and esters were different even thought the differences were small.

Consequently, when grape must was treated by PEF, the SO_2 concentration usually used in winemaking could be reduced to safer levels or even eliminated without an important effect on the volatile compounds content of the final product. Therefore absence of SO_2 should not have a negative impact on sensory characteristics of wine.

Keywords: PEF; *Saccharomyces cerevisiae*; Sulphur dioxide; White wines; Fatty acids; Amino acids; Nitrogen compounds; Biogenic amines; Volatile compounds.

INTRODUCTION

Fruit juices have become very popular commodities because consumers associate them to healthy products, so their commercialisation is increasing continuously. Among them, grape juice is one of the most important because it is consumed directly either as a final product or as a raw material (i.e. winemaking). In both manufacturing processes, grape juice is undergone to different treatments such as thermal processing which can affect its components. From the point of view of human consumption, lipid and nitrogen contents of grape juice are low and they have hardly nutritional interest in human diet. However, they are related with the sensorial quality of grape juice and wine. Therefore, a modification of the profile of these components could affect their flavour and taste. Such sensory changes come from collateral reactions, in which are involved amino acids and unsaturated fatty acids, occurred during the manufacturing process. These side reactions acquire more significance when the product temperature increases. Thus, amino acids produce reduced sulphur compounds like hydrogen sulphide [1], and they also participate in non-enzymatic browning of grape juice. Unsaturated fatty acids, by their side, can yield some volatile compounds by enzymatic splitting such as aldehydes, ketones and alcohols that confer undesirable flavour and taste to final products [2].

In addition, both lipids and nitrogen compounds play an important role in the fermentative steps of winemaking. Fatty acids and sterols have a great influence on the growth of fermentative yeast and thus, on the development of alcoholic fermentation. They have a remarkable influence on the transport of amino acids through the microbial membrane and the activity of the membrane-linked enzymes such as ATPase [3]. Moreover, the lack of unsaturated fatty acids decreases the yeast tolerance to ethanol [4]. Nitrogen compounds of grape juice are also essential in the metabolism of yeasts because nitrogen is, after carbon, the second element utilized during their growth. The content of nitrogen compounds also affects the kinetics of fermentation. Thus, a lack of nitrogen was related with some "sluggish" and "stuck" fermentation [5]. However, unless nitrogen compounds are completely consumed after the fermentation process they can promote microbiological instability because of the bacterial growing, and the production of ethyl carbamate, which is a carcinogenic compound [6]. Some factors affecting the yeast assimilation of nitrogen compounds from the must such as must composition [7, 8], must clarification [9], yeast strain [10], pH, temperature and ethanol content [11] have already been studied.

The compounds formed during the alcoholic fermentation have a decisive influence on the volatile composition of wine. The major volatile products of yeast metabolism such as ethanol, glycerol, and carbon dioxide have a relatively small but fundamental contribution to wine flavour. The main groups of compounds that form the *fermentation aroma* are esters, alcohols, and acids [12]. The formation of these compounds depends on several factors where yeast strain, fermentation conditions and type of vinification are the most important parameters [13-16]. Moreover, the concentration of amino acids of must can influence in a decisive way in the *fermentation aroma* of wine due to the fact that the main groups of volatile compounds that form this *aroma* are influenced to various degrees by the nitrogen source [17-20]. The catabolism of amino acids to yield the keto-acids and their corresponding alcohols are an example of the important relationship between nitrogen metabolism and these groups of volatile compounds.

Other chemical compounds to take into consideration when safety is of concern are biogenic amines. These compounds are aliphatic, aromatic or heterocyclic organic bases of low molecular mass with a basic behaviour that occur in plants and in fermented foods. These compounds are undesirable in all foods and beverages because if consumed at an excessively high concentration, they may induce headaches, respiratory distress, heart palpitation, hyper-hypotension, and several allergenic disorders in man [21]. Moreover, polyamides, spermine, spermidine, and putrescine, can react with nitrous acid and its salts to form nitrosamines, compounds of known carcinogenic action [21]. Furthermore, the volatile amines can have an influence on wine aroma. Due to the acidic pH of the wine these amines occur as odourless salts, but in the mouth they are partially converted in the acidic form and their flavour becomes apparent [22]. The variability in biogenic amines contents of wine could be explained on the basis of differents in winemaking processes, time and storage conditions, raw material quality, and possible microbial contamination during winery operations [23, 24]. The microorganisms responsible for biogenic amines production in the wine is still a matter of controversy. Several studies attribute their formation to the action of lactic acid bacteria during the malolactic fermentation [25, 26]. However, Landete et al. [27] observed that histamine was the only amine that increased its concentration during the malolactic fermentation. In this sense, Buteau at al. [28] question that the formation of biogenic amines is due to the action of the lactic acid bacteria and they attribute its formation to the action of spoilage microorganisms.

Sulphur dioxide is used in vinification as an antiseptic against undesirable microorganisms and as an antioxidant against the effects of the oxygen. It has also some effect on the activity of certain grape enzymes that promote the loss of quality of the juice and its derivatives. It is the case of polyphenoloxidases, including tyrosinase and peroxidase. These enzymes occur in the must, arising from the grape itself, or from fungi that have infected the grapes. SO_2 inactivates these enzymes by reducing their copper cofactor [29]. Once dissolved in water, sulphur dioxide is a weak acid that renders other inorganic compounds called generically SO_2-free forms. In addition, each form reacts with several components of the must to produce SO_2-combined forms. The concentrations of each product depend mainly on the temperature, pH and the initial concentration of sulphur dioxide since these factors have a strong influence on the equilibrium of the chemical reactions. In general, at low concentrations and high pH, sulphur dioxide has a fungistatic effect whereas at high concentrations and low pH acts as a fungicide. It is well accepted that yeast are mainly affected by SO_2-free forms that disturb essential biological paths after entering the yeast cells. Macris and Markakis [30] proposed that *S. cerevisiae* uptakes SO_2 by active transport although other study [31] suggested that diffusion could be bound to occur. Once inside the cell, SO_2 would induce changes in the tridimensional enzymatic conformations as well as cause depletion of the yeast's cellular ATP content due to its effects on glycolysis and respiratory chain phosphorylation [32]. Thus, the SO_2 could influence in the utilization of amino acids by the yeasts. Regarding bacteria, all SO_2-compounds have antibacterial activity and consequently it is possible to act selectively on the different microorganisms present in must [33]. However, sulphur dioxide could have negative effects on human health [29]. For that reason, several international organizations (WHO, FAO, OIV) have set down maximum limits for the vinification as well as promoted a reduction of its concentration in foodstuffs, specifically in wines. However, as far as we know, the combination of both PEF and SO_2 has not been considered previously in grape juice processing.

A convenient way to achieve the same effects of sulphur dioxide could be the thermal processing of grape juice after pressing although it is of general knowledge that thermal treatments modify not only the sensorial characteristics of food but also it could affect its composition and some physicochemical properties. Pulsed electric field (PEF) technology has been used to preserve fruit juices and to delay their spoilage by microorganisms [34-36]. Recently, this technology has been implemented for the production of commercial fruit juices in the USA whereas in the EU an integrated project named NovelQ try to promote this technology industrially (http://www.novelq.org/ANQ/ANQ_index.aspx). It has also been reported that PEF treatments also decreases the activity of enzymes as peroxidases and polyphenoloxidases in grape juice [37], apple and pear extracts [38], peach puree [39] and orange juice [40]. The proposed mechanism of enzymatic inactivation might be related with the change of specific structures of the enzymes [41]. However, few studies exist on the effects of this preservation treatment in the grape juice composition.

After what has been stated, the aims of this research were firstly evaluating the influence of pulsed electric fields (PEF) treatment on fatty acids and free amino acids contents of grape juice, and secondly assessing the effect of the sulphur dioxide content on the consumption of nitrogen compounds, on the evolution of biogenic amines and volatile compounds throughout the alcoholic fermentation of must processed by PEF and inoculated with *Saccharomyces cerevisiae*, which could lead to a reduction on the sulphur dioxide content of wines. Thus this study could be a starting point leading to an effective reduction of the sulphur dioxide content in wines. For this purpose, must of *Vitis vinífera* var. *Parellada* was stabilized by a PEF treatment and inoculated with *S. cerevisiae* Na33 strain. The fermentations were carried out with and without SO_2.

MATERIALS AND METHODS

Grape Juice Preparation

A local wine manufacturer, Raimat (Lleida, Spain), kindly provided grapes (*Vitis vinifera* L. variety *Parellada*). They were harvested at ripeness, washed, drained, split from bunches and frozen at –20 °C until processing during the following two months. The frozen grapes were thawed at 5 °C for 24 hours, afterwards they were manually pressed leading to approximately 15 l of grape juice that were de-aerated by stirring under reduced pressure for 30 minutes. A portion of 3 l of grape juice was kept as must control sample, and the other 12 l was treated by PEF. All recipients and materials, which were in contact with the samples, were previously sterilized.

Devices and Treatment Conditions of PEF Processing

A laboratory scale PEF unit (Ohio State University, Columbus, OH, USA) was used to treat grape juice by PEF. The pulse generator module consists of a high voltage generator (OSU-4F), which can produce potential differences of up to 12 kV, and a pulse generator unit model 9412A (Quantum Composers, Inc., Bozeman, MT, USA), which can render square wave pulses of up to 10 μs and 2000 Hz. The chamber module has eight equal treatment chambers composed of two stainless steel connectors, which act as electrodes, screwed into a Delrin® insulator and separated 0.292 cm (figure 1).

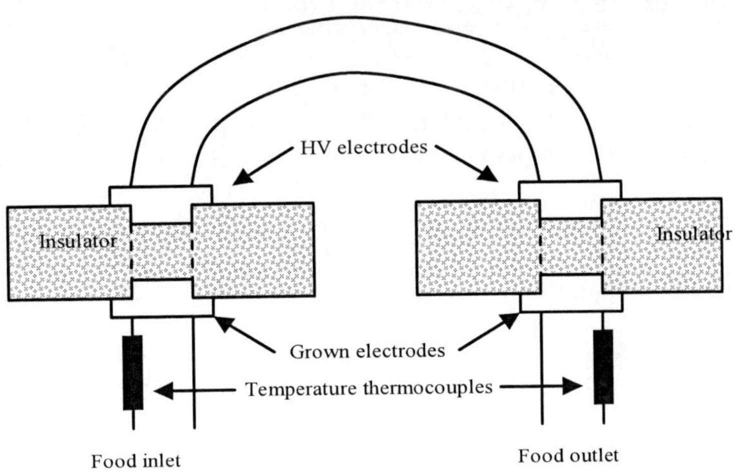

Figure 1. Scheme of a pair of treatment chambers of the PEF equipment used.

The total volume of each chamber is 0.012 cm^3 and the generated electric field between the electrodes had the same direction of the juice flow. A tubing system and a gear peristaltic pump model 75210-25 (Cole Palmer, Vernon Hills, IL, USA), allowed a continuous mode processing of grape juice (3.5 ml/s). Temperature probes attached just before and after each pair of chambers measured inlet and outlet juice temperatures. After each two chambers, grape juice was refrigerated in a tubular heat exchanger immersed into a water-ice bath to avoid temperatures higher than 40 °C, which was the highest temperature recorded by the thermocouples. PEF treatment was performed with bipolar electric field pulses of 4 μs width and with field strength of 35 kV/cm. The pulse repetition rate was 1000 Hz and the total PEF treatment time was 1 ms, which was calculated as the product of the pulse width and the number of pulses delivered to grape juice.

Microbial Culture and Inoculation

To evaluate the effects on microbial population of PEF treatment, 100 ml of freshly squeezed grape juice was inoculated with *S. cerevisiae* CECT 1383 (Spanish type culture collection, University of Valencia, Valencia, Spain). First, the yeast was cultured on dishes containing chloramphenicol glucose agar (CGA) (Biokar Diagnostics, Beauvais, France) for 48 hours at 30 °C to obtain cells in the stationary phase. Afterwards, cells were suspended in saline peptone solution (Biokar Diagnostics) and collected by centrifugation (JP Selecta, Barcelona, Spain) at 4000 rpm for 10 minutes at 4 °C. Cell pellet was added to the juice providing an initial yeast load of 2.7×10^7 cfu/ml. Microbial manipulation was performed with sterile material in a biological safety cabinet (Telstar, S.A., Terrassa, Spain).

Determination of the Microbial Inactivation

After sterile sampling, control and processed grape juice were serially diluted and 1 ml of each dilution was pour plated with chloramphenicol glucose agar (Biokar Diagnostics) for 5 days at 25 °C. The yeast surviving fraction logarithm of each treatment (Equation 1) was used to make comparisons.

$$\text{Log}\left(\text{Surviving fraction}\right) = \text{Log}\left(\frac{C}{C_0}\right) \tag{1}$$

Where C and C_0 are the recovered yeast concentration (cfu/ml) of the processed and non-processed grape juice, respectively, calculated as the average of the four dishes with a count of colony forming units ranging within 25-250.

Vinification

The PEF-processed must was divided into four batch of 3 l. Diammonium phosphate (DAP) was added to must until reaching approximately 55 mg N/l due to the low ammonium content of the must. Two lots of must were kept without any preservative and the other two lots were supplied with potassium metabisulphite up to a concentration of 20 mg/l of total SO_2. After that, all musts were inoculated with an active dry of the Na33 strain of *S. cerevisiae* subsp. *cerevisiae* selected from the Estación de Viticultura y Enología de Navarra (Olite, Spain) and commercialized by Lallemand España. Na33 strain was inoculated in the musts in a proportion of 0.2 g/l rehydrating 0.65 g of dry in a sterile flask with 7.5 ml of distilled water containing 0.07 g of sucrose for 30 min at 35 °C (number of viable cells/ml $\geq 2 \times 10^9$).

The fermentations took place, in duplicate, in glass fermentors with a capacity of 3.5 l and with a burnished lid with two outlets, one of them for sample extractions and the other with a CO_2 trap to eliminate it from the fermentative environment and prevent the entrance of air during fermentation. The hole for sample extraction was covered with a septum during the fermentation. The fermentors were placed over magnetic stirrers (Ikamag RCT basic, Milian SA, Geneve, Switzerland), to ensure a homogenous fermentation. The fermentations were carried out in a hot-cold incubator (Selecta, Barcelona, Spain) at a controlled temperature of 18 °C. The fermentations were daily measured for sugar concentration through their refractive index at 20 °C, using a refractometer ABBE model 325 (Misco, Cleveland, OH, USA) and through enzymatic measurements (reagents from Chema Italia, Rome, Italy) using a multi-parametric analyzer Enochem (Tecnología Difusión Ibérica, Barcelona, Spain). This is an automated device where the appropriate reactions take place. It automatically provides the necessary reactants and also performs the spectrophotometric measurement of the absorbance changes after the programmed incubation time. Samples were taken before the beginning of the fermentation, at 25, 50 and 75% of consumed sugars and at the end of fermentation (reducing sugars < 2.5 g/l). All recipients and materials, which were in contact with the samples, were previously sterilized.

Nitrogenous Fractions and Oenological Parameters

The ammonium content was analysed by enzymatic measurement of the ammonium cation present in the samples using the multi-parametric analyzer Enochem, using reactives from Chema Italia. The free amino acid content measured by HPLC was taken as the amino nitrogen value whereas the assimilable nitrogen was calculated as the sum of the ammonium and the amino nitrogen without taking into account the proline concentration. All the measurements were performed four times.

Determinations of acetic acid, total SO_2, acetaldehyde and total polyphenols were made in the multi-parametric analyzer Enochem by enzymatic and colorimetric methods [42]. The pH was determined by using a pH-meter Metrohm 702 (Metrohm, Herisau, Germany). The total acidity was determined following the method described by the Office International de la Vigne et du Vin [43]. The alcoholic level of the final wine was determined by using a Salleron-Dujardin ebulliometer (Paris, France). Of each one of the samples, the analysis of these parameters was carried out twice.

Extraction and Analysis of Fatty Acids

The lipid fraction of grape juice was extracted using the procedure of Darné and Madero-Tamargo [44]. Thus, 10 ml of ethanol (Merck, Darmstadt, Germany), and 10 ml of distilled water were added to 20 ml of sample and homogenised for 2 minutes at 8000 rpm using an Ultra-Turrax T25 (Rose Scientific, Edmonton, Canada). Afterwards, fatty acids were extracted 5 times with 20 ml of chloroform (Merck) at 0 °C by homogenising at 8000 rpm for 1.5 min with the Ultra-Turrax T25. All chloroform aliquots were combined before fatty acid derivatization, which was done following the method recommended in the Código Alimentario Español [45]. This method consists of generating methyl esters of the naturally occurring fatty acids by transesterification or esterification. Afterwards, these methyl esters were analysed with a GC-MS Shimadzu QP 5000 (Shimadzu, Kyoto, Japan), equipped with an automatic injector Shimadzu AOC-20i.

Helium (99.999% purity) was the carrier gas (41.1 cm/s). Samples of 1 μl were injected into an inlet at 230 °C where they were splitted using a 24:1 ratio. A DB-WAX capillary column (Cromlab, Barcelona, Spain) of 30 m length, 0.25 mm internal diameter and 0.25 μm film thickness with a bonded stationary phase of cross-linked polyethylene glycol was used to perform the separation of methyl esters. Oven temperature was raised from 40 °C up to 111 °C with a slope of 2 °C/min that was immediately followed by other constant increase of 3 °C/min up to 220 °C. This temperature was maintained for 5 minutes before the oven program returned to the initial conditions. The temperature of the detector was set at 230 °C. The ionisation of fatty acid methyl esters was achieved by electronic impact at 70 eV. The fragments analysed were in the range between 40 and 298 *m/z*. Undecanoate and heptadecanoate methyl esters (Aldrich, Gillingham, UK), were used as the internal standards. Identification of fatty acid methyl esters was made using the retention times and comparing either their mass spectra with a spectral library of known standard compounds. The quantification of the compounds was made in Full Scan. For the quantification of the compounds, the area of the corresponding peaks was normalized by that of the corresponding internal standard and was interpolated in a calibration graph made through the analysis of standard solutions in hexane. Of each one of the samples, fatty acids analysis was carried out 4 times.

Preparation and HPLC Analysis of Free Amino Acids

Analysis were performed with a Waters high-pressure liquid chromatography (Milford, MA, USA) equipped with two 510 pumps, a 717 Plus Autosampler, and a 996 Photodiode Array Detector used at 254 nm. A Pico·Tag reverse phase column (300 mm × 3.9 mm i.d.) with a stationary phase of dimethyloctadecylsilyl bonded to amorphous silica was used. Amino acid derivatization was performed using a Waters Pico·Tag workstation. The Pico·Tag method used for amino acid analysis is described in Garde-Cerdán et al. [42]. Samples were cleaned by ultra filtration with a Millipore Ultrafree MC cartridge (Billerica, MA, USA), and then L-norleucine and L-methionine sulfone (Aldrich) were added as internal standards. Afterwards, a precolumn derivatisation was carried out with phenylisothiocyanate (Pierce Biotechnology, Rockford, IL, USA). A Millennium 32 software package (Waters) was employed for chromatographic control. The amount of sample injected was 10 µl. The column was set at 46 °C. Mobile phase A: solution of 2.5% of acetonitrile (Scharlau, Barcelona, Spain) and 97.5% of a solution of sodium acetate (70 mM), with pH adjusted to 6.55 with acetic acid (10%) (Merck); mobile phase B: acetonitrile, water and methanol (Scharlau) (45:40:15, v/v/v). The mobile phases used were filtered through a 0.45 µm Millipore filter. Table 1 shows the elution gradient used to perform amino acid separation. Amino acids determination was repeated four times for each sample.

Table 1. Gradient elution program using a flow rate of 1 ml/min

Time (min)	Eluent A (%)	Eluent B (%)
0	100	0
13.5	97	3
24.0	94	6
30.0	91	9
50.0	66	34
62.0	66	34
62.5	0	100
66.5	0	100
67.0	100	0
87.0	100	0

HPLC Analysis of Biogenic Amines

Fifteen amines were studied (putrescine, spermine, phenethylamine, spermidine, histamine, tyramine, cadaverine, amylamine, hexylamine, dimethylamine, ethylamine, diethylamine, isopropylamine, isobutylamine, and pyrrolidine). The method used to determine biogenic amines is described in Ancín-Azpilicueta et al. [16]. Samples were cleaned by ultrafiltration with a Millipore Ultrafree MC cartridge. Subsequently, precolumn derivatization with 6-aminoquinolyl-N-hydroxysuccinimidyl carbamate (AQC) from AccQ-Fluor reagent kit (Waters) was carried out. Analyses of the derivatized amines were performed with a Waters high-pressure liquid chromatograph equipped with two 510 pumps, a 717 Plus autosampler, and a 474 fluorescence detector, using 250 and 395 nm as excitation and emission wavelengths, respectively. Millennium 32 software was employed for chromatographic control. The amount of sample injected was 10 µl. A reversed phase column (300 mm x 3.9 mm i.d.) was used, with a stationary phase of dimethyloctadecylsilyl bonded to amorphous silica. The column was set at 65 °C. The compositions of the mobile phases were as follows: phase A, solution of sodium acetate trihydrate (140 mM) (Scharlau) and triethylamine (17 mM) (Aldrich), with pH adjusted to 5.05 with phosphoric acid (85%) (Merck); phase B, methanol (Scharlau). The program used followed the sequence: initial isocratic elution at 80% phase A and 20% phase B for 5 min, followed by linear gradient elution from 20 to 80% phase B up to 25 min (constant total flow of 1 ml/min). Phenethylamine and spermidine could not be separated, and they were quantified as a single peak. The measures of biogenic amines were carried out in duplicate.

Analysis of Volatile Compounds by Gas Chromatography

For the analyses of the compounds of high volatility and high concentration (ethyl acetate, n-propanol, isobutanol, and isoamyl alcohols) the method outlined by Fraile et al. [46] was used. These compounds were analysed by direct injection of 0.5 μl of sample in a gas chromatograph Shimadzu GC-14B (Shimadzu) with a flame ionisation detector (FID). The DB-WAX capillary column with stationary phase of polyethylene glycol bonded and cross-linked was used. Chromatographic conditions were as follow: He as carrier gas (30.9 cm/s); injector and detector temperature, 180 °C; oven temperature, 80 °C. The standards were prepared with reagents from Aldrich at concentrations between 1 and 400 mg/l.

For the analyses of the middle-range volatility and, in general, present in lesser concentrations than the former ones the method outlined by Garde-Cerdán and Ancín-Azpilicueta [47] was used. To extract middle-range volatile compounds, solid-phase extraction (SPE) with cartridges LiChrolut EN resins (Merck) was used. The analysis of the extract was carried out in a GC-MS Finnigan (San Jose, USA) using the same DB-WAX capillary column. The chromatographic conditions were: He as carrier gas (30.9 cm/s); injector temperature, 240 °C; temperature of the transfer line, 240 °C. The middle-range volatile compounds were separated using a temperature program with initial oven temperature of 40 °C for 5 min, a temperature gradient of 2 °C/min to a temperature of 50 °C, maintained during 10 min, followed by a gradient temperature of 2 °C/min to a final temperature of 240 °C, and a final time of 20 min (total run time=135 min). The sample injected was 2.5 μl, using the spiltless technique. The ionisation was produced by electronic impact at 70 eV. Operation mode was Full Scan, between 35 and 300 amu. The dissolutions of the standards were prepared in dichloromethane HPLC quality (Panreac) from Aldrich reagents in concentrations between 0.1 and 250 mg/l, to which heptanoic acid (Aldrich) was added as internal standard in the same concentration as in the samples.

Identification of these compounds was made using the retention times and comparing either their mass spectra with a spectral library of known standard compounds. The standards of each compound were injected individually and thus a library was made of the characteristic mass spectra of each one of the compounds. The quantification of these compounds was made in Full Scan. For the quantification, the area of the corresponding peaks was normalized by that of the internal standard and was interpolated in a calibration graph made through the analysis of standard solutions in dichloromethane. The recovery values were always > 78%.

The compounds of the middle-range volatility and their retention time (in minutes) were: isoamyl acetate (11.44), ethyl hexanoate (21.14), ethyl lactate (31.23), n-hexanol (32.55), ethyl octanoate (38.40), ethyl 3-hydroxybutyrate (44.06), butyric acid (51.01), ethyl decanoate (52.07), diethyl succinate (54.00), 3-(methylthio)-1-propanol (56.09), 2-phenylethyl acetate (61.14), hexanoic acid (63.18), benzyl alcohol (64.38), 2-phenylethanol (66.41), internal standard (heptanoic acid, 68.48), diethyl malate (73.05), octanoic acid (74.14), 4-methoxyacetophenone (76.48), decanoic acid (83.49), ethyl acid succinate (88.10), dodecanoic acid (92.42), tetradecanoic acid (100.58), hexadecanoic acid (108.42), tyrosol (111.54), octadecanoic acid (115.56), 9,12-octadecadienoic acid (116.56), vanillic acid (126.39), and tryptophol (129.44).

Each determination was performed 4 times and the results averaged.

Statistical Analysis

All the results are expressed as mean and standard deviation. The differences between means were compared using the least significant difference (LSD) method with a significance level of 5%. All data processing was performed with a SPSS software package (SPSS Inc., Chicago, IL).

RESULTS AND DISCUSSION

Oenological Parameters

Table 2 shows the measured properties of the fresh and processed *Parellada* grape juice. Reducing sugar content in all the samples was below the usual values for this parameter in wine grape juice varieties, which are between 180 and 288 g/l. Therefore, *Parellada* is commonly used to be mixed with others to elaborate sparkling low alcohol or fizzy wines with pale colour and a freshly and floral taste [33]. There were no significant changes in the reducing sugar content, pH and total acidity of grape juice when *Parellada* must was processed by PEF (table 2). These results widen the outcome obtained when tomato and orange juices were treated by PEF, as they did not show significant changes of these parameters [48, 49].

Table 2. Physicochemical properties measured on fresh and processed *Parellada* grape juice

Measured parameter	Control	PEF
Reducing sugar (g/l)	131 ± 2 a	131 ± 2 a
pH	3.84 ± 0.02 a	3.83 ± 0.02 a
Total acidity (g/l)*	2.37 ± 0.04 a	2.43 ± 0.05 a

* Expressed as g/l tartaric acid.

Values were reported in mean ± standard deviation (n = 4). Different letters indicate significant differences between the samples ($p < 0.05$).

The wines obtained from the inoculated must fermented with or without SO_2 did not show the presence of acetic acid (table 3). This result could be due to the fact that the inoculated yeast (*S. cerevisiae* Na33 strain) produces a very low concentration of acetic acid [47]. In general, *Saccharomyces* yeasts produce less acetic acid than other yeasts [50]. The total concentration of SO_2 decreases during the fermentation, so that the half of the initial concentration of SO_2 was observed in the wines (table 3). The concentration of acetaldehyde was higher at the beginning of the fermentation in the samples fermented in presence of SO_2 than in those fermented without SO_2, which is known to enhance the production of acetaldehyde [51]. The addition of SO_2 induced significantly higher acetaldehyde production by yeast because this molecule binds SO_2 and in this form the toxicity of SO_2 is reduced. At the end of the fermentation, higher concentration of acetaldehyde was observed in the wine obtained from the fermentation without SO_2 (table 3).

During the alcoholic fermentation, the concentration of total polyphenols decreased in the studied samples. Polyphenols (including catechins, proanthocyanidins, cinnamic acids and their derivatives) are subject to oxidation so that the initial straw yellow colour of white wines turns into the deep golden yellow typical of browned wines [52]. The wines obtained from both fermentations with or without SO_2 presented similar levels of total polyphenols (table 3), therefore the SO_2 content did not affect to the final polyphenol concentration.

Table 3. Oenological parameters at 25%, 50% and 75% of consumed sugars and of the final wines obtained from fermentation with SO_2 (20 mg/l) and without SO_2. All parameters are given with their standard deviation (n = 4).

Sample	pH	Acetic acid (g/l)	Total acidity (g/l)*	Total SO_2 (mg/l)	Acetaldehyde (mg/l)	Total polyphenols (mg/l)	Alcohol (v/v %)
25% of consumed sugars							
With SO_2	3.19 ± 0.04 a	-	3.48 ± 0.09 a	10 ± 0 a	28 ± 1 a	243 ± 3 a	2.2 ± 0.2 a
Without SO_2	3.17 ± 0.03 a	-	4.67 ± 0.04 b	- b	7.3 ± 0.5 b	192 ± 4 b	2.1 ± 0.2 a
50% of consumed sugars							
With SO_2	3.22 ± 0.04 a	-	3.5 ± 0.2 a	13 ± 1 a	17.5 ± 0.2 a	203 ± 4 a	4.2 ± 0.2 a
Without SO_2	3.17 ± 0.02 a	-	4.1 ± 0.1 b	- b	11 ± 1 b	189.5 ± 0.6 b	4.1 ± 0.1 a
75% of consumed sugars							
With SO_2	3.20 ± 0.04 a	-	3.88 ± 0.06 a	10.8 ± 0.5 a	9.8 ± 0.5 a	180 ± 8 a	6.3 ± 0.5 a
Without SO_2	3.17 ± 0.03 a	-	4.21 ± 0.06 b	- b	12 ± 1 b	190.5 ± 0.6 a	6.1 ± 0.1 a
Wine							
With SO_2	3.24 ± 0.02 a	-	4.1 ± 0.1 a	8 ± 1 a	1.7 ± 0.5 a	122 ± 2 a	8.3 ± 0.2 a
Without SO_2	3.25 ± 0.01 a	-	4.33 ± 0.07 a	- b	8 ± 1 b	122 ± 4 a	8.5 ± 0.5 a

* Expressed as g/l tartaric acid.

Different letters indicate significant differences between the samples with and without SO_2 ($p < 0.05$).

Kinetics of Fermentations

To characterize the kinetics, the process rate has been calculated from fermentation curves, as an average percentage of the daily-consumed sugar in the ranges of 5-50% ($vf_{5\text{-}50}$) and 0-99% ($vf_{0\text{-}99}$) of total sugars [53]. These results are shown in table 4. The inoculated fermentation with SO_2 showed a daily consumption of sugars somewhat lower than in the inoculated fermentations without SO_2, probably because the SO_2 destroyed part of the population of inoculated yeasts.

Table 4. Features of the fermentation kinetics in the samples

	dt_{5-50}[a] (days)	dt_{0-99}[b] (days)	Vf_{5-50}[c] (%/day)	Vf_{0-99}[d] (%/day)
With SO_2	2	4	22.5	24.80
Without SO_2	2	3	22.5	33

[a] Days needed to ferment from 5 to 50% of sugars. [b] Days needed to ferment from 0 to 99% of sugars. [c] Average percentage of sugar used daily during the fermentation time required from 5% to 50% of the total. [d] Average percentage of sugar used daily during the fermentation time required from 0% to 99% of the total.

Effects of PEF Processing on *Saccharomyces cerevisiae*

The average of *S. cerevisiae* recovered from *Parellada* grape juice after 1 ms of square waved pulses of 4 μs width and 35 kV/cm electric field strength in bipolar mode using a continuous PEF equipment (figure 1) was 2.7 x 10^3 cfu/ml that means 4.0 ± 0.4 decimal logarithmic reductions at a maximum temperature of 40 ºC [42]. The lessening of survival fraction of yeast obtained after PEF processing is within the range of values reported in other juices inoculated with *S. cerevisiae*. A similar PEF treatment was effective enough to reach up to 5.1 and 5.8 logarithmic reductions of *S. cerevisiae* and *Lactobacillus brevis* population in orange juice using the same equipment [34, 35]. Cserhalmi et al. [54] achieved a maximum reduction of 3.4 logarithms when apple juice was treated with square wave pulses of 2 μs and 28 kV/cm for 100 μs in a similar PEF. All these results show how microbial destruction and its rate might vary with a large number of factors such as the processing conditions, the media and the microorganism characteristics. In this context, the effects of using several combination of treatments (thermal and PEF treatments and antimicrobials) to reduce yeast population of red and white grape juice have recently been published [55]. Wu et al. [55] reported 3.9 log microbial reductions combining a thermal treatment of 50 ºC for 30 s with a PEF treatment of 20 adjacent triangular shaped pulses of 1 μs width and 40 kV/cm in bipolar mode using a batch PEF equipment. They also reported up to 5.2 log reductions when these treatments were combined with 4 g/l of lysozyme.

Effects of PEF Processing on Grape Juice Fatty Acids and Free Amino Acids

The fatty acid concentrations of control and processed grape juice are showed in table 5. Comparing *Parellada* grape juice with other varieties such as *Cortese* and *Garnacha*, the total fatty acid values are similar or quite lower, respectively, [9, 56] evincing that composition of grape juice is variety dependent. The total fatty acid content in the PEF treated grape juice (51 mg/l) was slightly lower than in the control juice (54.1 mg/l). These values show that the processing treatment has little effect on total fatty acid content. The PEF treatment made that the concentration of lauric acid in the grape juice diminished (table 5).

Table 5. Concentration of fatty acids (mg/l) measured on fresh and processed *Parellada* grape juice

Fatty acid	Control	PEF
Caprilic acid (C8)	-	-
Capric acid (C10)	-	-
Lauric acid (C12)	0.32 ± 0.01 a	0.19 ± 0.03 b
Myristic acid (C14)	0.37 ± 0.05 a	0.38 ± 0.03 a
Palmitic acid (C16)	14.55 ± 0.08 a	13.8 ± 0.4 a
Palmitoleic acid (C16:1)	-	-
Stearic acid (C18)	1.07 ± 0.01 a	1.11 ± 0.09 a
Oleic acid (C18:1)	2.296 ± 0.003 a	2.3 ± 0.1 a
Linoleic acid (C18:2)	25.38 ± 0.04 a	24.2 ± 0.8 a
Linolenic acid (C18:3)	10.073 ± 0.009 a	9.4 ± 0.4 a
Total fatty acids	54.1 ± 0.1 a	51 ± 1 b

Values were reported in mean ± standard difference (n = 8).
Different letters indicate significant differences between the samples ($p < 0.05$).

This result is in agreement with those obtained by Zulueta et al. [57]. Provably, the degasification chamber of the PEF equipment could makes a little release of C12, due to the volatile characteristic of this molecule. The presence of short chain fatty acids (C12, C14) in the yeasts is only given in occasions and in trace levels. On the other hand, linolenic and oleic acid contents were unaffected by the treatment. These are the most necessary fatty acids during the normal growth of yeasts. In addition, both fatty acids act as survival factors at the end of fermentation [58]. In a similar way, the processing treatment did not modify the long chain saturated fatty acids (C14 and C16), which affect the degree of saturation of the plasma membrane of yeast [59]. Actually, grape juice treatments should keep unaltered the total concentration of fatty acids since a low level could lead to slow fermentations and an increase of volatile acidity of wine because of an incorrect development of the yeast along the fermentative process. Some of these troubles have been reported when other treatments have been carried out on other varieties of grapes [9].

Table 6 shows the concentrations of free amino acids found in *Parellada* grape juice before and after processing. All *Parellada* grape juice samples, either treated or untreated, showed a higher amino acid content (control 1394 mg/l, PEF 1424 mg/l) than the described for *Garnacha* (678 mg/l), *Cabernet Sauvignon* (782 mg/l), and *Pinot Noir* (857 mg/l). The treatment applied to the grape juice did not affect the total concentration of amino acids (table 6). On the other hand, the preservative treatment showed few effects on free amino acids content. In PEF treated grape juice, the concentrations of histidine, tryptophan, asparagine, phenylalanine and ornithine were superiors than in the control. These amino acids probably were released through the pores formed in the plasmatic membrane of the grape juice indigenous yeasts [60]. The conditions of PEF treatment could cause organelle disruptions, so vacuoles were destroyed too allowing the proteases to have a free access to the cytoplasmic enzymes [61]. These proteases could cause cellular protein degradation into smaller peptides and amino acids. It is remarkably that PEF treatment at least did not change significantly the natural amino acid content because, as noted previously, it is directly linked with the fermentation rate, the yeast population and with the global quality of the resulting wine [7, 17].

Table 6. Concentration of amino acids (mg/l) measured on fresh and processed *Parellada* grape juice

Amino acid	Control	PEF
Proteic amino acids		
Arginine (Arg)	774 ± 69 a	772 ± 52 a
Proline (Pro)	119 ± 11 a	101 ± 6 a
Alanine (Ala)	82 ± 7 a	87 ± 6 a
Leucine (Leu)	28 ± 2 a	25 ± 2 a
Serine (Ser)	29 ± 3 a	29 ± 4 a
Threonine (Thr)	16 ± 1 a	14 ± 3 a
Tryptophan (Trp)	30 ± 2 a	46 ± 3 b
Glutamic acid (Glu)	31 ± 2 a	31 ± 2 a
Aspartic acid (Asp)	26 ± 2 a	23 ± 2 a
Valine (Val)	22 ± 2 a	30 ± 5 a
Asparagine (Asn)	24 ± 2 a	37 ± 3 b
Tyrosine (Tyr)	8.6 ± 0.3 a	11 ± 2 a
Histidine (His)	26.5 ± 0.9 a	33 ± 4 b
Methionine (Met)	28 ± 3 a	20 ± 4 a
Phenylalanine (Phe)	12.9 ± 0.7 a	18 ± 1 b
Isoleucine (Ile)	7.3 ± 0.2 a	6.3 ± 0.9 a
Lysine (Lys)	5.2 ± 0.5 a	8 ± 2 a
Glycine (Gly)	3.5 ± 0.3 a	3.2 ± 0.4 a
Non-proteic amino acids		
γ-Amino butyric acid (Gaba)	38 ± 3 a	32 ± 2 a
Cystathionine (Cyst)	37 ± 1 a	39 ± 12 a
Creatinine (Creat)	13 ± 1 a	12 ± 2 a
Ornithine (Orn)	9 ± 1 a	18 ± 3 b
Hydroxyproline (Hyp)	16 ± 2 a	20 ± 2 a
Phosphoserine (Pser)	8.3 ± 0.4 a	8.1 ± 0.5 a
Total amino acids	1394 ± 71 a	1424 ± 54 a

Values were reported in mean ± standard difference (n = 8).
Different letters indicate significant differences between the samples ($p < 0.05$).

Utilization of Nitrogen Nutrients during the Alcoholic Fermentations

The highest uptake of all nitrogen fractions occurred in the first half of the fermentation (table 7), likely due to the exponential growth phase of yeast where nitrogen is used for biomass production [62]. The ammonium nitrogen was almost entirely consumed either with SO_2 (96%) or without SO_2 (94%). Regarding amino nitrogen, it was reduced up to a 76% when the fermentation was carried out with sulphur dioxide and a 67% in absence of SO_2 (table 7). Thus, the total consumption of assimilable nitrogen was 328 mg N/l (95%) during the fermentation carried out with SO_2 and 315 mg N/l (91%) when SO_2 was not present.

Arginine and proline, together with alanine were the most abundant amino acids in PEF treated must (table 6). They accounted for 68% of the total amino acids content of must. This fact agrees with data reported by other authors [7, 11, 16]. The concentration of arginine in the initial must is the greatest by far accounting for 56% of total amino acids. This result is similar to those reported by other authors [63]. *Parellada* variety had a low proline/arginine ratio, what means that the must contained a high quantity of assimilable nitrogen for the yeasts [64]. This ratio is influenced mainly by the grape variety, and the grape ripeness [65].

Table 7. Nitrogenous fractions of the initial PEF treated must, at 50% of consumed sugars and of the final wines obtained from fermentation with SO_2 (20 mg/l) and without SO_2. All parameters are given with their standard deviation (n = 8).

Samples	Ammonium nitrogen (mg N/l)	Amino nitrogen (mg N/l)	Assimilable nitrogen (mg N/l)
Must			
	57.9 ± 0.5	300 ± 1	347 ± 1
50% of the consumed sugars			
With SO_2	3.7 ± 0.7 a	129 ± 1 a	27 ± 1 a
Without SO_2	5 ± 0 b	175 ± 4 b	68 ± 8 b
Wine			
With SO_2	2.3 ± 0.6 a	71 ± 3 a	18.8 ± 0.6 a
Without SO_2	3.7 ± 0.7 a	100 ± 6 b	31.7 ± 0.7 b

Different letters indicate significant differences between the samples with and without SO_2 ($p < 0.05$).

It is well known that the availability and metabolism of nitrogen compounds is among the key components of both, fermentation development and final wine quality. As can be seen in tables 6 and 8, amino acids are taken up by *S. cerevisiae* mainly during the first half of the fermentation. Besides, in this phase, the consumption of amino acids by yeasts was greater in the fermentation carried out with SO_2 (1198 mg/l) than in that performed without this substance (1048 mg/l). It is well known that SO_2 decreases the yeast population, so that is capable to damage the yeasts plasmatic membrane, as well SO_2 is reactive to some enzymes and can degrade the sulphur bonds needed for structural stability. Once these bonds are broken the enzyme is inactive. SO_2 resistant yeast (Na33) is used in these fermentations. Probably one mechanism of resistance of this yeast against SO_2 was the consumption of more quantity amino acids to replace the damaged enzymes and proteins, which were necessary for their grown in this phase of fermentation.

The most consumed amino acid was the most abundant, that is, arginine; this amino acid presented a higher consumption in the fermentation carried out in presence of SO_2 (769 mg/l) than in the fermentation without SO_2 (676 mg/l) (table 8). Arginine and ammonium ions were the yeasts' principal source of nitrogen during fermentation. Alanine was consumed in a great extension by yeasts during both fermentations (with SO_2, 83.2 mg/l; without SO_2, 79.8 mg/l). Leucine, threonine, tryptophan, tyrosine, isoleucine, γ-amino butyric acid, and citrulline were completely consumed in this phase of fermentation in both cases since they are suitable nitrogen sources [11]. Glutamic acid was not consumed in none of the two fermentations (tables 6 and 8), though this amino acid is a preferred source for the yeasts. This phenomenon could be attributed to the fact that the arginine consumption was very high and glutamate anion is among the final products of arginine metabolism, so yeasts did not need to take glutamic acid from the medium.

The lysine and glycine contents did not decrease in this step of the fermentations because these amino acids are not considered good nitrogen sources for *S. cerevisiae* although they could be metabolised by microorganisms in other fermentations [66]. Yeasts did not consume proline during the initial stage of fermentation because this amino acid is uptaken by the yeasts only under severe nitrogen stress conditions [7, 64], and the presence of ammonium in the medium will inhibit or repress the uptake of proline [67]. The liberation of proline to the medium might be due to the metabolism of arginine since it is an intermediate product in the degradation of arginine [6]. It is thought that, at the beginning of fermentation, *S. cerevisiae* obtain the necessary nitrogen compounds for cellular division from the medium without performing any modification on them. Once the first necessities of each amino acid are satiated, yeasts usually take those amino acids in excess in the medium to use them as nitrogen source [68].

In the second half of fermentation, the amino acid uptake was the same in both types of fermentation (466 mg/l), so that the concentration of SO_2 did not affect to the amino acids consumption in this phase of fermentation (table 8). The total decrease of amino acids was lower than the achieved in the first part of the fermentation. Conversely to the first stage, proline was the most consumed amino acid accounting for 49% (428 mg/l) and 36% (328 mg/l) of the total in the fermentation with and without SO_2, respectively (table 8). Yeasts could use this amino acid in this phase of the fermentation since there were less good nitrogen sources in the medium than at the beginning of the fermentation (table 8). When the good nitrogen sources depleted, the general amino acid permeases and the specific permeases such as proline permease allow the accumulation of the poorer nitrogen sources as proline [65]. The remaining amino acids underwent few variations in their concentrations except arginine, glutamic acid and glycine, which were significantly reduced their concentrations in the fermentation without SO_2, and alanine, which was excreted in both types of fermentation (table 8). Non-proteic amino acids were consumed in greater extension through the second half of the fermentation (table 8).

At the end of the fermentation, high ethanol concentration usually alters the structure and permeability of the plasmatic cell membrane accelerating the passive entry of protons as the electrochemical gradient between both membrane faces decreases in a similar way [69]. While this process takes place, some yeasts also release amino acids into the wine by a passive process of desorption. All these processes are the physiological response to the exhaustion of sugars [70]. However, the yeast strain used in our study was resistant to the presence of ethanol, which is a specific strain characteristic [71]. Thus, the yeasts did not release amino acids at the end of the fermentation but they continued consuming amino acids. At the end of the vinification process, the wine obtained from the fermentation with SO_2 had less concentration of amino acids (532 mg/l) than the wine obtained from the fermentation without SO_2 (728 mg/l).

Formation of Biogenic Amines During the Alcoholic Fermentations

In figure 2 is shown the evolution of the concentration of biogenic amines formed throughout the alcoholic fermentations, with and without SO_2. We only show in this figure the results of the amines found in the analyzed samples (putrescine, spermine, phenethylamine + spermidine, dimethylamine and ethylamine). The other amines (histamine, tyramine, cadaverine, amylamine, hexylamine, diethylamine, isopropylamine, isobutylamine and pyrrolidine) were not detected in the must and they were not formed during the alcoholic fermentation. In the musts, amines were not detected (figure 2). The concentration of amines in the musts is very low [72] and their presence is function of the grape variety, of the soil fertilization and of the climatic conditions [24, 73]. The synthesis of putrescine took place after the consumption of the first 25% of sugars (figure 2a), after the stage of more consumption of nitrogenous compounds (tables 6-8). During winemaking, putrescine can originate from the microbial decarboxylation of arginine and of ornithine, which may be formed by microbial metabolism of arginine [74]. Spermine (figure 2b) and phenethylamine + spermidine (figure 2c) were formed in the second half of the fermentations. This could be because spermine and spermidine are formed from putrescine, which was formed mainly between 25% and 75% of consumed sugars.

Table 8. Concentration of amino acids (mg/l) at 50% of consumed sugars and in the final wines obtained from fermentation of PEF treated must, with SO_2 (20 mg/l) and without SO_2

	50% of consumed sugars		Wine	
Amino acids	With SO_2	Without SO_2	With SO_2	Without SO_2
Proteic amino acids				
Arginine (Arg)	3.0 ± 0.1 a	96 ± 7 b	3.03 ± 0.09 a	13 ± 1 b
Proline (Pro)	874 ± 33 a	919 ± 40 a	446 ± 12 a	591 ± 25 b
Alanine (Ala)	3.8 ± 0.1 a	7.2 ± 0.2 b	8.7 ± 0.2 a	11.9 ± 0.7 b
Leucine (Leu)	-	-	- a	1.2 ± 0.1 b
Serine (Ser)	3.1 ± 0.1 a	2.7 ± 0.2 a	2.4 ± 0.4 a	2.5 ± 0.6 a
Threonine (Thr)	-	-	-	-
Tryptophan (Trp)	-	-	-	-
Glutamic acid (Glu)	21 ± 1 a	34 ± 2 b	22.1 ± 0.2 a	22 ± 1 a
Aspartic acid (Asp)	3.2 ± 0.1 a	8.2 ± 0.5 b	4.2 ± 0.2 a	5.3 ± 0.3 a
Valine (Val)	- a	1.7 ± 0.1 b	- a	1.5 ± 0.2 b
Asparagine (Asn)	2.8 ± 0.1 a	7.4 ± 0.3 b	3.7 ± 0.3 a	7.2 ± 0.2 b
Tyrosine (Tyr)	-	-	- a	2.0 ± 0.1 b
Histidine (His)	1.7 ± 0.3 a	- b	1.9 ± 0.1 a	2.6 ± 0.2 b
Methionine (Met)	- a	5.3 ± 0.3 b	- a	4.0 ± 0.2 b
Phenylalanine (Phe)	0.81 ± 0.01 a	- b	- a	0.45 ± 0.03 b
Isoleucine (Ile)	-	-	-	-
Lysine (Lys)	8 ± 1 a	4.8 ± 0.4 b	3.0 ± 0.1 a	3.1 ± 0.2 a
Glycine (Gly)	4.8 ± 0.2 a	16 ± 2 b	3.0 ± 0.2 a	7.0 ± 0.7 b
Non-proteic amino acids				
γ-Amino butyric acid (Gaba)	-	-	-	-
Cystathionine (Cyst)	15 ± 1 a	21 ± 2 b	11 ± 1 a	13 ± 1 a
Creatinine (Creat)	27 ± 1 a	36 ± 1 b	18.7 ± 0.1 a	27 ± 1 b
Ornithine (Orn)	1.9 ± 0.1 a	11 ± 1 b	1.0 ± 0.1 a	8 ± 1 b
Hydroxyproline (Hyp)	22 ± 2 a	18 ± 1 b	0.76 ± 0.03 a	2.6 ± 0.1 b
Phosphoserine (Pser)	6.7 ± 0.1 a	5.9 ± 0.1 b	2.9 ± 0.1 a	2.4 ± 0.2 b
Total amino acids	999 ± 33 a	1194 ± 41 b	532 ± 12 a	728 ± 25 b

The concentrations are shown with their standard deviations (n = 8).
Different letters indicate significant differences between the samples with and without SO_2 ($p < 0.05$).

At the end of the alcoholic fermentation the concentration of these amines was low, what indicates that the yeasts are little producers of these compounds during the alcoholic fermentation. These results agree with those found by other authors in white wines after the alcoholic fermentation. In this way, Leitao et al. [75] found concentrations of putrescine in the wines between 0 and 2500 μg/l; Romero et al. [76] did not find spermine and spermidine in the wines and Landete et al. [27] found concentrations of phenethylamine smaller than 2500 μg/l. Of all them the most abundant was putrescine (figure 2a), majority amine in the wines [22, 24, 27]. In none of our samples, the concentration of phenethylamine was above the concentration considered as toxic for the man (3000 μg/l) [77]. Differences were not observed in the formation profile neither in the concentration of these amines in function of the level of SO_2 ($p<0.05$) (figures 2a-c). This indicates that the concentration of SO_2 did not affect the formation of these compounds, result that it agrees with that found by Vidal-Carou et al. [23], in white wines, for histamine and tyramine.

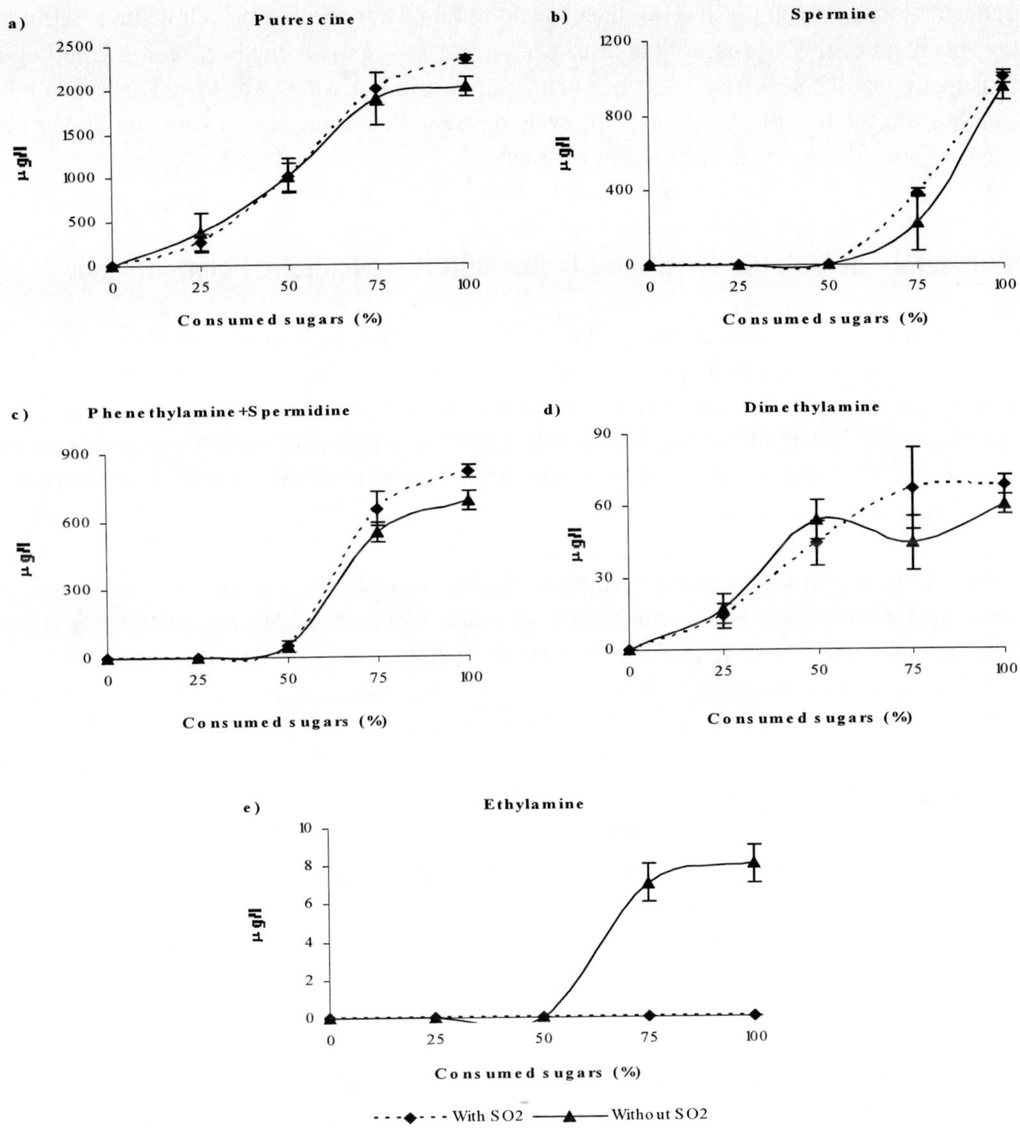

Figure 2. Evolution of biogenic amines (μg/l) during the wine alcoholic fermentations with (20 mg/l) and without SO_2. All parameters are given with their standard deviation (n=4).

In the alcoholic fermentations, with and without SO_2, dimethylamine was formed mainly between 25% and 50% of consumed sugars (figure 2d). The formation of this compound was not affected by the concentration of SO_2 ($p<0.05$). Ethylamine was only formed in the fermentation without SO_2 (figure 2e). Its synthesis took place in the second half of the fermentation but in low quantities so that the effect of the SO_2 it can be considered minimum. The concentration of dimethylamine was above 50 μg/l, above which this amine can have negative effects in the beer aroma [78]. As for ethylamine, in all the samples its concentration was below the concentrations found by Soleas et al. [79] in white wines after the alcoholic fermentation (150-300 μg/l). Also, the concentration of this amine was below the level found by Palamand et al. [78] susceptible of causing negative impact in the beer aroma (2000 μg/l). It is likely that the sensorial effect of volatile amines in our wines was low. This assumption comes from the fact that the threshold levels of organoleptic impact on wine are higher than those of beer, due to the grater content of ethanol.

Formation of Volatile Compounds through the Alcoholic Fermentation

Figure 3 shows the evolution of alcohols (n-propanol, isobutanol, isoamyl alcohols, 2-phenylethanol, tyrosol, tryptophol, 3-methylthio-1-propanol, n-hexanol, and benzyl alcohol) through the alcoholic fermentation. It is clear that the formation of alcohols was higher during the first half of the fermentation, because the consumption of amino acids was greater in this stage of the fermentation [64]. The process with presence of sulphur dioxide hardly modified its content after middle fermentation whereas the increase of alcohols in samples without preservative was smooth from the beginning to the end (figure 3a). Final alcohol content (160 mg/l) of wines fermented without sulphur dioxide was around a 20% lower than in those fermented with it. This value corresponds to a half of the threshold for affecting adversely wine aroma that has been settled above 300 mg/l [80].

Total alcohol concentration followed the same trend that isoamyl alcohols content since they are the main alcohols of wines [81, 82] (figure 3d). The isoamyl content found was well above 60 mg/l, which is the sensory detection level of this compound [83]. A similar pattern was observed for 2-phenylethanol and tyrosol (figures 3e-f). The yeasts consume amino acids to use them to form proteins as well as a nitrogen source. Although higher alcohols may originate via synthesis from sugars, the deamination of certain amino acids from yeast, originate the release of higher alcohols into the fermentative medium. As noted previously, the consumption of the amino acids, which are principal precursors of the mentioned above leucine, isoleucine, phenylalanine and tyrosine, was completely in both fermentations (table 8). The higher production of these alcohols was probably because the yeast population in the fermentation with SO_2 presented more anabolic activity than the yeast population in the fermentation without SO_2, and used more quantity of these amino acids as a nitrogen source than in the fermentation without SO_2. 2-Phenylethanol could contribute positively to the aroma of wine obtained from the fermentation with SO_2 because it found around its perception threshold (14 mg/l) [84].

No differences were observed in the release of tryptophol, and 3-methyltio-1-propanol (figures 3g-h), between both fermentations, although the consumption of tryptophol precursor, tryptophan, was completely in both fermentations and the consumption of methionine was lesser in the fermentation without SO_2 addition (table 8). The production of n-propanol and n-hexanol by yeast was practically the same either using or not sulphur dioxide (figures 3b and 3i). The production of these alcohols is not related with the anabolic routes of amino acids, the same as benzyl alcohol which was the only compound whose content was higher in the fermentation without preservative than with its presence (figure 3j) even though its effect on sensory properties is not important due to its high sensory threshold (200 mg/l) [85].

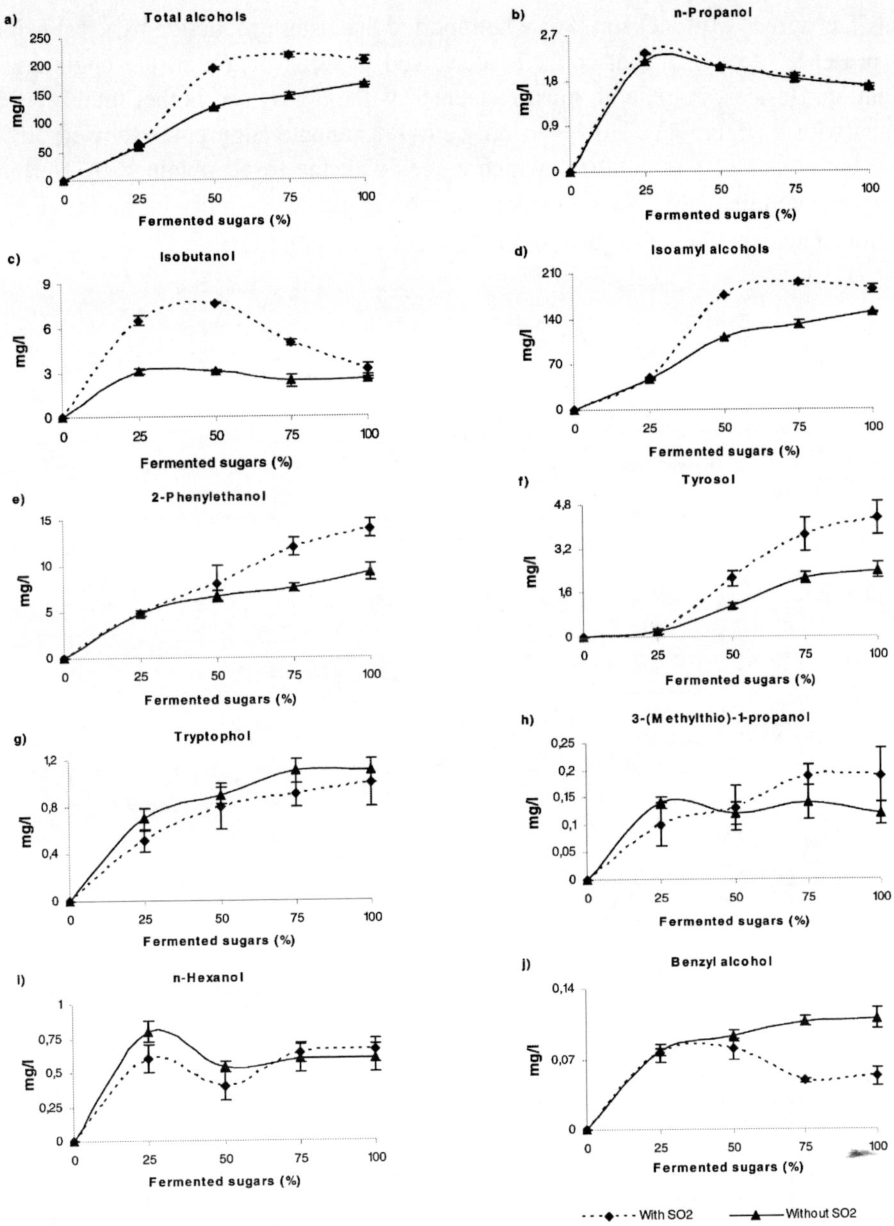

Figure 3. Evolution of alcohols concentrations (mg/l) during the wine alcoholic fermentations with (20 mg/l) and without SO2. All parameters are given with their standard deviation (n=8).

As for volatile esters (ethyl acetate, isoamyl acetate, 2-phenylethyl acetate, ethyl hexanoate, ethyl octanoate, and ethyl decanoate) produced during fermentation, their evolution throughout the process is gathered in figure 4 where figure 4a collects the general behaviour except for ethyl acetate. Ethyl acetate (figure 4b) is considered separately due to its different contribution to wine flavour. Anyway, it is obvious that, independently of the use of sulphur dioxide, the evolution profile for all of them was very similar having a substantial rise after 25% of consumed sugars followed by a gradual increase up to reaching the maximum at the end of the fermentation.

This fact agrees with Jackson [86] who reported that ester production by yeast is inhibited by the presence of oxygen that could be dissolved in some degree at the beginning of the fermentation. Besides, in general, must fermented without SO_2 had higher total ester content than must with it (figure 4a). However, only ethyl hexanoate (figure 4e) showed differences between both types of fermentation, which agrees with the result obtained by Herraiz [87]. This author found that ethyl hexanoate was formed in greater quantity in the fermentation of *Verdejo* must made without SO_2 than in the fermentation with SO_2.

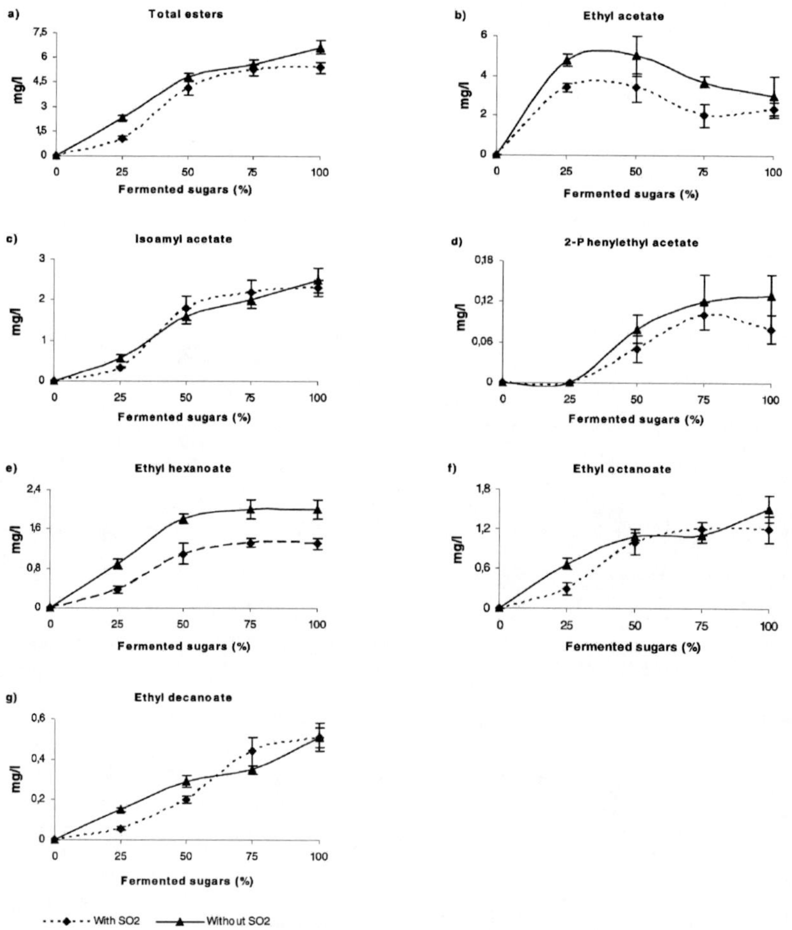

Figure 4. Evolution of esters concentrations (mg/l) during the wine alcoholic fermentations with (20 mg/l) and without SO_2. All parameters are given with their standard deviation (n=8).

Ethyl acetate confers complexity to the wine fragrance below 50 mg/l whereas above 150 mg/l it is bound to add vinegar off-odours to the wine [88]. Both types of fermentation yielded a similar final concentration, which was less than 50 mg/l, despite being the most abundant ester produced [12]. The final concentration of ethyl acetate was lower than concentrations commonly found in wines [89-92], since the inoculated yeast (Na33) produces a low concentration of this ester [16, 47]. Isoamyl acetate, ethyl hexanoate, ethyl octanoate, and ethyl decanoate concentrations (figures 4c and 4e-g), which play a significant role in wine flavour, were above their sensory threshold levels (1, 0.08, 0.58 and 0.51 mg/l, respectively) [83, 93]. This data suggests that the absence of sulphur dioxide should not decrease the quality of wine.

Fatty acids (butyric acid, hexanoic acid, octanoic acid, decanoic acid, dodecanoic acid, tetradecanoic acid, hexadecanoic acid, and ethyl acid succinate) were the third group of substances analysed (figure 5). They showed a more homogeneous behaviour between fermentations with and without sulphur dioxide than the previous compounds since both, the trend and the measured concentrations, were practically the same throughout the process. Similar outcomes have been reported by other authors [46, 47].

Final concentration of fatty acids was 15 mg/l regardless the presence of sulphur dioxide (figure 5a). These compounds produce changes in wine flavour depending on their concentrations and it has been described that the limit of perception is around 20 mg/l [94]. At this level, fatty acids add a fresh flavour to wine increasing the appreciation of other taste sensations whereas higher values confer an unpleasant flavour. Consequently, the obtained results indicate that the elimination of the preservative during fermentation did not produce any damage to the typical notes that fatty acids give to the wine flavour when must is stabilized by PEF.

CONCLUSION

PEF treatment led to four logarithmic reductions of the microbial population of *Parellada* must and did not modify the total content of fatty acids and free amino acids of *Parellada* grape juice. This is important since these compounds are essential for the development of the yeast during fermentation. As far as the development of the wine alcoholic fermentation, results showed that yeast consumed preferably the amino acids in the first half of fermentation in presence of SO_2. The final concentration of amino acids in the wines obtained using PEF was greater when the must fermented without SO_2 than when the latter compound was present. Therefore, it could be stated that the presence of SO_2 facilitated the consumption of amino acids and, hence, the wine may have higher microbiological stability than that obtained from fermentation without SO_2.

Regarding the biogenic amines, they were mainly synthesized after the consumption of the first 25% of sugars and their formation was qualitative and quantitatively low. The SO_2 concentration did not affect the formation of biogenic amines during the alcoholic fermentation. On the other hand, the evolution of the volatile compounds profile throughout the fermentations with and without SO_2 was similar. The content of volatile acids in the wine obtained using SO_2 was not significantly different than that fermented without adding this compound. However, the final content of total alcohols and esters were different even thought the differences were small. Thus, when grape must was treated by PEF, the SO_2 concentration usually used in winemaking could be reduced to safer levels or even eliminated without an important effect on the volatile compounds content of the final product.

Consequently, PEF treatments together with the inoculation of a selected strain of yeast may lead to a reproducible fermentation process of must to wine. Besides, this approach should allow reducing or even eliminating the use of sulphur dioxide, so on the labels of wine bottles may appear that the wines are "free of sulfites added".

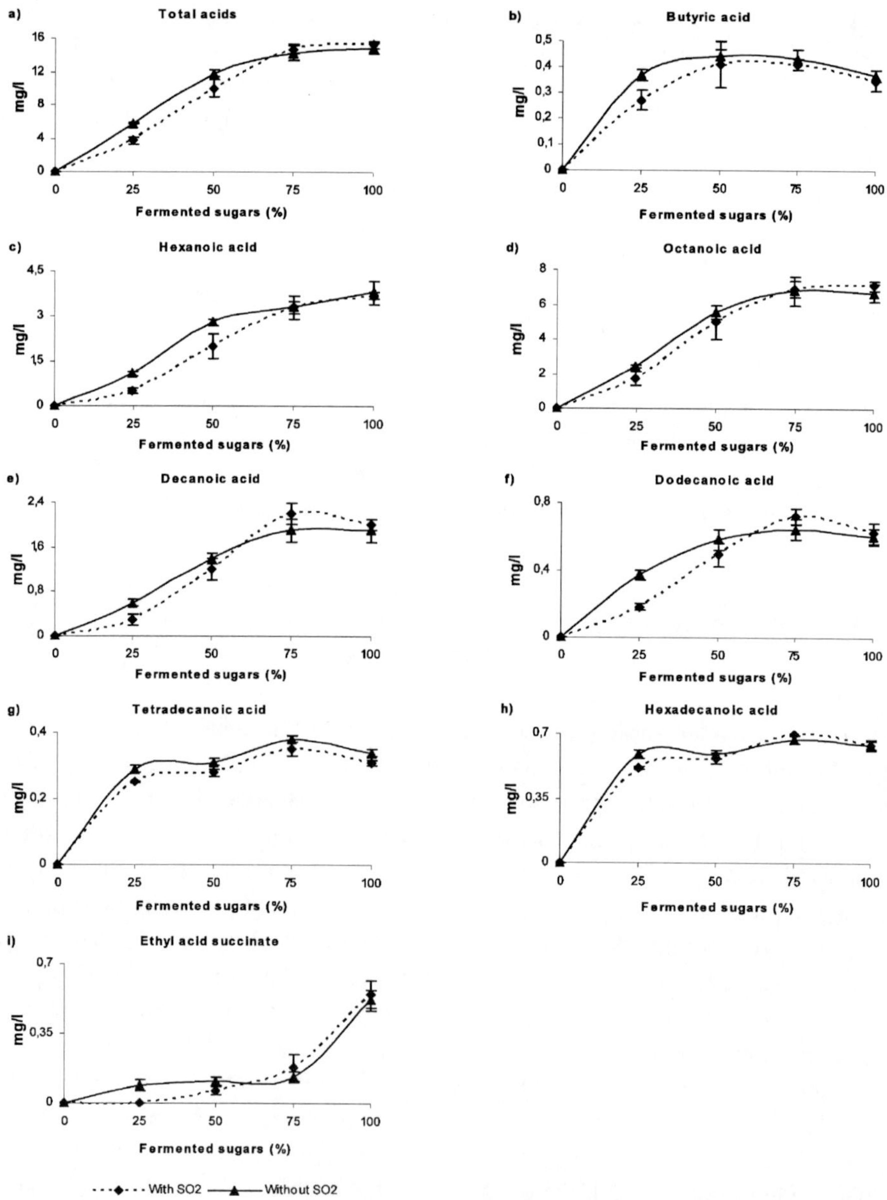

Figure 5. Evolution of acids concentrations (mg/l) during the wine alcoholic fermentations with (20 mg/l) and without SO_2. All parameters are given with their standard deviation (n=8).

ACKNOWLEDGEMENTS

This work was supported by the *Ministerio de Ciencia y Tecnología* through the project AGL2002-04399-C02-02. A. R. Marsellés-Fontanet would like to thank the *Ministerio de Ciencia y Tecnología* for his pre-doctoral grant, M. Arias-Gil would like to thank the *Gobierno de Navarra* for her formation scholarship and T. Garde-Cerdán would like to thank the *Ministerio de Educación y Ciencia* for the Juan de la Cierva contract.

REFERENCES

[1] Henschke, P. A., and Jiranek, V. (1991). Hydrogen sulfide formation during fermentation: effect of nitrogen composition in model grape must. In J. Rantz (Ed.), *International Symposium on Nitrogen in Grapes and Wines*, (pp. 172-184). Davis (USA): American Society for Enology and Viticulture.

[2] Rapp, A., Hastrich, H., and Engel, L. (1976). Gaschromatographische untersuchungen uber du aromastoffe von weinbeeren I Anreicheung und kapillar chromatograshiche auftrennung. *Vitis*, *15*, 29-36.

[3] Prasad, R., and Rose, A. H. (1986). Involvement of lipids in solute transport in yeasts. *Yeast*, *2*, 205-220.

[4] Pilkington, B. J., and Rose, A. H. (1989). Accumulation of sulphite by *Saccharomyces cerevisiae* and *Zygosaccharomyces bailii* as affected by phospholipid fatty-acyl unsaturation and chain length. *Journal of General Microbiology*, *135*, 2423-2428.

[5] Kunkee, R. E. (1991). Relationship between nitrogen content of must and sluggish fermentation. In J. Rantz (Ed.), *International Symposium on Nitrogen in Grapes and Wines*, (pp. 148-155). Davis (USA): American Society for Enology and Viticulture.

[6] Ough, C. S., Crowel, E. A., and Mooney, L. A. (1988). Formation of ethyl carbamate precursors during grape juice (chardonnay) fermentation. I. Addition of amino acid, urea, and ammonia: effects of fortification on intercellular and extracellular precursors. *American Journal of Enology and Viticulture*, *39*, 243-249.

[7] Arias-Gil, M., Garde-Cerdán, T., and Ancín-Azpilicueta, C. (2007). Influence of addition of ammonium and different amino acids concentrations on nitrogen metabolism in spontaneous must fermentation. *Food Chemistry*, *103*, 1312-1318.

[8] Jiranek, V., Langridge, P., and Henschke, P. A. (1990). Nitrogen requirement of yeast during wine fermentation. In P. J. Williams, D. M. Davidson, and T. H. Lee (Eds.), *Proceedings of the Seventh Australian Wine Industry Technical Conference* (pp. 166-171). Adelaida (Australia): Australian Industrial Publishers.

[9] Ancín-Azpilicueta, C., Torrea-Goñi, D., and Garde-Cerdán, T. (2001). Effects of the clarification of must in the development of the alcoholic fermentation. In S. G. Pandalai (Ed.), *Recent Research Development of Agricultural and Food Chemistry*, vol. 5 (pp. 231-249). Kerala (India): Research Signpost.

[10] Ough, C. S., Huang, Z., An, D., and Stevens, D. (1991). Amino acid uptake by four commercial yeasts at two different temperatures of growth and fermentation: effects on urea excretion and reabsorption. *American Journal of Enology and Viticulture*, *42*, 26-40.

[11] Henschke, P. A., and Jiranek, V. (1993). Metabolism of nitrogen compounds. In G. H. Fleet (Ed.), *Wine Microbiology and Biotechnology* (pp. 77-164). Victoria (Australia): Harwood Academic Publishers.

[12] Lambrechts, M. G., and Pretorius, I. S. (2000). Yeast and its importance to wine aroma. A review. *South African Journal of Enology and Viticulture*, *21*, 97-129.

[13] Lema, C., García-Jares, C., Orriols, Y., and Angulo, L. (1996). Contribution of *Saccharomyces* and non-*Saccharomyces* populations to the production of some components of Albariño wine aroma. *American Journal of Enology and Viticulture*, *47*, 206-216.

[14] Egli, C. M., Edinger, W. D., Mitrakul, C. M., and Henick-Kling, T. (1998). Dynamics of indigenous and inoculated yeast populations and their effect on the sensory character of Riesling and Chardonnay wines. *Journal of Applied Microbiology*, *85*, 779-789.

[15] Ancín, C.; Torrea, D., Fraile, P., and Garde, T. (2004). Amino acids and volatile compounds in the fermentation of inoculated musts: biogenic amines in the wines. In F. Shahidi, and D. K. Weerasinghe (Eds.), *Nutraceutical Beverages. Chemistry, Nutrition, and Health Effects. ACS Symposium Series 871* (pp. 302-313). Washington (USA): American Chemical Society.

[16] Ancín-Azpilicueta, C., Fraile-Jiménez de Maquirriain, P., Garde-Cerdán, T., and Torrea-Goñi, D. (2005). Influence of inoculation of selected yeast on the quality of rosé and white wines. In A. P. Riley (Ed.), *Food Research, Safety and Policies* (pp. 57-92). New York (USA): Nova Science Publishers, Inc.

[17] Garde-Cerdán, T., and Ancín-Azpilicueta, C. (2008). Effect of the addition of different quantities of amino acids to nitrogen-deficient must on the formation of esters, alcohols, and acids during alcoholic fermentation. *LWT-Food Science and Technology*, *41*, 501-510.

[18] Hernández-Orte, P., Ibarz, M. J., Cacho, J., and Ferreira, V. (2005). Effect of the addition of ammonium and amino acids to musts of Airen variety on aromatic composition and sensory properties of the obtained wine. *Food Chemistry*, *89*, 163-174.

[19] Hernández-Orte, P., Bely, M., Cacho, J., and Ferreira, V. (2006). Impact of ammonium additions on volatile acidity, ethanol, and aromatic compound production by different *Saccharomyces cerevisiae* strain during fermentation in controlled synthetic media. *Australian Journal of Grape and Wine Research*, *12*, 150-160.

[20] Hernández-Orte, P., Ibarz, M. J., Cacho, J., and Ferreira, V. (2006). Addition of amino acids to grape juice of the Merlot variety: Effect on amino acid uptake and aroma generation during alcoholic fermentation. *Food Chemistry*, *98*, 300-310.

[21] Silla-Santos, M. H. (1996). Biogenic amines: their importance in foods. *International Journal of Food Microbiology*, *29*, 213-231.

[22] Lehtonen, P. (1996). Determination of amines and amino acids in wine. A review. *American Journal of Enology and Viticulture*, *47*, 127-132.

[23] Vidal-Carou, M. C., Codony-Salcedo, R., and Mariné-Font, A. (1990). Histamine and tyramine in Spanish wines: relationships with total sulfur dioxide level, volatile acidity and malolactic fermentation intensity. *Food Chemistry*, *35*, 217-227.

[24] Bover-Cid, S., Izquierdo-Pulido, M., Mariné-Font, A., and Vidal-Carou, M. C. (2006). Biogenic mono-, di- and polyamine contents in Spanish wines and influence of a limited irrigation. *Food Chemistry*, *96*, 43-47.

[25] Moreno-Arribas, V., Torlois, S., Joyeux, A., Bertrand, A., and Lonvaud-Funel, A. (2000). Isolation, properties and behaviour of tyramine producing lactic acid bacteria from wine. *Journal of Applied Microbiology, 88*, 584-593.

[26] Moreno-Arribas, M. V., Polo, M. C., Jorganes, F., and Muñoz, R. (2003). Screening of biogenic amine production by lactic acid bacteria isolated from grape must and wine. *International Journal of Food Microbiology, 84*, 117-123.

[27] Landete, J. M., Ferrer, S., Polo, L., and Pardo, I. (2005). Biogenic amines in wines from three Spanish regions. *Journal of Agricultural and Food Chemistry, 53*, 1119-1124.

[28] Buteau, C., Duitschaever, C. L., and Ashton, G. C. (1984). A study of the biogenesis of amines in a Villard noir wine. *American Journal of Enology and Viticulture, 35*, 228-236.

[29] Romano, P., and Suzzi, G. (1993). Sulfur dioxide and wine microorganisms. In G. H. Fleet (Ed.), *Wine Microbiology and Biotechnology* (pp. 373-393). Victoria (Australia): Harwood Academic Publishers.

[30] Macris, B. J., and Markakis, P. (1974). Transport and toxicity of sulphur dioxide in Saccharomyces cerevisiae var. ellipsoideus. *Journal of the Science of Food and Agriculture, 25*, 21-29.

[31] Stratford, M., and Rose, A. H. (1986). Transport of sulphur dioxide by Saccharomyces cerevisiae. *Journal of General Microbiology, 132*, 1-6.

[32] Maier, K., Hinze, H. and Leuschel, L. (1986). Mechanism of sulfite action on the energy metabolism of Saccharomyces cerevisiae. *Biochimica et Biophysica Acta, 848*, 120-130.

[33] Hidalgo-Togores, J. (2002). *Tratado de Enología*. Madrid (Spain): Mundi-Prensa.

[34] Elez-Martínez, P., Escolà-Hernàndez, J., Soliva-Fortuny, R. C., and Martín-Belloso, O. (2004). Inactivation of *Saccharomyces cerevisiae* suspended in orange juice using high-intensity pulsed electric fields. *Journal of Food Protection, 6*, 2596-2602.

[35] Elez-Martínez, P., Escolà-Hernández, J., Soliva-Fortuny, R. C., and Martín-Belloso, O. (2005). Inactivation of *Lactobacillus brevis* by high-intensity pulsed electric fields. *Food Microbiology, 22*, 311-319.

[36] Sen Gupta, B., Masterson, F., and Magee, T. R. A. (2005). Inactivation of *E-coli* in cranberry juice by a high voltage pulsed electric field. *Engineering in Life Sciences, 5*, 148-151.

[37] Marsellés-Fontanet, A. R., and Martín-Belloso, O. (2007). Optimization and validation of PEF processing conditions to inactivate oxydative enxymes of grape juice. *Journal of Food Engineering, 83*, 452-462.

[38] Giner, J., Gimeno, V., Barbosa-Cánovas, G. V., and Martín, O. (2001). Effects of pulsed electric fields processing on apple and pear polyphenoloxidases. *Food Science and Technology International*, 7, 339-345.

[39] Giner, J., Ortega, M., Mesegué, M., Gimeno, V., Barbosa-Cánovas, G. V., and Martín, O. (2002). Inactivation of peach polyphenoloxidase by exposure to pulsed electric fields. *Journal of Food Science*, 67, 1467-1472.

[40] Elez-Martínez, P., Aguiló-Aguayo, I., and Martín-Belloso, O. (2006). Inactivation of orange juice peroxidase by high-intensity pulsed electric fields as influenced by process parameters. *Journal of the Science of Food and Agriculture*, 86, 71-81.

[41] Zhong, K., Wu, J., Wang, Z., Chen, F., Liao, X., Hu, X., and Zhang, Z. (2007). Inactivation kinetics and secondary structural change of PEF-treated POD and PPO. *Food Chemistry*, *100*, 115-123.

[42] Garde-Cerdán, T., Arias-Gil, M., Marsellés-Fontanet, A. R., Ancín-Azpilicueta, C., and Martín-Belloso, O. (2007). Effects of thermal and non-thermal processing treatments on fatty acids and free amino acids of grape juice. *Food Control*, *18*, 473-479.

[43] Office International de la Vigne et du Vin (1990). Recueil des Méthodes Internationales d'Analyse des Vins et des Moûts. Paris, France.

[44] Darné, G., and Madero-Tamargo, J. (1979). Mise au point d'une méthode d'extraction des lipides solubles totaux, des glucides solubles totaux et des composés phénoliques solubles totaux des organes de la vigne. *Vitis*, *18*, 221-228.

[45] Código Alimentario Español. Análisis. Métodos Oficiales de aceites, grasas, cereales y derivados, productos lácteos y derivados de la uva. *Boletín Oficial del Estado* (BOE) del 17 de julio de 1977 y del 27 de julio de 1977.

[46] Fraile, P., Garrido, J., and Ancín, C. (2000). Influence of a *Saccharomyces cerevisiae* selected strain in the volatile composition of rosé wines. Evolution during fermentation. *Journal of Agricultural and Food Chemistry*, *48*, 1789-1798.

[47] Garde-Cerdán, T., and Ancín-Azpilicueta, C. (2006). Contribution of wild yeasts to the formation of volatile compounds in inoculated wine fermentations. *European Food Research and Technology*, *222*, 15-25.

[48] Min, S., Min, S. K., and Zhang, Q. H. (2003). Inactivation kinetics of tomato juice lipoxygenase by pulsed electric fields. *Journal of Food Science*, *68*, 1995-2001.

[49] Yeom, H. W., Streaker, C. B., Zhang, Q. H., and Min, D. B. (2000). Effects of pulsed electric fields on the quality of orange juice and comparison with heat pasteurisation. *Journal of Agricultural and Food Chemistry*, *48*, 4597-4605.

[50] Rojas, V., Gil, J. V., Piñaga, F., and Manzanares, P. (2003). Acetate ester formation in wine by mixed cultures in laboratory fermentations. *International Journal of Food Microbiology*, *86*, 181-188.

[51] Herraiz, T., Martin-Alvarez, P. J., Reglero, G., Herraiz, M., and Cabezudo, M. D. (1989). Differences between wines fermented with and without sulphur dioxide using various selected yeasts. *Journal of the Science of Food and Agriculture*, *49*, 249-258.

[52] Margheri, G., Tonon, D., and Trepin, P. (1980). I polifenoli dei vini bianchi come potenziali di ossidazione. *Vignevini*, *7*, 35-44.

[53] Houtman, A. C., and du Plessis, C. S. (1985). Influence du cépage et de la souche de levure sur la vitesse de fermentation et sur la concentration des composants volatils du vin. *Bulletin de l'O.I.V.*, *648-649*, 234-246.

[54] Cserhalmi, Z. S., Vidács, I., Beczner, K., and Czukor, B. (2002). Inactivation of *Saccharomyces cerevisiae* and *Bacillus cereus* by pulsed electric fields technology. *Innovative Food Science and Emerging Technologies*, *3*, 41-45.

[55] Wu, Y., Mittal, G. S., and Griffiths, M. W. (2005). Effect of pulsed electric field on the inactivation of microorganisms in grape juice with and without antimicrobials. *Biosystems Engineering*, *90*, 1-7.

[56] Delfini, C., Conterno, L., Giacosa, D., Cocito, C., Ravaglia, S., and Bardi, L. (1992). Influence of clarification and suspended solid contact on the oxygen demand and long-chain fatty acid contents of free run, macerated and pressed grape musts, in relation to

acetic acid production. *Die Wein-Wissenschaft. Viticultural and Enological Sciences, 47,* 69-75.

[57] Zulueta, A., Esteve, M. J., Frasquet, I., and Frígola, A. (2007). Fatty acid profile changes during orange juice-milk beverage processing by high-pulsed electric field. *European Journal of Lipid Science and Technology, 109,* 25-31.

[58] Quain, E. D. (1988). Studies on yeast physiology impact fermentation performance and product quality. *Journal of the Institute of Brewing, 95,* 315-323.

[59] Ness, W. D., Adler, J. H., and Ness, W. R. (1984). A structure-function correlation for fatty acids in *Saccharomyces cerevisiae*. *Experimental Mycology, 8,* 55-62.

[60] Teissié, J., Eynard, N., Vernhes, M. C., Bénichou, A., Ganeva, V., Galutzov, B., and Cabanes, P. A. (2002). Recent biotechnological developments of electropulsation. A prospective review. *Bioelectrochemistry, 55,* 107-112.

[61] Harrison, S. L., Barbosa-Cánovas, G. V., and Swanson, B. G. (1997). *Saccharomyces cerevisiae* structural changes induced by pulsed electric field treatment. *LWT-Food Science and Technology, 30,* 236-240.

[62] O'Connor-Cox, E. S. C., and Ingledew, W. M. (1989). Wort nitrogenous sources. Their use by brewing yeasts: a review. *The Journal of the American Society of Brewing Chemists, 47,* 102-108.

[63] Valero, E., Millán, C., Ortega, J. M., and Mauricio, J. (2003). Concentration of amino acids in wine after the end of fermentation by *Saccharomyces cerevisiae* strains. *Journal of the Science of Food and Agriculture, 83,* 830-835.

[64] Garde-Cerdán, T., Marsellés-Fontanet, A. R., Arias-Gil, M., Martín-Belloso, O., and Ancín-Azpilicueta, C. (2007). Influence of SO_2 on the consumption of nitrogen compounds through alcoholic fermentation of must sterilized by pulsed electric fields. *Food Chemistry, 103,* 771-777.

[65] Bell, S.-J., and Henschke, P. A. (2005). Implications of nitrogen nutrition for grapes, fermentation and wine. *Australian Journal of Grape and Wine Research, 11,* 242-295.

[66] Cooper, T. G. (1982). Transport in Saccharomyces cerevisiae. In J. N. Strathern, E. W. Jones, and J. B. Broach (Eds.), *The Molecular Biology of the Yeast Saccharomyces. Metabolism and Gene Expression* (pp. 399-461). New York (USA): Cold Spring Harbor Laboratory.

[67] Ough, C. S., and Stashak, R. M. (1974). Further studies on proline concentration in grapes and wines. *American Journal of Enology and Viticulture, 25,* 7-12.

[68] Bisson, L. F. (1991). Influence of nitrogen on yeast and fermentation of grapes. In J. Rantz (Ed.), *Proceedings of the International Symposium on Nitrogen in Grapes and Wine* (pp. 78-89). Davis (USA): American Society for Enology and Viticulture.

[69] Cartwright, C. P., Juroszek, J. R., Beaven, M. J., Ruby, F. M. S., de Morais, S. M. F., and Rose, A. H. (1986). Ethanol dissipates the proton-motive force across the plasma membrane of Saccharomyces cerevisiae. *Journal of General Microbiology, 132,* 369-377.

[70] Bidan, P., Feuillat, M., and Moulin, J. P. (1986). Les vins mousseux. Rapport francais. 65ème Assemblée Générale de l'OIV. *Bulletin de l'OIV, 663-664,* 563-626.

[71] Jones, R. P. (1989). Biological principles for the effects of ethanol. *Enzyme and Microbial Technology, 11,* 130-153.

[72] Radler, F., and Fäth, K. P. (1991). Histamine and other biogenic amines. In J. A. Rantz (Ed.), *Proceedings of the International Symposium on Nitrogen in Grapes and Wine* (pp. 185-195). Davis (USA): American Society of Enology and Viticulture.

[73] Sass-Kiss, A., Szerdahelyi, E., and Hajós, G. (2000). Study of biologically active amines in grapes and wines by HPLC. *Chromatographia*, *51*, S-316-S-320.

[74] Arena, M., and Manca de Nadra, M. (2001). Biogenic amine production by *Lactobacillus*. *Journal of Applied Microbiology*, *90*, 158-162.

[75] Leitao, M. C., Marques, A. P., and San Romao, M. V. (2005). A survey of biogenic amines in commercial Portuguese wines. *Food Control*, *16*, 199-204.

[76] Romero, R., Sánchez-Viñas, M., Gázquez, D., and Gracia Bagur, M. (2002). Characterization of selected Spanish table wine samples according to their biogenic amine content from liquid chromatographic determination. *Journal of Agricultural and Food Chemistry*, *50*, 4713-4717.

[77] Glória, M. B. A., Watson, B. T., Simon-Sarkadi, L., and Daeschel, M. A. (1998). A survey of biogenic amines in Oregon Pinot noir and Cabernet sauvignon wines. *American Journal of Enology and Viticulture*, *49*, 279-282.

[78] Palamand, S. R., Hardwick, W. A., and Markl, K. S. (1969). Volatile amines in beer and their influence on beer flavor. In *Proceedings of the American Society of Brewing Chemists* (pp. 54-58).

[79] Soleas, G. J., Carey, M., and Goldberg, D. M. (1999). Method development and cultivar-related differences of nine biogenic amines in Ontario wines. *Food Chemistry*, *64*, 49-58.

[80] Rapp, A., and Mandery, H. (1986). Wine aroma. *Experientia*, *42*, 873-884.

[81] Torrea, D., Fraile, P., Garde, T., and Ancín, C. (2003). Production of volatile compounds in the fermentation of chardonnay musts inoculated with two strains of *Saccharomyces cerevisiae* with different nitrogen demands. *Food Control*, *14*, 565-571.

[82] Garde-Cerdán, T., Marsellés-Fontanet, A. R., Arias-Gil, M., Ancín-Azpilicueta, C., and Martín-Belloso, O. (2008). Influence of SO_2 on the evolution of volatile compounds through alcoholic fermentation of must stabilized by pulsed electric fields. *European Food Research and Technology*, in press. DOI: 10.1007/s00217-007-0734-5.

[83] Simpson, R. F. (1979). Some important aroma components of white wines. *Food Technology in Australia*, *31*, 516-522.

[84] Ferreira, V., López, R., and Cacho, J. F. (2000). Quantitative determination of the odorants of young red wines from different grape varieties. *Journal of the Science of Food and Agriculture*, *80*, 1659-1667.

[85] Gómez-Míguez, M. J., Cacho, J. F., Ferreira, V., Vicario, I. M., and Heredia, F. J. (2007). Volatile components of *Zalema* white wines. *Food Chemistry*, *100*, 1464-1473.

[86] Jackson, R. S. (1994). *Wine Science. Principles and Applications*. New York (USA): Academic Press.

[87] Herraiz Tomico, T. (1990). Formación de compuestos volátiles por distintas levaduras vínicas. Influencia del SO_2 y de los hollejos utilizados durante la fermentación. Thesis, Universidad Complutense de Madrid, Madrid, Spain.

[88] Amerine, M. A., and Roessler, E. B. (1983). *Wines. Their Sensory Evaluation*. New York (USA): Freeman.

[89] Salinas, M. R., Garijo, J., Pardo, F., Zalacain, A., and Alonso, G. L. (2005). Influence of prefermentative maceration temperature on the colour and the phenolic and volatile

composition of rosé wines. *Journal of the Science of Food and Agriculture*, *85*, 1527-1536.

[90] Cabrita, M. J., Costa Freitas, A. M., Laureano, O., Borsa, D., and Di Stefano, R. (2007). Aroma compounds in varietal wines from Alentejo, Portugal. *Journal of Food Composition and Analysis*, *20,* 375-390.

[91] Lorenzo, C., Pardo, F., Zalacain, A., Alonso, G. L., and Salinas, M. R. (2008). Complementary effect of Cabernet Sauvignon on Monastrell wines. *Journal of Food Composition and Analysis*, *21*, 54-61.

[92] Masa, A., and Vilanova, M. Flavonoid and aromatic characterisation of cv. Albarín blanco (*Vitis vinifera* L.). *Food Chemistry*, in press. DOI: 10.1016/j. foodchem.2007.08.014.

[93] Etiévant, P. X. (1991). Wine. In H. Maarse (Ed.), *Volatile Compounds in Foods and Beverages* (pp. 483-546). New York (USA): Marcell Dekker Inc.

[94] Pozo-Bayón, M. A., Alegría, E. G., Polo, M. C., Tenorio, C., Martín-Álvarez, P. J., Calvo de la Banda, M. T., Ruiz-Larrea, F., and Moreno-Arribas, M. V. (2005). Wine volatile and amino acid composition after malolactic fermentation: effect of Oenococcus oeni and Lactobacillus plantarum starter cultures. *Journal of Agricultural and Food Chemistry*, *53*, 8729-8735.

In: Progress in Food Chemistry
Editor: E. N. Koeffer, pp. 105-138
ISBN: 978-1-60456-303-0

Chapter 4

CHEMISTRY OF DEFECTIVE COFFEE BEANS

Adriana S. Franca* and Leandro S. Oliveira
Programa de Pós-Graduação em Ciência de Alimentos/UFMG
Av. Antônio Carlos, 6627 – 31270-901 – Belo Horizonte, MG – Brasil

ABSTRACT

The term "coffee" is usually employed in reference to the consumable beverage obtained by extracting roasted coffee with hot water, but it actually comprises a wide range of intermediate products, starting from the freshly harvested fruit (coffee cherries), then to green beans and to the final product of consumption (roasted coffee). Green coffee beans are the main item of international trade, and their quality is evaluated according to a wide variety of criteria, including bean size, color, and shape, processing method, crop year and flavor (cup quality). Among these, flavor is the most important criterion, and it is directly affected by the presence of the so-called defective coffee beans. The presence of defective beans is usually a consequence of problems that occur during harvesting and pre-processing operations. The most important defects are black, sour or brown, immature, bored or insect-damaged, and broken beans. Both black and sour defects are associated with bean fermentation and play a major role in downgrading coffee flavor. Immature beans (from immature fruits) contribute to beverage astringency. Such defective beans are usually present in the coffee produced in Brazil, due to the strip-picking harvesting and processing practices adopted by the coffee producers. They are separated (color sorting) from the non-defective beans prior to commercialization in external markets, and the majority of these beans are dumped on the Brazilian internal market. Thus, the roasting industry in Brazil has been using these defective beans in blends with healthy ones, and, overall, a low-grade roasted coffee is consumed in the country. Currently there are no analytical methodologies that allow for detection and quantification of defective beans in roasted coffee, and thus an assessment of chemical attributes that could provide differentiation between defective and healthy coffee beans is of relevance. Thus, a review on physical and chemical attributes of defective coffee beans in comparison to healthy ones is herein provided, for both green and roasted coffees. Physical attributes include bean size, volume, density, color and water activity. Chemical attributes include proximate composition, acidity, pH, sucrose levels, caffeine,

*E-mail:adrianafranca@pesquisador.cnpq.br.Tel:+55-31-34096910.Fax:+55-31-34096989

trigonelline, chlorogenic acids, amines and volatile substances. The evaluation of such attributes indicates that, in the case of green coffee, it is possible to differentiate defective and non-defective (healthy) beans by color, size, acidity levels, sucrose levels, and the presence of histamine. In the case of roasted coffee, only an evaluation of the volatile profile will effectively provide the means for differentiation.

1. Introduction

The quality of coffee used for beverages is strictly related to the chemical composition of the roasted beans, which in turn is affected by the composition of the green beans and post-harvesting processing conditions (handling, drying, storage, roasting and grinding). The criteria commonly used to evaluate the quality of coffee beans include bean size, color, shape, roast potential, processing method, crop year, flavor or cup quality and presence of defects (Banks et al., 1999). Among those, the last two are the most important criteria and are employed worldwide in coffee trading. Flavor is the main and most important criterion for evaluating coffee quality. Brazilian coffees are officially categorized by reference to the following flavor scale (Clarke and Macrae, 1987; Banks et al., 1999):

1) Strictly soft: low acidity, mellow sweetness, pleasant feel of the mouth easiness;
2) Soft: same characteristics as strictly soft, only less accentuated;
3) Softish: same characteristics as soft, only less accentuated;
4) Hard: lacks sweetness and softness;
5) Rioysh: iodine, inky flavor from microbe-tainted beans; and

Rio: same characteristics as Rioysh, only more accentuated

This classification, also known as 'cup quality', is assessed using the brewing method of steeping (10 g of roast and ground coffee per 150 ml boiling water left for 5 min), with a medium roast coffee prepared in a sample roaster and with a relatively fine grind. The term defect is used in commercial practice in reference to the presence of defective (black, sour or brown, immature, insect-damaged or bored) beans and also of extraneous matter (twigs, husks, skins and stones) in a given coffee sample. The New York Coffee and Sugar Exchange devised a type-classification system in which a rank is assigned to the coffee type based on the number of defects counted in a sample (table 1). A system, known as the ''black bean count basis'', was also devised in which all defects, intrinsic and foreign, are accounted for in

Table 1. Summary description of the NY type classification system (Franca et al., 2005a)

Type Number	Maximum allowable number of defects per 300 g sample
NY 2	6
NY 3	13
NY 4	30
NY 5	60
NY 6	120
NY 7	240
NY 8	450

terms of equivalence to black beans (table 2). For example, five insect-damaged beans correspond to one black bean, which is equivalent to one defect.

Table 2. Equivalence ratings (number of defects) for type classification according to the count of defective beans in a sample (Freitas, 2001)

Count	**Intrinsic defect**	Equivalence rating (number of defects)
1	Black bean	1
2	Brown or sour	1
2 to 5	Insect-damaged	1
3	Shells	1
5	Immature	1
5	Broken	1
5	Malformed	1
	Foreign defect	
1	Large rock or stick	5
1	Medium rock or stick	2
1	Small rock or stick	1
1	Dried cherry	1
2	Floater	1
1	Large skin or husk	1
3	Medium skin or husk	1
5	Small skin or husk	1

The presence of defects is quite relevant in establishing coffee quality, since they could be associated with specific problems during harvesting and post-harvest processing operations (figure 1). Black beans result from dead beans within the coffee cherries (Clarke and Macrae, 1987) or from beans that fall naturally on the ground by action of rain or over-ripening (Mazzafera, 1999). The presence of sour beans can be associated with 'overfermentation' during wet processing (Clarke and Macrae, 1987) and with improper drying or picking of overripe cherries (Sivetz and Desrosier, 1979). Immature beans come from immature fruits. Immature-black beans are those that fall on the ground while immature, remaining in contact with the soil and thus subject to fermentation (Mazzafera, 1999). Typical defects, such as black, sour and immature beans, are known to negatively affect beverage quality. According to Clarke and Macrae (1987), the black bean is usually associated with a heavy flavor; sour beans contribute to sour and oniony tastes, while immature beans will impart astringency to the beverage.

Brazil is the largest coffee producer in the world and, currently, about 15 to 20% of its production consists of defective beans, which upon roasting decrease beverage quality (Oliveira et al., 2006). Regardless of growth, harvest and processing conditions, some defects are intrinsic in nature and will always be present and black, brown and immature beans are the ones that affect beverage quality the most. Usually, these beans are mechanically separated from the non defective beans prior to commercialization in international markets. However, since to coffee producers they represent an investment in growing, harvesting, and handling, these defective beans are commercialized both in the international trade market and internal market in Brazil, where the roasting industries uses them in blends with non defective beans.Thus, the overall quality of the roasted coffee consumed worldwide is depreciated.

After separation from the exportable portion, defective beans may be representing more than 50% of the coffee consumed in Brazil (Oliveira et al., 2008). In order to eliminate these defective beans from the trade market, thus improving the quality of the beverage consumed worldwide, there is a need for proposals of more attractive alternative uses for them. In view of that, an assessment of chemical attributes that could allow for differentiation between defective and non-defective beans prior and after processing is of relevance (Oliveira et al., 2006). Only a few studies have addressed physical and chemical attributes of defective coffee beans in comparison to non-defective ones and it is the aim of this work to present a compilation of the literature reports so far.

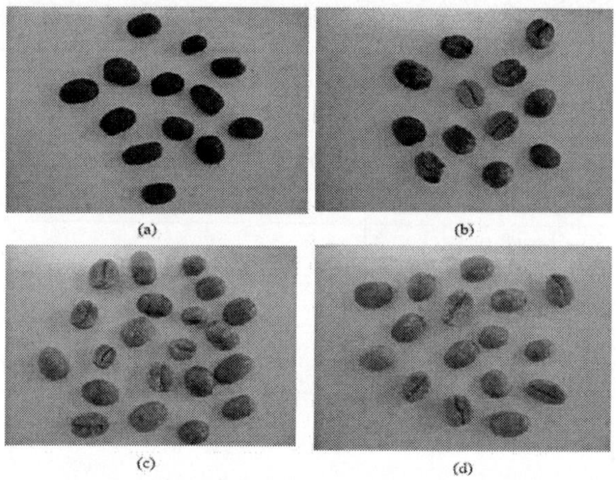

Figure 1. Coffee beans: (a) black; (b) sour; (c) immature; (d) non-defective.

2. Physical Attributes

Physical attributes such as size, density and color of coffee beans are influenced by botanical species and variety, growth and post-harvest processing conditions and, to some extent, are employed for grading and separation between defective and non-defective coffee beans. Furthermore, such parameters present significant variations during roasting and specifically bean color and weight loss are employed for determination of the roasting degree of the final product. Thus, discussion of each of these parameters will be first presented for green (crude) coffee, in relation to discrimination between defective and non-defective beans prior to roasting. Then, the effect of roasting will be discussed.

2.1. Size/Shape

The coffee bean shape can be described as oval with one flat face or, in terms of a geometric form, as half a triaxial ellipsoid (Dutra et al., 2001), as shown in figure 2 (a). Some beans, called peaberries, do not present the flat size because they come from coffee cherries bearing only one seed and are usually smaller than the common beans (figure 2 (b)). The coffee bean size is usually assessed in order to ensure uniformity and when a size is specified for a given coffee sample or lot, it means that over 85% of the beans should be in the same size range (Sivetz and Desrozier, 1979). For commercialization purposes, coffee beans size and shape are commonly assessed by sieving. Screen apertures are either round (for regularly shaped beans) or oblong (for peaberries), with diameters varying from 12/64 to 18/64 inches (round) or from 8/64 to 13/64 inches (oblong) at increments 1/64 inches (Vincent, 1987; Freitas, 2001).

Coffee bean sizes can also be evaluated in terms of measurements of major, minor and intermediate diameters of individual beans (see figure 3). A compilation of volume measurements data for defective and non-defective coffee beans from the same origin is displayed in table 3. Such results show that Arabica beans are larger than Robusta and that all types of defective beans are smaller than non-defective ones, for both coffee species. Also, the smaller beans are the ones that underwent fermentation (sour and black). These results confirm that Arabica and Robusta coffees can be separated by size, as previously reported in the literature (Martín et al., 1999; Casal et al., 2000) and also indicate that sieving could be employed for separation of non-defective and defective coffee beans of a given coffee species. Sieving is also efficient for separation of broken and cut beans (Ramalakshmi et al., 2007).

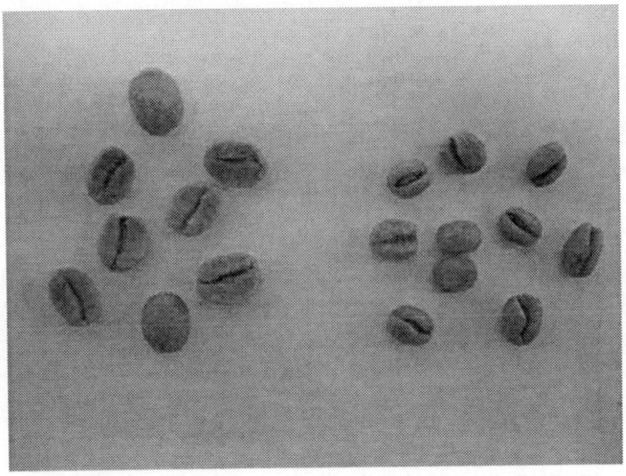

Figure 2. Coffee beans photograph: (a) regular; (b) peaberries.

Coffee bean size, and in consequence its volume, increases during roasting as a result of the softening of the cellulose bean structure coupled to the increase in pressure from the release of pyrolysis products. Franca et al. (2005a) presented volume measurements for defective and non-defective beans prior to and after roasting. An evaluation of the percentage increase in volume after roasting showed that defective beans presented lower degrees of swelling (35-41%) in comparison to non-defective coffee beans (65%). Such results can be associated to the fact that beans that swell less should roast more slowly (Clarke, 1987a), fact later corroborated by weight loss data presented by Franca et al. (2005a). Such results are an indication that defective beans will attain a lighter roasting degree than non-defective ones under the same roasting conditions. Also, aside from their inherent physico-chemical characteristics affecting their degree of roast, Cristo et al. (2006), in their study of flow regimes in rotating coffee roasters, discussed that smaller beans will tend to migrate to the low velocity core of the bed transverse section. Thus, due to poor mixing (low heat transfer rates) in that region these beans will necessarily roast to a lesser degree, which would be the case of smaller black and sour beans in a mixture with larger non-defective beans.

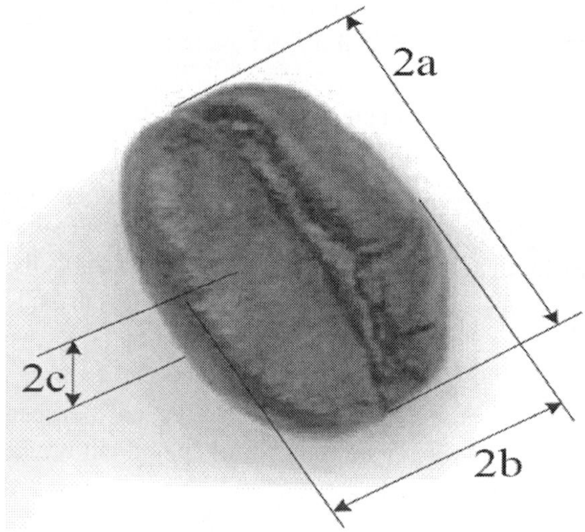

Figure 3. Coffee bean dimensions - 2a, 2b and 2c correspond to major, intermediate and minor diameter measurements, respectively.

Table 3. Green (crude) coffee beans volumes and densities – Compilation of measurement data from coffees from Minas Gerais State, Brazil (Franca et al., 2005a; Mendonça, 2006)

	Volume x 10^9 (m^3)		Density (kg m^{-3})	
	Arabica	Robusta	Arabica	Robusta
Non-defective	111-119	72-76	1210-1310	1246-1250
Immature	94-105	50-54	1234-1297	1272-1278
Light Sour	90-105	69-71	1231-1267	1295-1299
Dark Sour	87-93	62-70	1230-1274	1261-1269
Black	62-79	40-45	1133-1236	1182-1192

2.2. Density

A compilation of density measurements data for defective and non-defective coffee beans from the same origin is also displayed in table 3. No significant variations in bean density were observed, indicating that this parameter alone does not provide the means for separation between defective and non-defective coffees, prior to roasting. Ramalakshmi et al. (2007) evaluated samples of Arabica and Robusta coffees from India and reported that good quality coffee beans were heavier than low quality coffees (mixture of defects) from the same origin. However, such differences were attributed to the presence of broken beans and were not associated with the presence of specific defects such as black, sour or immature beans. Coffee bean density decreases considerably during roasting, due to the simultaneous increase in volume and decrease in weight associated to the loss of water and volatile components (Dutra et al., 2001; Rodrigues et al., 2003). The percent density reduction will depend on the degree of roast, with average reported values of 45 and 60% for light to medium and medium to dark roasts, respectively (Sivetz and Desrozier, 1979; Clarke, 1987a; Dutra et al., 2001). Franca et al. (2005a) reported that black beans were the only defects that presented higher density values in comparison to non-defective ones, after roasting under the same conditions. This can be attributed to the fact that such defects present lower weight loss values and swell less than non-defective beans during roasting, i.e., roast to a lighter degree. As a consequence, the beans will be heavier and smaller than non-defective ones, and therefore will present higher density.

2.3. Weight Loss

Another important physical aspect that is commonly monitored during coffee roasting is weight loss. This parameter can be employed to assess the degree of roast (Clarke, 1987a). According to the literature on weight loss variation during roasting, the weight loss curve can be represented by two lines of different slopes, as shown in figure 4 (a) (Sivetz and Desrosier, 1979; Dutra et al., 2001; Rodrigues et al., 2003; Oliveira et al., 2005). The smaller slope of the first line representing weight loss is attributed to the slow release of water and green coffee volatile components and it is known as the "drying phase" of the roasting process. The increase in weight loss that occurs afterwards can be attributed to the intensive release of organic compounds and CO_2 associated to the pyrolysis reactions, and therefore this is the so called "pyrolysis phase". The onset of pyrolysis is then associated with the transition between the two slopes, which has been reported to occur in the range of 7 to 12% weight loss, depending on processing conditions (Sivetz and Desrosier, 1979; Rodrigues et al., 2003; Oliveira et al., 2005). It is noteworthy to mention that this behavior seems to be related to roasting temperature. A recent study (Mancha Agresti et al., 2008) reported a logarithmic model fit (figure 4 (b)) for weight loss behavior when roasting coffee in a convective oven at 200°C. However, when temperature was raised to 300°C (unpublished data), the weight loss behavior changed to the one presented in figure 4 (a). Such variation in weight loss behavior with roasting temperature can be perceived as an indication that the roasting temperature is affecting the production of volatile components by favoring different reactions and removal pathways at different processing temperatures.

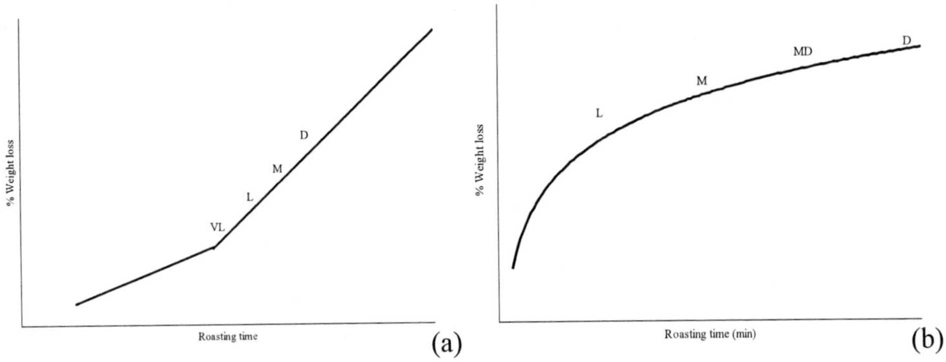

Figure 4. Weight loss behavior during coffee roasting at (a) high and (b) low temperatures. VL = very light roast, L=light roast, M=medium roast, MD=medium/dark roast, D=dark roast.

Since the weight loss is a direct measure of the roasting degree, the evolution of this parameter during roasting was investigated for both non-defective and defective coffee beans (Franca et al., 2005a; Vasconcelos et al., 2007; Mancha Agresti et al., 2008). The data presented in those studies showed that non-defective beans presented higher weight loss values than defective ones, in the following order: non-defective > immature > sour > black. Also, a comparison of the logarithmic (Mancha Agresti et al., 2008) or linear model coefficients (Franca et al., 2005; Vasconcelos et al., 2007) indicates that non-defective coffee beans roast slightly faster than defective coffee beans and that, among the defects, black beans are the ones that roast slower. Such results confirm that defective beans roast to a lesser degree than non-defective ones, under the same processing conditions.

2.4. Color

Bean color is an important attribute for classification of green coffee, due to its direct impact on appearance. It will vary considerably depending on coffee species, origin and processing conditions such as dry vs. wet processing, drying time, exposure to light, storage conditions, etc. Variations on the external color of the coffee beans can be also be associated to aging (see table 4) and non uniform coloration of a given coffee lot is usually taken as a sign of non-uniform quality. For Arabica coffees, blue to gray green is the most desirable color, based on correlation of visual inspection and cupping results (Sivetz and Desrozier, 1979; Freitas, 2001). Good quality Robusta coffees, on the other hand, present a brownish color, whereas for Arabica, brown coloration is usually associated with aging, fermentation or improper drying.

Color sorting is the major procedure employed for separation of defective and non-defective coffee beans prior to roasting. In Brazil, manual sorting is usually employed for type classification and electronic sorting is employed in farms and cooperatives of producers for the actual removal of defective beans. In the electronic sorters, coffee beans pass, one by one, by an electronic eye or camera system, and depending on wavelength measurements, the bean is either allowed to pass or it is shot with a puff of air into a reject pile. The sorting systems employ either monochromatic or bichromatic light measurements, and can be adjusted to eliminate more or less defects. Monochromatic machines will be able to remove black, grey and some beans attacked by insects and the more specific bichromatic color sorting machines detect and eliminate coffee beans that are white, immature, broken, insect damaged, brown (sour) and black (Sivetz and Desrosier, 1979; Clarke, 1987b). Even though color sorting is the procedure employed in the farms, cooperatives and industries for separation of defective beans, there are only a few literature data on color measurements for defective or low quality coffees (Franca et al., 2005a; Vasconcelos, 2005; Mendonça, 2006; Ramalakshmi et al., 2007). Most reported data on measurements of color (L*a*b*) of coffee beans prior to or after roasting are either restricted to good quality coffee or do not make reference to coffee quality (Mendes et al., 2001; Cirilo et al., 2003; Marcone, 2004; Gokmen and Senyuva, 2006; Summa et al., 2007).

Table 4. Association between aging and external bean color for Arabica coffees (Freitas, 2001)

Coffee bean age	Color (based on visual inspection)
Recent	green, blue to gray green (wet processed)
1-2 years	greenish
3-4 years	whitish
5-10 years	yellowish
+ 10 years	brownish

Franca et al. (2005a) presented color measurements data for both whole and ground defective and non-defective coffee beans, prior to and after roasting. Regarding whole green beans, it was observed that luminosity values were higher for non-defective and immature beans in comparison to sour and black defects, with the lowest luminosity values measured for black beans. Such results raise the question to whether monochromatic separation will be effective in separating immature and sour beans from non-defective ones. Actually, in order make sure that such defects are effectively removed from a specific coffee lot, color sorting machines are usually set up to allow some non-defective coffees to be also removed if their color is similar to that of sour or immature beans. As a consequence of this, PVA mixtures of Arabica coffees usually present a high percentage of non-defective coffees, as pointed out in studies employing machine sorted PVA mixtures or low quality Arabica coffees from different origins and crops (Franca et al., 2005ab; Farah et al., 2006; Vasconcelos et al., 2007). Franca et al. (2005a) also reported that luminosity values were higher for ground beans compared to whole ones (surface measurements), indicating that the bean surface is darker than its interior, and that differences in luminosity between surface and interior were more significant for defective beans in comparison to non-defective ones. Regarding chroma (color saturation) and hue angle (color hue) measurements for whole beans, only black beans presented significant differences in comparison to other coffee samples. Black beans presented the highest hue value, corresponding to a dark green, whereas the other beans presented a yellowish green hue. After grinding, no significant differences in chroma and hue angle were detected.

Mendonça (2006) compared defective and non-defective Arabica and Robusta green (crude) coffees from the same origin and crop in terms of L*a*b* color measurements. Sour coffees were separated into two categories, light and dark, based on manual separation by visual inspection. These authors reported no significant differences between Arabica and Robusta coffees, in terms of luminosity measurements. However, black and dark sour beans presented lower luminosity values than the other samples, for both Arabica and Robusta species. It was also reported that, for a specific type of bean, healthy or defective, Robusta coffees presented higher chroma values than Arabica. Also, black beans presented the lowest chroma values among the defects, for both Arabica and Robusta species. These authors did not find significant variations in color hue (hue angle) between Arabica/Robusta and defective/non-defective coffees. This was attributed to aging of the beans, since external bean color tends to become yellowish/brownish with time. This was observed even for the immature beans. Based on color difference calculations, which takes into account all color measurements in one parameter, it was concluded that, in the case of Robusta coffees, color separation between defective (black, immature, dark sour and light sour) and non-defective coffees can be safely accomplished. However, the results obtained for Arabica coffee indicate that separation will not be effective in the case of immature and light sour beans. This study also concluded that color parameters can be employed as a criterion for separation between Arabica and Robusta coffees, only in the case of good quality samples, since no significant color differences between the two species were observed for low quality (defective) beans. An evaluation of color reflectance results presented by Ramalakshmi et al. (2007) for green Arabica and Robusta coffees from India, of good (graded) and low (mixture of defects) qualities corroborates such conclusions.

The most obvious physical change that takes place during roasting is the variation of the bean color from green to yellow to brown to dark brown as roasting becomes more intense. The effect of roasting on color parameters of defective and non-defective coffee beans is discussed by Franca et al. (2005a). Luminosity values decreased as expected and black/sour beans still presented lower luminosity values than non-defective and immature beans (surface measurements). However, for measurements taken after grinding the coffee beans, luminosity values for black and sour beans increased in comparison to surface measurements, and this was not observed for non-defective and immature beans. These results reinforced the conclusion that black/sour beans were roasted to a lighter degree than the others, since uniformity of color between surface and interior is expected as roasting progresses. The bean surface was still darker than its interior after roasting, thus indicating that these beans were roasted to a lighter degree than the others. Non-defective and immature beans did not present significant differences in luminosity values between whole and ground beans, indicating that the beans attained a uniform color after roasting. Chroma values diminished after roasting, except for black beans. Also, whole black beans still presented the highest values of hue angle after roasting, maintaining a greenish hue, whereas the other beans became brown. After grinding, no significant differences in hue angle were detected.

Similar measurements and conclusions were found in another study (Vasconcelos, 2005) employing Arabica coffees from the same origin but a later crop (See table 5). In this case, the effect of roasting on color was further investigated, and measurements were taken at different degrees of roast. As expected, luminosity decreases as roasting progresses. However, a comparison of luminosity values for defective and non-defective beans at a specific degree of roast shows that, after roasting, defective beans are actually lighter than non-defective ones, since they roast less than non-defective ones. An evaluation of the data presented in table 5 indicates that, after roasting, even though there are differences in color attributes between defective and non-defective beans from a statistical point of view, there is no difference in attributes between the PVA mixture and non-defective beans, except for luminosity of green coffee. These results indicate that color separation is only feasible for green coffee (i.e., prior to roasting) and other parameters should be sought for discrimination between defective and non-defective coffee after roasting.

Table 5. CIE L*a*b parameters for crude (green) and roasted coffees (ground coffees) (Vasconcelos, 2005)

	Black	Immature	Sour	PVA mixture	Non-defective
Green					
L*	41,59±1,59^{d,w}	66,05±1,01^{a,w}	60,92±0,76^{c,w}	63,22±0,16^{b,w}	67,52±1,63^{a,w}
a*	- 6,32±0,95^{b,z}	-2,82±1,88^{a,z}	-2,6±1,37^{a,z}	-1,77±1,09^{a,z}	-3,16±1,52^{a,z}
b*	35,56±0,44^{a,x}	30,66±1,33^{abc,x}	32,33±2,39^{ab,x}	28,81 ± 2,25^{c,x}	30,37±1,92^{bc,x}
c*	36,18±0,49^{a,w}	30,87±1,50^{bc,x}	32,76±2,42^{b,x}	28,91±2,30^{c,x}	30,61±1,87^{bc,w}
h_{ab}	99,86±1,49^{w}	95,13±3,32^{w}	94,32±2,25^{w}	93,22±1,99^{w}	95,97± 2,80^{w}
Light Roast					
L*	36,55±1,12^{b,x}	35,65±0,22^{b,x}	38,70±0,94^{a,x}	32,21±1,24^{c,x}	30,03±1,41^{d,x}
a*	3,47±1,18^{b,wx}	10,05±0,13^{c,w}	8,12±1,57^{a,w}	8,76±0,82^{a,w}	7,91±1,39^{a,w}
b*	37,69±1,81^{b,w}	38,09± 0,44^{b,w}	42,8 ± 1,63^{a,w}	33,43± 1,91^{c,w}	30,06±2,14^{d,w}
c*	38,15 ±1,84^{b,w}	39,94 ± 0,45^{b,w}	44,53 ±1,39^{a,w}	34,65 ±1,69^{c,w}	31,10±1,90^{d,w}
h_{ab}	84,20 ±2.96^{a,x}	75,54±1,68^{bc,x}	79,74±2,12^{b,x}	74,03 ± 1,85^{c,x}	75,36±2.76^{bc,y}
Medium Roast					
L*	33,06±1,46^{a,y}	30,89±1,93^{a,y}	32,77±2,11^{a,y}	26,67±0,68^{b,y}	25,46±0,76^{b,y}
a*	4,53±0,84^{c,w}	8,72±0,65^{a,w}	8,40±0,98^{a,w}	6,72±0,61^{b,x}	5,26±0,99^{c,x}
b*	33,23±1,87^{a,x}	30,55±2,65^{a,x}	33,53±3,27^{a,x}	24,35±1,18^{b,y}	22,61±1,30^{b,x}
c*	33,85±1,86^{a,x}	31,87±2.53^{a,x}	34,77±3,21^{a,x}	24,89 ±1,36^{b,y}	22,43 ±1,47^{b,x}
h_{ab}	82,21±1,69^{a,y}	74,38± 2,73^{b,x}	75,93 ±2,74^{b,x}	75,42 ±1,22^{b,x}	77,35±1,82^{b,xy}
Dark roast					
L*	29,35±0,45^{a,z}	26,70±0,09^{bc,z}	27,30±1,24^{b,z}	24,97±0,70^{cd,z}	23,97±0,23^{d,y}
a*	2,76±0,07^{c,x}	6,22 ± 0,71^{a,x}	5,80±0,46^{ab,x}	4,85 ± 0,92^{b,y}	3,54 ± 0,63^{c,x}
b*	28,20±0,96^{a,z}	24,73±0,22^{b,y}	25,75±2,21^{b,y}	21,89± 1,19^{c,y}	19,93±0,51^{c,x}
c*	28,19±0,78^{a,y}	25,07± 0,34^{b,y}	25,81±2,21^{b,y}	21,51±1,34^{c,z}	19,30 ±0,63^{c,y}
h_{ab}	84,19±0,60^{a,xy}	75.49 ± 1,10^{c,x}	77,49 ±1,05^{c,x}	76,97 ± 1,79^{c,x}	79.87± 0,94^{b,x}

Average value±Standard Deviation. Values followed by the same letter in the same line (a,b,c,d) or for a specific parameter in the same column (w,x,y,z) do not differ significantly by the Duncan test at 5% probability. Values without letters in the same line do not differ significantly by variance analysis at 5% probability.

3. Chemical Attributes

Green coffee is devoid of the pleasant aroma and flavor appreciated worldwide in association with the coffee beverage. Such desired aroma and flavor are developed in the roasting process, where the beans undergo a series of reactions leading to the corresponding changes in chemical composition. These changes will affect sensory attributes and therefore the way the consumer perceives coffee quality. They are affected by roasting conditions, and are dependent on the chemical composition of green coffee beans, which is in turn influenced by several factors such as species, variety, growth and post-harvest processing conditions, and of course the presence of defective coffee beans. At this point it is clear that separation of defective and non-defective coffee beans prior to roasting can be satisfactorily accomplished by sieving and/or color sorting, in the case of black and sour coffees. Separation of immature beans by means of physical attributes does not seem feasible. Furthermore, detection and quantification of defective coffee beans in roasted coffee still poses a problem, and in this case an evaluation of chemical attributes, which are directly related to the chemical changes taking place during roasting, could provide the means for that. Therefore, a discussion of chemical attributes of defective and non-defective coffee beans is herein presented, for both green and roasted coffees.

Average data on the proximate composition of green and roasted coffee is displayed in table 6. The observed variations are mostly related to variations in species/variety and to a lesser extent to other factors including origin, agricultural practices, growth and storage conditions and maturation degree (Clarke and Macrae, 1985). There are extensive changes in chemical composition with roasting, as a result of pyrolysis reactions. However, the proximate composition remains approximately the same, since changes occur within a specific class of compounds. For example, protein results are based on the determination of crude nitrogen and multiplication by the factor 6.25, so they include all nitrogenous compounds. In view of the high temperatures attained during roasting, a decrease in total protein levels is expected. However, the degradation into polypeptides and the formation of volatile (pyrroles, pyridines, pyrazines, etc) and non-volatile (pigments, such as melanoidins, and others) nitrogenous components during roasting (Homma, 2001) also contributes to protein nitrogen determination by Kjeldahl and therefore the protein results for roasted coffee remain practically unaltered on an as is basis.

Table 6. Proximate composition of green and roasted Arabica and Robusta coffee beans (g/100 g dry basis green coffee)[a]

	Arabica		Robusta	
	Green	Roasted	Green	Roasted
Water	8-13	1-3	12-13	1-2
Protein	11-17	12-15	11-13	13-15
Lipids	9-18	15-20	9-13	11-16
Minerals	4-5	4-5	4-5	5
Carbohydrate[b]	60-76	40-79	69-76	64-71

[a] Compilation of data presented by Sivetz and Desrosier, 1979; Clarke and Macrae, 1985; Clarke and Macrae, 1987; Speer and Kölling-Speer, 2001; Reh et al., 2006; Mendonça et al., 2007.
[b] Determined by difference.

Average data on the proximate composition of green and roasted, defective and non-defective Arabica coffee from Brazil are displayed in table 7. Reported values for defective and non-defective coffee beans are in the same range reported in the coffee literature in general (See table 6). Also, there are no significant variations in proximate composition of defective and non-defective coffee beans, both green and roasted. Only small variations have been reported. For example, non-defective beans presented slightly lower moisture contents than healthy ones, prior to roasting (Mazzafera, 1999; Oliveira et al., 2006; Vasconcelos et al., 2007). Slightly higher average protein levels are reported for black beans in comparison to the other samples (Oliveira et al., 2006; Vasconcelos et al., 2007). However, this was actually due to caffeine and trigonelline contribution to protein determination based on crude nitrogen. No differences were detected between defective and non-defective coffee beans after protein levels were corrected by subtracting both caffeine and trigonelline contents. Healthy coffee beans presented slightly higher oil contents than both black and sour beans whereas ash contents were slightly lower (Mazzafera, 1999; Oliveira et al., 2006; Vasconcelos et al., 2007). The proximate composition did not vary considerably after roasting, with the obvious exception of moisture content. In view of that, and of the fact that there were no significant variations between defective and non-defective coffees in terms of the general classes of compounds, a discussion on specific substances in each class is presented as follows.

Table 7. Proximate composition of green and roasted coffee beans (g/100 g dry basis green coffee)[a]

	Black	Immature	Sour	Non-defective
Green				
Water	9-13	9-10	8-10	9-12
Protein	16-17	15	15-16	14-15
Lipids	8-10	10	8-9	10-11
Ash	6	5-6	5-6	5
Carbohydrate[b]	59-70	62-70	61-71	60-72
Roasted				
Water	1	1-2	1	1
Protein	14-16	13-15	14-15	13-14
Lipids	10-12	9-11	10-12	9-11
Ash	6	5	5	4-5
Carbohydrate[b]	66-69	68-71	67-71	68-73

[a] Compilation of data presented by Mazzafera, 1999; Oliveira et al., 2006; Vasconcelos et al., 2007.
[b] Determined by difference.

3.1. Water Content

Water content is a critical parameter for evaluation of green coffee quality, in the sense that it affects mold growth, mycotoxin production, fermentation, physical, chemical and sensory parameters. As water is quite cheap compared to coffee, its amount within the beans is also of interest from a commercial point of view (Mendonça et al., 2007). Its ammount is usually controlled by processing conditions, and, for green coffee, it is kept at about 12% to allow for safe transportation and storage (Clarke, 1985; Reh et al., 2006). Immediately after roasting, coffee moisture content can be as low as zero moisture, especially for dark roasts (Clarke, 1985) when water quenching is not employed. However, measured values can increase up to 3% as the coffee beans tend to absorb water from the surrounding air.

Reported data on moisture content of defective vs. non-defective coffee beans indicated that non-defective green coffees presented slightly higher moisture contents than defective ones (Mazzafera, 1999; Oliveira et al., 2006; Vasconcelos et al., 2007). The same behavior was reported in terms of water activity measurements in green coffee, with average values of

0.44 and 0.48 for defective and non-defective coffees, respectively (Vasconcelos et al., 2007). Such differences could be attributed to defective beans presenting smaller water diffusion coefficients, but further studies are needed in order to validate such hypothesis. Both moisture content and water activity decreased with roasting, without significant differences between defective and healthy coffee beans.

3.2. Nitrogen-Based Compounds

Such class of substances will be discussed in terms of protein contents and also with respect to other nitrogenous substances of relevance in terms of coffee and/or defective coffee beans.

3.2.1. Protein

The reported values of green coffee protein contents are usually based on the determination of crude nitrogen and multiplication by the factor 6.25 (Macrae, 1985) and are in the range of 11 to 17% dry basis, without significant differences between Arabica and Robusta. True protein values are in the range of 8 – 9%, with the difference being mainly attributed to caffeine and trigonelline nitrogen.

Protein data on defective coffees are based on crude nitrogen (Oliveira et al., 2006; Vasconcelos et al., 2007) or NaOH extraction (Mazzafera, 1999; Ramalakshmi et al., 2007). Mazzafera (1999) reported that the total protein content was higher for black beans in comparison to immature and immature-black. However, this could not be correlated to amino acid content, which was higher for immature beans in comparison to black and immature-black coffees, with the main amino acids in immature beans being asparagine, followed by tyrosine, alanine, lysine, serine and glutamic acid. Although immature-black and black coffees presented similar contents of total amino acids, qualitative changes were observed. Lysine, tyrosine and alanine were the main amino acids for immature-black coffee, as opposed to glutamic acid, asparagine, alanine, aspartic acid and lysine for black beans. Oliveira et al. (2006) and Vasconcelos et al. (2007) presented data on Arabica coffees from the same origin but subsequent crops and both reported higher protein contents for black beans in comparison to other defects and to non-defective coffee. However, such higher contents were actually due to caffeine-nitrogen. Ramalakshmi et al. (2007) reported slightly lower protein contents for low quality coffees.

3.2.2. Caffeine

This compound has been historically accredited with most of the physiological effects of coffee and therefore it is the single most frequently determined compound in coffee (Macrae, 1985). The caffeine content of green coffees varies considerably, especially with respect to species and also within the same species. Robusta coffees have approximately twice the amount of caffeine presented in Arabica coffees, with reported average values being 1.2% db for Arabica (0.6–1.9% range) and 2.2% db for Robusta.

Comparison of caffeine levels between defective coffees have been reported by Mazzafera (1999), for black, immature-black and immature coffees, and by Franca et al. (2005a), for black, sour and immature defects. No significant differences in caffeine levels were found among the defective beans, with an average of 1.3% caffeine in defective coffees reported by both studies. However, Franca et al. (2005a) found that non-defective beans presented lower caffeine contents (0.9%) than the defective ones. A few recent studies have also compared caffeine levels for samples of different sensory qualities (Franca et al., 2005b; Farah et al., 2006). According to Franca et al. (2005b), the highest (1.1%) and lowest (0.7%) caffeine levels corresponded to the highest (soft) and lowest (rio) quality samples, respectively. Farah et al. (2006) also reported that the highest caffeine level (1.2%) was determined for the highest quality sample (soft), but found the lowest caffeine level (1.0%) for a good quality sample (hard), that consisted of 97% non-defective beans. Ramalakshmi et al. (2007) also reported slightly lower caffeine levels for low quality coffees. These results seem to be in contradiction with the fact that higher caffeine levels have been associated to defective or low quality coffees (Mazzafera, 1999; Franca et al., 2005a). However, the studies by Franca et al. (2005b), Farah et al. (2006) and Ramalakshmi et al. (2007) did not employ coffees from the same origin/crop, thus the highest caffeine levels in good quality coffees may be associated to variations in growth and processing conditions.

Roasting was reported to cause approximate reductions of 30% (Franca et al., 2005a,b) in caffeine content. Since the solubility of this compound in water increases with temperature, the caffeine loss was attributed to a drag by water vapor released during roasting, and this compound has been detected in the exhaust gas from roasting (Dutra et al., 2001). Roasting did not significantly affect caffeine levels of either black or sour beans (Franca et al., 2005a). The fact that the caffeine content remained relatively constant for both black and sour beans upon roasting was interpreted as an indication that black and sour beans were roasted to a lesser extent than the other types of coffee beans (immature and non-defective).

3.2.3. Trigonelline

Together with caffeine, this compound has received considerable attention in coffee chemistry research, given that its thermal degradation products are important in terms of sensory and nutritional aspects (Macrae, 1985). Nicotinic acid is the major non-volatile component resulting from demethylation of trigonelline during roasting. The amount of nicotinic acid present in roasted coffee (10-40 mg/100g) coupled to the fact that it is readily available for biological conversion indicates that roasted coffee should be considered a significant source of this vitamin (Macrae, 1985). The sensory importance of trigonelline is associated to the fact that approximately half of the volatile substances generated during its thermal degradation consist of pyridines and pyrroles. Both classes of compounds have been detected in roasted coffee. Pyrroles have been associated to medicine and cereal flavours (Mancha Agresti et al., 2008) whereas pyridines are associated with adstringent/hazelnut (2-methylpyridine) and buttery/caramel (3-ethylpyridine) aromas (Dart and Nursten, 1985).

Evaluations of trigonelline levels correlation with coffee quality are available from studies presented by Franca et al. (2005a) (defective vs non-defective coffee), Franca et al. (2005b) and Farah et al. (2006) (low vs high quality coffees). Franca et al. (2005a) reported trigonelline levels of approximately 1% in non-defective, immature and sour coffee beans and lower values (~0.8%) for black beans. Franca et al. (2005b) did not find significant differences in trigonelline levels between high and low quality coffees, whereas Farah et al. (2006) reported a decrease in trigonelline levels as coffee quality worsened, and also verified a strong negative correlation of trigonelline levels with poor quality and with the Rio-off-flavor. Trigonelline levels were significantly reduced by roasting, with such reduction attaining higher values for darker roasts. After roasting, trigonelline levels did not show significant correlations with cup quality or the presence of defective coffee beans. Slightly higher trigonelline levels were observed for black/sour beans and lower quality samples (rio/rioysh/rio zona), in association with such beans attaining lighter roasting degrees in comparison to high quality ones.

3.2.4. Amines

Amines are organic bases encountered in both raw and processed food products. They can be formed either by natural metabolic pathways or by action of decarboxylase-positive microorganisms (Fernandes and Ferreira, 2000; Oliveira et al., 2005). Amine levels and distribution will vary considerably among different foodstuffs and also for a specific food product (Kalač and Krausová, 2005). In non-fermented foods, the presence of biogenic amines above a certain level has been associated with undesired microbial activity. Furthermore, several amines are known to be vasoactive and psychoactive, and ingestion of high quantities has been associated to food poisoning cases. Thus, amine levels could be indicative of microbial spoilage and have been employed as a criterion for quality evaluation and spoilage detection in a wide variety of food products (Bardócz, 1995; Santos, 1996). In view of this, it could also be considered a quality parameter for coffee and thus the studies that present an evaluation of amines in green and roasted coffees are discussed below.

Only a few studies have addressed the presence of amines in green and roasted coffee (Amorim et al., 1977; Casal et al., 2004; Cirilo et al., 2003; Oliveira et al., 2005), and only the study by Vasconcelos et al. (2007) dealt with the presence of amines in defective coffee beans. A brief review on the major findings from these studies is presented as follows.

Amorim et al. (1977) investigated the presence of polyamines in coffee, before and after roasting at 240 °C for 10 (light roast) and 12 (dark roast) min. Their experiments were conducted with Arabica coffees of the same variety (*Coffea Arabica L.* var. Mundo Novo) harvested in the same year, but classified as of different cup qualities. They compared high quality samples (mild flavor, cup classification as soft) to low quality ones (strong medicinal flavor, cup classification as rio). Prior to roasting, putrescine was the prevailing amine in green coffee (64%), followed by spermidine (23%) and spermine (12%), regardless of sample quality. These authors reported that only putrescine was present after a light roast and no amines were detected in the samples submitted to a dark roast. Given that no significant differences were found in amine levels between the high and low quality coffee samples, it was concluded that polyamine content did not present correlation with the Rio off-flavor.

Cirilo et al. (2003) investigated the presence of amines in coffees submitted to two degrees of roasting, herein designated as light (American roast, 6 min roasting at 300°C) and dark (French roast, 12 min roasting at 300°C). These authors encountered serotonin, putrescine, spermine and spermidine in green coffee and the reported amine levels were quite different from the ones presented by Amorim et al. (1977). Cirilo et al. (2003) found both serotonin (35%) and putrescine (32%) as the prevailing amines, followed by spermidine (19%) and spermine (14%). Roasting caused a significant decrease in amine content. However, total amine contents after the dark roast were twice the ones observed after the light roast. According to this study, both putrescine and spermine were not present after roasting, whereas spermidine and serotonine were still detected in low concentrations. Agmatine was only detected for the sample that was submitted to dark roasting and the authors suggested that its formation could be associated to the decarboxylation of arginine or to the release of this amine from conjugated forms.

Casal et al. (2004) evaluated the levels of biogenic amines (putrescine, cadaverine, serotonin, tyramine, spermidine, and spermine) in Robusta and Arabica coffees. These authors reported putrescine as the most abundant amine in both species, followed by spermidine, spermine and serotonin (see figure 5). They also detected small amounts of cadaverine and tyramine. Their results indicated that putrescine levels could be used as a criterion for the discrimination between Arabica and Robusta coffees. These authors also mentioned that amines could be used for discrimination between green coffees subjected to different postharvest processes (wet vs. dry). They reported variations in biogenic amine levels after roast, but the statistical significance for species discrimination was reduced.

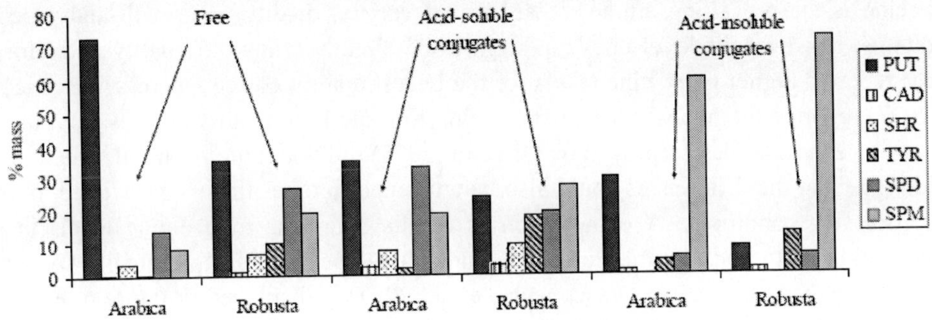

Figure 5. Percent mass distribution of biogenic amines in Arabica and Robusta green coffees based on the data from Casal et al. (2004). PUT = putrescine; CAD = cadaverine; SER = serotonin; TYR = tyramine; SPD = spermidine; SPM = spermine.

Oliveira et al. (2005) evaluated the effect of roasting on the levels of amines in high and low quality coffees, classified by cup as soft and rio, respectively. Results with respect to amines distribution in green coffee were similar to those presented by Amorim et al. (1977) and Casal et al. (2004), given that putrescine was the prevailing amine (75%), followed by spermine (12%) and spermidine (12%). These authors also reported that putrescine levels were significantly higher for the low quality sample and that both histamine and tryptamine were only present in the low quality sample. Their results indicated that both amine levels and profiles could be related to coffee quality. In this study, amine levels were also monitored during roasting and a significant decrease in total amine content occurred with an increase in roasting time. Based on weight loss monitoring during roasting and comparison to other literature reports (Amorim et al., 1977; Cirilo et al., 2003), these authors concluded that amine degradation takes place mainly during the drying stage of the roasting process, which precedes the pyrolysis stage. Thus, even after a mild roast, total amine levels are expected to be quite small.

Vasconcelos et al. (2007) investigated the presence of amines in defective and non-defective coffee beans, green and submitted to three different levels of roasting at 200°C: light (30 min roasting), medium (60 min roasting), and dark (120 min roasting). Seven of the ten evaluated amines were detected in green coffee: putrescine, cadaverine, histamine, serotonin, spermidine, spermine and tryptamine. Among those, only putrescine, the prevailing amine in all samples, was detected in all samples above trace levels. Prevalence of putrescine followed by spermine and spermidine was observed for all coffee samples with the exception of black beans, for which histamine levels corresponded to approximately 50% of putrescine levels, and both spermine and spermidine were present in smaller quantities. Histamine was detected, above trace levels, only in the samples that consisted purely of defective coffee beans. This corroborated the study by Oliveira et al. (2005), who reported that histamine was detected only in low sensory quality coffee. The results obtained in both studies are an indication that the detection of histamine in green coffee could be associated with the presence of defective beans. After roasting to a light degree, only traces of serotonin were detected and no amines were detected after roasting to medium and dark degrees, also in accordance with the data by Oliveira et al. (2005) regarding amine degradation before pyrolysis reactions.

Based on the reviewed literature on amines in green coffee, it can be concluded that putrescine is the prevailing amine, regardless of variety, quality or growth and processing conditions. However, its level does not seem to be directly related to quality. Oliveira et al. (2005) reported higher putrescine levels for the lowest quality coffee whereas Vasconcelos et al. (2007) reported the opposite when comparing low and high quality coffees from the same origin. Since the samples employed by Oliveira (2005) did not come from the same crop, one could argue that the differences could also be attributed to other factors associated to growth and processing conditions. A compilation of results regarding total amine levels in green coffees, taking into consideration only the studies that specified sample quality (Amorim et al., 1977; Oliveira et al., 2005; Vasconcelos et al., 2007) is displayed in figure 6. From these results it is clear that only black coffee beans presented a significantly lower amount of amines in comparison to other coffees. Since such defective beans are present in much lower amounts than the other types of defects, regardless of coffee quality, the variations in total amine contents between coffee samples will probably be due to variations in crop and processing conditions rather than be related to sample quality.

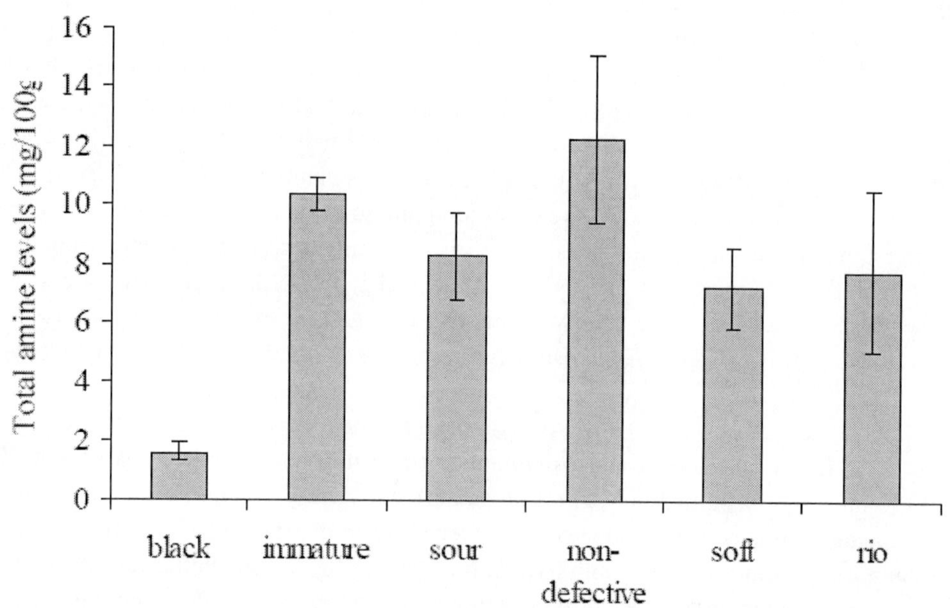

Figure 6. Total amine levels in Arabica green coffees of different qualities, based on the data published by Amorim et al. (1974), Oliveira et al. (2005) and Vasconcelos et al. (2007).

The results obtained by Oliveira et al. (2005) and Vasconcelos et al. (2007) indicate that histamine is a potential marker for detection of defective beans in green coffee, since this amine was detected either in defective beans or low quality coffee. However, histamine levels in coffee are quite low compared to other amines, ranging from 0.1 to 1.0 mg/100g. Also, histamine levels found in coffee do not pose a concern in terms of intoxication. The toxicological levels of amines are not easily established, because they depend on individual characteristics of each amine, as well as on interactions among amines and also with the food substract. Nevertheless, the highest histamine value reported in the literature for green coffee (Vasconcelos et al., 2007) corresponds to approximately 10% of the suggested limit for histamine toxicity (Halász et al., 1994; Santos, 1996). Furthermore, histamine was not detected after roasting of the low quality samples (Oliveira et al., 2005; Vasconcelos et al., 2007).

3.3. Lipids

The lipids (fat) of coffee beans are comprised of coffee oil, mainly present in the endosperm, and of coffee wax, located in the outer layers of the beans in small amounts (Folstar, 1985). The chemical composition of both green and roasted coffee oils is similar to those of edible oils (Sivetz and Desrosier, 1979) with the non-glyceride fraction, which can amount up to 25% (w/w) of the oil, being comprised mainly of free and esterified diterpene alcohols and sterols (Speer and Kölling-Speer, 2001). Considering the bulk of the literature data on coffee oil, the total oil content in green coffee beans, determined by a diversity of methodologies, falls in the range of 9 to 15% (w/w) db for arabicas and in the range of 7 to 12% (w/w) db for robustas (Folstar, 1985; Nikolova-Damyanova et al., 1998; Speer and Kölling-Speer, 2001; Turatti, 2001; Vila et al., 2005; Oliveira et al., 2006). The values for oil content in roasted coffees are higher than those for green beans due to the beans dry matter loss during roasting, which in turn varies with the degree of roast (Speer and Kölling-Speer, 2001). Comprehensive reviews on coffee lipids content and composition were presented by Folstar (1985) and Speer and Kölling-Speer (2001). However, specific information on the content and composition of the lipids in defective coffee beans is scarce and is discussed next.

Mazzafera (1999) reported a study on the chemical composition of defective coffee beans in which the total lipid content was determined by Soxhlet extraction with hexane. In this study, black beans presented the highest average value for oil content (~13%) and immature beans presented no significant differences in oil content when compared to immature-black beans. Oliveira et al. (2006) determined the lipid contents of Arabica coffees in their study of the proximate composition of green and roasted defective coffee beans and the respective values (dry green basis) are 9.2±0.6 g/100g for sour, 9.6±0.7 g/100g for immature, 10.0±0.3 for black and 10.8±0.3 g/100g for non-defective beans. The method employed was that of Soxhlet extraction with petroleum ether. The lipid contents were found to be significantly different among non-defective and defective beans according to the Duncan test at 5% probability. Non-defective mature coffee beans presented higher oil contents than those for defective beans. Amongst the defective beans, black beans presented higher oil contents than those for immature and sour beans, corroborating the results presented by Mazzafera (1999). There were no significant differences among the oil contents for roasted non-defective and sour beans. Regarding the effect of the roasting process on the oil content, there was a slight decrease (in dry green basis) in the oil content of non-defective mature beans while the content of the other types remained constant. This fact corroborates the observation that defective beans are roasted to a lesser degree than non-defective mature beans for the same processing conditions (Franca et al., 2005a). The lipid contents determined by Oliveira et al. (2006), be it for non-defective or defective beans, fall within the range encountered in the literature (9–15%) for unspecified types of arabica coffee (regarding the amount of defects) (Folstar, 1985; Speer and Kölling-Speer, 2001; Turatti, 2001; Vila et al., 2005). The solvent extracted coffee oils obtained for each separate sample of black, immature, sour and non-defective beans, and the screw-pressed coffee oil obtained from a mixture (PVA) containing 31.2% non-defective, 40.5% sour, 21.1% immature and 3.2% black beans were analyzed for the fatty acids profile. There were no significant differences in the amounts of all fatty acids for green and roasted non-defective and defective beans, based on the Duncan test at 5% probability. Linoleic and palmitic acids were the predominant fatty acids, with averages of 44% and 34%, respectively. The oil samples were comprised of moderate quantities of oleic (9%) and estearic (7%) acids and low quantities of araquidic (3%), linolenic (1.5%), behenic (0.7%) and eicosenoic (0.3%) acids. Miristic and palmitoleic acids were present in trace amounts.

The factors that are usually employed to define the quality of edible oils were determined by Oliveira et al. (2006) for coffee oils obtained by screw pressing of the mixture of defective beans (PVA). These factors are represented by the following parameters: saponification value, unsaponifiable matter, free fatty acids, free acidity, iodine value, and refractive index. The unsaponifiable matter was determined for both screw-pressed and solvent-extracted PVA oil in order to verify the effects of the extraction method on this quantity. The unsaponifiable matter content determined for the solvent-extracted oil was 9.2 g/100 g oil, a value significantly smaller than that for the screw-pressed oil (12.8 g/100 g oil). This was somewhat expected, since the screw-pressing is not a selective process, thus extracting with the oil other matter than exclusively the lipidic fraction. The value obtained by Oliveira et al. (2006) for the pressed oil is within the range published in the literature of 9–13 g/100 g oil for green (crude) coffee oil (Ravindranath et al., 1972; Turatti, 2001).

Oliveira et al. (2006) also obtained high values for free fatty acids contents of screw-pressed coffee oils: 4.9±4 g oleic acid/100 g oil. High values for free fatty acids content can be attributed either to inadequate storage conditions or long periods of storage of the beans (Vila et al., 2005) or to the fact that the oil was extracted by more than one pressing cycle (Rossell and Pritchard, 1991). Spiz et al. (1989) also found high values for free fatty acids in coffee oil (1.9–6.7 g oleic acid/100 g oil). The calculated value for free acidity (9.7±0.8% w/w expressed as oleic acid) was also high since it is based on the value for free fatty acids. The saponification value determined for the green coffee oil presented a value of 192.0±1.4 mg KOH/g oil that lies within the range encountered in the literature which is 180–200 mg KOH/g oil for coffee oil (Lago, 2001) and also within standards established for the trading of other edible oils, such as virgin olive oil (184–196 mg KOH/g oil). The iodine value (Wijs) was determined to be 95.5±5.6 and also falls within the range published in the literature for coffee oil (84.6–98.5; Lago, 2001). The refractive index determined for the coffee oil in this study was 1.468±0.001 and falls outside the range determined by Lago (2001), which was 1.458–1.462. This can be attributed to the facts that the crude oil used in the study by Oliveira et al. (2006) presented a high value of unsaponifiable matter and also contained fine particulate matter in it.

In their study of the evaluation of the potential of coffee oil as a feedstock for biodiesel production, Oliveira et al. (2008) used oils extracted from a batch of exclusively non-defective beans and also from a mixture of defective (34% w/w) and non-defective beans (66% w/w). The extraction was in a Soxhlet apparatus (20 kg solids capacity) with hexane for 16 h. The compositions of the oils from the non-defective and the PVA mixture were determined by a thermogravimetric procedure, adapted from that proposed by Goodrum and Geller (2002), to be comprised of 81 and 76% (w/w) of triglycerides, respectively. The titrated acidities of the oils of non-defective and defective beans were 2.62±0.29 and 10.04±0.03% (w/w), respectively. The contribution of the defective beans to the acidity of the oil was fairly high, since these beans were partially comprised of fermented beans (black and brown, ~20% w/w).

3.4. Ash (Minerals)

Mineral content represents 4-5% of coffee weight on a dry basis (Clarke, 1985). Potassium is the main constituent, representing approximately 40% of total mineral content, followed by calcium and magnesium in much smaller amounts (Clarke, 1985). Other minerals are present in small quantities (iron, cesium, manganese, sodium, vanadium and aluminum; Santos and Oliveira, 2001; Vega-Carrillo et al., 2002). Regarding mineral content in roasted coffee, literature data are scarce and show a small increase associated to weight loss during roasting (Ferreira et al., 1971; Clarke, 1985). There are evidences that both the mineral content and profile in coffee could be affected by growth conditions (e.g. fertilizers, maturity state), pre-processing operations (dry vs. wet processing) and fermentation (Clarke, 1985). Since the mineral content of coffee is not affected by roasting and it is known to vary with bean maturity state, elemental analysis could be a potential candidate for differentiation between defective and non-defective beans in roasted coffee.

Oliveira et al. (2006) and Vasconcelos et al. (2007) evaluated the total mineral content of defective coffee beans in comparison to non-defective ones. Both studies reported higher mineral contents for defective beans (~6% d.b.) in comparison to non-defective ones (~5% d.b.), prior to and after roasting. Among the defects, black beans presented the highest mineral content. The only reported data on the mineral profile of defective and non-defective coffees, based on atomic absorption spectrometry, was presented by Custódio et al. (2005) and are displayed in tables 8 and 9.

Table 8. Mineral profile in green coffee beans (g/100 g dry basis)

	Calcium	Magnesium	Potassium	Zinc
Non-defective	0.448±0.093[a]	0.257±0.005[a]	1.335±0.047[c]	0.0027±0.0004[a]
Immature	0.307±0.016[b]	0.261±0.035[a]	1.545±0.065[b]	0.0001±0.0001[a]
Black	0.335±0.022[b]	0.274±0.010[a]	1.838±0.074[a]	0.0028±0.0026[a]
Sour	0.301±0.025[b]	0.258±0.017[a]	1.635±0.110[b]	0.0028±0.0040[a]

Average value±Standard deviation. Mean values with the same letter in the same column do not differ significantly by the Duncan test at 5% probability

Table 9. Mineral profile in roasted coffee beans (g/100 g dry green basis)

	Calcium	Magnesium	Potassium	Zinc
Non-defective	0.227±0.024[b]	0.246±0.005[bc]	1.240±0.025[b]	ND
Immature	0.250±0.012[ab]	0.254±0.010[ab]	1.360±0.042[b]	ND
Black	0.267±0.008[a]	0.268±0.006[a]	1.645±0.094[a]	ND
Sour	0.263±0.016[a]	0.232±0.020[c]	1.563±0.084[a]	ND

Average value±Standard deviation. Mean values with the same letter in the same column do not differ significantly by the Duncan test at 5% probability. ND=non detected.

Potassium was found to be the main constituent of the ashed mineral content, in agreement with literature data on coffee mineral content (Clarke, 1985). Significant differences were detected among some samples. For green beans, potassium levels were the highest for black beans and the lowest for non-defective ones. Intermediate values were obtained for both the immature and sour beans. A small decrease in potassium levels was observed after roasting. The highest levels were found in both black and sour samples, whereas the lowest were observed for non-defective and immature beans. Calcium levels, about 80% lower than potassium, were higher for the non-defective coffee beans in comparison to the defective ones, prior to roasting. Calcium levels decreased approximately 30% after roasting, with the highest levels presented by black and sour beans and the lowest by non-defective ones. Such behavior could be attributed to the fact that both black and sour coffee beans are known to roast to a lesser degree than non-defective ones (Franca et al., 2005a). No significant differences were found in magnesium and zinc levels, prior to and after roasting. Also, a comparison of mineral profiles among both coffees from different crops, green and roasted did not show significant variations (see table 10). The obtained data showed that high potassium levels could be perceived as a marker for black and sour coffees, even after roasting. However, given the expressive amounts of non-defective beans usually found in PVA mixtures, such attribute can not be employed for separation of defective/non-defective coffees after roasting. These results suggest that a more sensitive analysis should be performed for minerals that are present in low quantities, in order to find specific markers for defective coffees.

Table 10. Mineral profile of the PVA mixture (g/100 g dry green basis)

		Calcium	Magnesium	Potassium
Crop 1	Green	0.212±0.015	0.238±0.004	1.605±0.049
	Roasted	0.233±0.012	0.241±0.003	1.725±0.034
Crop 2	Green	0.210±0.014	0.217±0.002	1.541±0.051
	Roasted	0.213±0.007	0.230±0.015	1.719±0.136

Average value±Standard deviation. Values did not differ significantly by Analysis of Variance at 5% probability.

3.5. Carbohydrates

Green coffee contains a wide range of carbohydrates, including poly-, tri-, di- and monosaccharides. Such class of substances is quite important for flavor development and several studies confirm that carbohydrate degradation is directly linked to the formation of several substances that affect coffee flavor and aroma (De Maria et al., 1994 ; De Maria et al., 1996; Alcázar et al., 2005; Murkovic & Derler, 2006). According to Oosterveld et al. (2003), approximately 20 to 40% of the total carbohydrates in coffee are degraded during roasting. The roasting process is responsible for opening the cell-wall matrix resulting in the solubilization of polysaccharides upon extraction. Then, the hydrolysis of the polysaccharides results in a release of oligosaccharides and monosaccharides, which in turn are converted into their degradation products through Maillard and Strecker reactions (Oosterveld et al., 2003). Such products, including furans, aldehydes, aliphatic and carboxylic acids, are aroma precursors and also play a major role on sensory perception in association with acidity (Ginz et al., 2000; Farah et al., 2006). Reactions between sucrose and aminoacids produce pyrazines and carbonilic substances that also affect coffee flavors (De Maria et al., 1996).

Sucrose is the main free sugar present in green coffee, in amounts varying according to species, maturity, origin and growth conditions, with averages of 6-9% db and 4-6% db for Arabica and Robusta, respectively (Trugo, 1985; Murkovic & Derler, 2006). Sucrose levels are expected to increase with coffee maturation and, since this is the main free sugar avalaible, its levels will naturally decrease if fermentation occurs. Therefore, this parameter is a potential candidate for separation of defective and non-defective beans and some reports are available with respect to correlation with the presence of defects (Mazzafera, 1999; Bradbury, 2001; Vasconcelos et al., 2007).

Mazzafera (1999) compared the amount of reducing sugars and sucrose of immature, black and immature-black coffees, and encountered lower sugar and sucrose contents for immature beans, so it was concluded that the amount of sugar is primarily associated with the developmental stage. It was also observed that the ratio between sucrose and reducing sugars increased almost four times from immature-black to black beans. According to this study, such difference can be attributed to the fact that, during seed filling, most of the carbohydrate metabolism is directed to accumulation of storage polysaccharides in the coffee seed. According to Bradbury (2001), the occurrence of black beans was associated to low carbohydrate accumulation during coffee bean development, which resulted in approximately 50% and 75% lower sucrose levels in black beans compared to non-defective coffees of the Arabica (from India) and Robusta (from Vietnam) species, respectively. Vasconcelos et al. (2007) compared sucrose levels of non-defective, immature, sour and black beans. Average reported levels were 1, 5 and 8% dry basis for black, immature/sour and non-defective, respectively. A comparison of these results with the ones presented by Mazzafera (1999) indicates that sucrose levels will be affected by both bean maturation stage and fermentation and therefore it can not be accertained which factor will be predominant. Only traces of sucrose were detected by Vasconcelos et al. (2007) in the light roasted coffee samples and no sucrose was detected for the other roasting degrees. This behavior is in agreement with literature data on sucrose degradation during roasting, ranging from 97% to 100% from light to dark roasts (Trugo, 1985).

The literature data on the correlation between sugar levels and coffee quality is still scarce. Chagas (1994) reported a positive association between coffee quality and content of reducing and non-reducing sugars in coffee beans from Brazil. Farah et al. (2006) did not find a direct correlation between sucrose levels and coffee quality and reported both the highest (~8 % db) and lowest (~5 % db) sucrose levels for low quality samples. However, the sample with the highest sucrose content contained only 8% defective beans whereas the amount of defective beans in the sample with less sucrose was almost 40%. Ramalakshmi et al. (2007) reported lower sucrose level for a mixture of defective beans in comparison to non-defective ones. These results confirm that the presence of defective coffees will have a direct impact on lowering sucrose levels of a given coffee sample.

3.6. Chlorogenic Acids

Chlorogenic acids (CGA) is the denomination given to a group of phenolic esters that correspond to approximately 6 to 12% mass of green coffee. They are the main phenolic compounds present in coffee and comprise esters of *trans*-cinnamic acids, such as caffeic, ferulic and *p*-coumaric acids, with (−)-quinic acid (Farah et al., 2005). Such substances are known to be responsible for coffee pigmentation, aroma formation, astringency and bitterness (Clifford, 1985; De Maria et al., 1995; Farah et al., 2005; Farah et al., 2006). The major CGA subgroups in coffee are the caffeoylquinic acids (CQA), feruloylquinic acids (FQA) and dicaffeoylquinic acids (diCQA) (Clifford, 1985). Caffeoylquinic acids, specifically 3- 4- and 5-CQA, correspond to approximately 85% of the total CGA in green coffee, with 5-CQA representing approximately 75% of the total CCA.

According to Farah et al. (2005) such class of compounds (CGA) in coffee has received much attention lately due to various pharmacological activities observed in vitro and in vivo studies. Examples include vascular activity (Bonita et al., 2007), antioxidant activity (Castilho et al., 2002), inhibition of the mutagenicity of carcinogenic compounds (Stich, 1982), glucose reduction in type 2 diabetes pacients (Van Dam, 2006), and others. Robusta coffees are reported to have higher CGA contents (7-10%) than Arabica (5-8%) (Clifford, 1985; Perrone et al., 2008). Martín et al. (1998) reported that the ratio between chlorogenic acids and caffeine levels provides a good separation between Arabica and Robusta coffees of different origins. According to Clifford (1985), there is an increase in total CGA content with maturity, with the higher levels being attained approximately four weeks before full maturity. Also, diCQA contents are reported to decrease with bean maturity.

CGA play an important role in the formation of roasted coffee flavor (Perrone et al., 2008). CGA are partially degraded during roasting, producing phenolic lactones and other derivatives. According to Clifford (1985) a decrease of approximately 8-10% of the original CGA content is observed for every 1% weight loss (dry matter basis). They are first hydrolyzed to quinic and caffeic acids, which then form phenolic volatiles during pyrolysis (Homma, 2001). Given the fact that such compounds affect coffee flavor, in association with their antioxidant and other physiological effects, some studies have investigated the relation of such class of compounds with coffee quality (Franca et al., 2005b; Farah et al., 2006; Ramalakshmi et al., 2007) and defective beans (Mazzafera, 1999; Franca et al., 2005a).

Mazzafera (1999) compared the levels of 5-CQA (by HPLC) and soluble phenols (colorimetricaly) of immature, black and immature-black green coffees and reported that the contents of soluble phenols and 5-CQA were approximately 35% higher in immature coffees compared to black and immature-black. Franca et al. (2005a) evaluated 5-CQA levels of non-defective, black, immature and sour coffee beans. It was observed that black beans had significantly lower levels of 5-CQA (~1.8% db) compared to the other samples (~3.2% db). Also, no significant differences in 5-CQA levels were observed for non-defective, immature and sour beans. It is noteworthy to point out that 5-CQA levels reported in this study were on the lower limit of the range reported by Clifford (1985): 3-5%. It was also reported that degradation of 5-CQA occurred to a smaller extent for black beans, which was attributed to the lighter roasting degree attained by these defects as previously discussed in terms of other attributes. The same research group (Franca et al., 2005b) evaluated 5-CQA levels of Arabica coffees of different cup qualities (soft, hard, rioysh and rio), prior to and after roasting. The highest (~2.5% db) and lowest (~2.3% db) 5-CQA contents were observed for the rioysh and rio samples, respectively, which represented the low cup quality samples. However, it was pointed out that the methodology employed in this study for evaluation of 5-CQA levels needed revision, since average values were quite low compared to coffee literature data on 5-CQA (Clifford, 1985; Farah, 2004; Farah et al., 2005). It is noteworthy to mention that the sample with the highest 5-CQA levels was also the one presenting the highest amount of immature beans. After roasting, 5-CQA levels presented slight variations among the samples, without correlation with cup quality.

Farah et al. (2005) identified eight CGA in Brazilian coffees of different cup qualities: 3-CQA, 4- CQA, 5-CQA, 3,4-diCQA, 3,5- diCQA, 4,5-diCQA, 4-FQA and 5-FQA, and reported that the CQA accounted for approximately 83% of the total CGA in green beans. In terms of total CGA, they reported the highest (~7.0% db) and lowest (~5.8% db) contents for the worst and best quality samples, respectively. It was also observed that 5-CQA and 5-FQA levels correlated strongly with poor cup quality, and 4-CQA, 5-CQA, 4-FQA and 5-FQA levels correlated strongly with the Rio-off-flavor. Furthermore, the amount of immature beans also correlated with poor cup quality and Rio-off-flavor. It was also reported that immature and immature-black defective beans contained significantly higher levels of all CGA, but mostly CQA and FQA, comparing to healthy and black defective beans (data not shown). Such results are in agreement with the high percentage of immature beans in the low quality samples employed in that study. The average loss of total CGA during roasting was 93%. Correlations between CQA and FQA levels and cup quality became less significant with roasting. Ramalakshmi et al. (2007) reported slightly higher CGA levels in low quality coffees (mixture of defective beans) in comparison to high quality ones (non-defective beans).

An evaluation of the published works on CGA in relation to coffee quality indicates that high CGA levels, mainly 5-CQA, seem to be associated to the presence of immature beans. However, since 5-CQA levels decrease as roasting progresses, such correlation is not significant for roasted coffees.

3.7. Acidity and pH

The acidity of coffee brews has been considered an important sensory attribute, and a certain level of acidity, that is quickly removed from the palate, is usually associated with good cup quality (Freitas, 2001). Lightly roasted good quality coffees should present a “clean” and “fine” acidity whereas such characteristic is not well perceived for dark roasts (Woodman, 1985). Acidity, in its strict sense, is determined by the hydrogen ion concentration related to the ionization degree of a given acid (or acids) present in an aqueous solution. Presence of acids will affect flavor, either through the acid taste in the tongue associated with the hydrogen ions, or through aroma perception if the undissociated acid is volatile enough (Woodman, 1985). Adstringency effects on the tongue may be also encountered in association with high acidity, and it will be clearly perceived if the coffee is not properly roasted. Furthermore, the term sour is employed in coffee tasting in association with an undesirable form of acidity. Given the significant effect of acidity on coffee flavor and quality, and the fact that both pH and titrable acidity can be correlated to perceived acidity (sensory), such parameters have also been investigated in terms of defective coffee beans (Mazzafera, 1999; Vasconcelos et al., 2007) and cup quality (Franca et al., 2005b).

Mazzafera (1999) presented pH and acidity measurements for immature, black and immature-black green (crude) coffees. Although significant differences were not reported for pH measurements (~5.9), the lowest pH value corresponded to the highest acidity found in immature beans (~3.5 mL NaOH g^{-1}). Both black and immature-black beans presented similar acidity (~2.5 mL NaOH g^{-1}). Franca et al. (2005b) evaluated both pH and total acidity levels of Arabica coffees of different cup qualities (soft, hard, rioysh and rio). It was reported that acidity increased (and pH decreased) as cup quality worsened, i.e., as both the amount of immature and sour beans increased. Ramalakshmi et al. (2007) also reported slightly higher acidity levels for a mixture of defective beans in comparison to non-defective beans, and attributed this to the presence of sour beans. High acidity of sour beans can be associated with bean fermentation. Acidity levels presented a significant decrease with roasting (50-60% reduction), and no significant differences were detected among the samples, even though the tendency for increase in acidity with decrease in cup quality could still be observed. pH values increased after roasting, with the highest values corresponding to the lowest quality samples.

Vasconcelos et al. (2007) presented both acidity and pH measurements for defective beans in comparison to non-defective ones, prior to and after light, medium and dark roasts. Before roasting, acidity values were the highest for sour beans and the lowest for black beans. The lowest acidity values observed for black beans were attributed to loss of acids during soil contact. pH values were higher for defective beans in comparison to non-defective ones, with the highest pH values encountered for black beans (~6). Acidity values decreased after roasting, without differences among samples. Regarding pH measurements, values remained higher for defective beans in comparison to non-defective ones, after roasting.

3.8. Volatile Components

A considerable amount of research has been done on the characterization of flavor related substances in coffee (Grosch, 2001; Rocha et al., 2003). The most common classes of compounds reported include acids, alcohols, aldehydes, alkanes, alkenes, benzenic compounds, esters, furans, ketones, lactones, oxazoles, phenolic compounds, pyridines, pyrazines, pyrroles, sulfur compounds, thiazoles, and thiophenes (Dart & Nursten, 1985; Sanz et al., 2001; Yeretzian et al., 2003; Mondello et al., 2004; Ryan et al., 2004). Given the direct impact of such components on flavor characteristics of roasted coffee, some recent studies have focused on the comparison of the volatile profiles of roasted Arabica and Robusta coffees and also of roasted coffees from different origins (Costa Freitas & Mosca, 1999; Costa Freitas et al. 2001; Rocha et al., 2003; Zambonin et al., 2005). It was concluded that the volatile profiles provided the means for separation of Arabica and Robusta coffees after roasting. Also, recent studies by Costa Freitas et al. (2001) and Zambonin et al. (2005) showed that gas chromatography-mass spectrometry analysis (GC-MS) of the volatile components of the coffee headspace concentrated by solid-phase micro-extraction (SPME) in combination with principal component analysis (PCA) also allowed for discrimination of Arabica/Robusta blends having different geographical origins.

The successful application of chemometrics for discrimination between coffee varieties and geographical origins indicated that this tool could also be evaluated for discrimination between defective and healthy coffee beans and, thus, a recent study was presented to that objective (Mancha Agresti et al., 2008). The coffee headspace volatiles profile was evaluated for defective coffee beans (black, immature and sour) in comparison to non-defective ones, after roasting to light, medium and dark degrees (roasting at 200°C for 30, 60 and 120 min, respectively). Volatiles extraction and concentration were performed by solid phase micro-extraction (SPME) of the roasted coffee headspace and analysis of the volatile profiles was performed by GC-MS. Detection of approximately 250 volatile compounds was reported, with only 2% (5 substances) being detected in all defects and not in the healthy coffee samples. Sour beans presented the highest amount of substances not detected in healthy coffee, followed by black and immature beans. Pyrazines and pyrroles were detected in greater quantities in sour/black coffee beans in comparison to immature ones. Principal component and hierarchical cluster analysis showed that the data could be separated into two groups, one containing immature and black beans and the other containing healthy and sour coffee beans. Such results are an indication that black and sour beans can be associated to fermentation of immature and non-defective coffees, respectively. Some separation between fermented/non fermented samples and also between roasting degrees was also observed.

4. Conclusion

Coffee is deemed as a commodity ranking second only to petroleum in terms of currency (usually US dollars) traded worldwide (Illy, 2002). Brazil is the largest coffee producer and exporter in the world and is the second largest consumer. As such this commodity is quite relevant to the country economy. This is also true for other countries which are relevant producers/exporters, such as Vietnam, Colombia, Ethiopia, Indonesia, Mexico and India. As an agricultural product, the produced coffee is prone to present a parcel that does not fit to established quality parameters and this parcel is denominated "defects". Currently, in Brazil, this category of beans amounts to 15 to 20% of the total production. Since such defects negatively affect the beverage quality, it is desirable not to have them in the trading and roasting markets. However, since these defects are intrinsic to production, harvesting and processing of coffee, although separated from non-defective coffee in farms and cooperatives, they are necessarily commercialized, because they represent an investment for the producers and, also, because currently there are no alternative uses for them. In order to propose alternative uses and to provide a means for the consumer awareness of quality, it is necessary to understand what are the underlying physical-chemical differences between defective and non-defective beans, green or roasted. Although coffee can be assuredly considered one of the most studied food products in the last two centuries, only recently the physical-chemical characterization of defective beans has been addressed for the purpose of discrimination/differentiation.

Regarding physical attributes, it can be concluded that crude black and sour beans can be satisfactorily discriminated from non-defective beans by size and color, while immature beans cannot. Upon roasting, it was demonstrated by several studies that defective beans will roast to a lesser degree than non defective ones. As a consequence, only black beans, which when crude are usually smaller than other beans, may be discriminated from the others, since they swell less and thus present higher density values than those for other beans under the same roasting conditions. Hence, as a general conclusion, discrimination of immature beans by means of physical attributes does not seem feasible and discrimination by color is only feasible for green coffee.

As for chemical attributes, no significant differences in proximate compositions were determined for defective and non defective coffee beans, both green and roasted. Again, black beans were the ones that presented the most pronounced differences in specific chemical components (caffeine, trigonelline, potassium) or classes of compounds (amines, lipids). However, since this type of beans is usually encountered in small amounts within a sample (2-3% w/w) it makes it difficult to detect and quantify it by means of specific chemical markers. Histamine was deemed a potential marker for defective beans in green coffee since it was detected only in those types of beans. However, since it was present in very small amounts, its detection and quantification in a large sample of a mixture of defective and non defective beans cannot be considered practical. A high CGA content was associated to the presence of immature beans in mixtures with other beans and, thus, with further studies, considering different crops and geographic regions, it could be considered as a potential marker for the detection of this type of defect in green coffee samples. However, since both CGA and histamine contents significantly decrease upon roasting, the use of these chemical markers was demonstrated not to be feasible for discrimination of defective and non defective beans in roasted coffees. The only promising alternative for discrimination of defective and non defective beans in roasted coffees was the multivariate statistical analysis of the volatile components of coffee headspace that allowed for separation between defective and non defective coffees together with roasting degrees. There is still a lot to be done in terms of research in regard to being capable of both qualitatively and quantitatively discriminating defective from non defective coffee beans, preferably after roasting. In regard to qualitative discrimination, geographic origin and crop year are parameters to be studied since they were demonstrated to affect the chemical profile of coffees. As for quantitative discrimination, the identification of chemical markers for each specific type of defect is imperative.

Acknowledgements

The authors gratefully acknowledge financial support from the following Brazilian Government Agencies: CNPq and FAPEMIG.

References

Alcázar, A., Jurado, J.M., Martín, M. J., Pablos, F. and González, A.G. (2005) Enzymatic-spectrophotometric determination of sucrose in coffee beans. *Talanta*, 67, 760-766.

Amorim, H.V., Basso, L.C., Crocomo, O.J. and Teixeira, A.A. (1977) Polyamines in green and roasted coffee, *Journal of Agricultural and Food Chemistry,* 25, 957–958.

Banks, M., McFadden, C. and Atkinson, C. (1999) *The World Encyclopaedia of coffee* , London: Anness Publishing Limited.

Bardócz, S. (1995) Polyamines in food and their consequences for food quality and human health, *Trends in Food Science and Technology,* 6, 341–346.

Bonita, J.S., Mandarano, M., Shuta, D. and Vinson, J. (2007). Coffee and cardiovascular disease: In vitro, cellular, animal, and human studies, *Pharmacological Research*, 55, 187-198.

Bradbury, A.G.W. (2001) Carbohydrates – Chemistry I: Non-volatile compounds. In R.J.Clarke e O.G.Vitzthum (Eds.), *Coffee Recent Developments* (pp.1-17), London: Elsevier Applied Science.

Casal, S., Mendes, E., Alves, M.R., Alves, R.C., Oliveira, M.B.P.P. and Ferreira, M.A. (2004) Free and conjugated biogenic amines in green and roasted coffee beans, *Journal of Agricultural and Food Chemistry,* 52, 6188–6192

Casal, S., Oliveira, M.B. and Ferreira, M.A. (2000) HPLC/diode array applied to the thermal degradation of trigonelline, nicotinic acid and caffeine in coffee, *Food Chemistry*, 68, 481-485.

Castillo, D.M., Ames, J.M. and Gordon, M.H. (2002). Effect of Roasting on the Antioxidant Activity of Coffee Brew, *Journal of Agricultural and Food Chemistry,* 50, 3698 – 3703.

Chagas, S. J. R. (1994). Caracterização química e qualitativa de cafés de alguns municípios de três regiões produtoras de Minas Gerais (Chemical and qualitative characterization of coffees from three regions in Minas Gerais State) MSc thesis, Universidade Federal de Lavras (in portuguese).

Cirilo, M.P.G., Coelho, A.F.S., Araujo, C.M., Goncalves, F.R.B., Nogueira, F.D. and Gloria, M.B.A. (2003). Profile and levels of bioactive amines in green and roasted coffee, *Food Chemistry*, 82, 397-402.

Clarke, R.J. (1987a). Roasting and Grinding. In R.J. Clarke and R. Macrae (Eds.), *Coffee Vol. 2: Technology* (pp. 73- 107), London: Elsevier Applied Science.

Clarke, R. J. (1987b). Grading, Storage, Pre-treatments and Blending. In R.J. Clarke and R. Macrae (Eds.), *Coffee Vol. 2: Technology* (pp. 35-58.), London: Elsevier Applied Science.

Clarke, R. J. (1985). Water and mineral contents. In R.J. Clarke and R. Macrae (Eds.), *Coffee Vol. 1: Chemistry* (pp. 42–82), London: Elsevier Applied Science.

Clarke, R. J. and Macrae, R. (1987). *Coffee Vol. 2: Technology.* London: Elsevier Applied Science.

Clarke, R. J. and Macrae, R. (1985) *Coffee Vol. 1: Chemistry.* London: Elsevier Applied Science.

Clifford, M.N. (1985) Chlorogenic Acids. In R.J. Clarke and R. Macrae (Eds.), *Coffee Vol. 1: Chemistry* (pp. 153-202), London: Elsevier Applied Science.

Costa Freitas, A. M., Parreira, C. and Vilas-Boas, L. (2001). The Use of an Electronic Aroma-sensing Device to Assess Coffee Differentiation - Comparison with SPME Gas Chromatography-Mass Spectrometry Aroma Patterns, *Journal of Food Composition and Analysis,* 14, 513-522.

Costa Freitas, A.M. and Mosca, A. I. (1999). Coffee geographic origin - an aid to coffee differentiation, *Food Research International*, 32, 565-573.

Cristo, H.P., Martins, M.A., Oliveira, L.S. and Franca, A.S. (2006). Transverse flow of coffee beans in rotating roasters, *Journal of Food Engineering,* 75, 142-148.

Custódio, B. M. O., Magalhães, F. S., Mansur, M. B., Franca, A. S. and Oliveira, L.S. (2005). Elemental analysis of defective and non-defective beans in green and roasted coffee. In: 2005 ASAE Annual International Meeting, 2005, Tampa, FL. ASAE Paper no. 056085, 8p.

Dart, S.K. and Nursten, H.E. (1985) Volatile components. In R.J. Clarke and R. Macrae (Eds.), *Coffee Vol. 1: Chemistry* (pp. 223-265), London: Elsevier Applied Science.

De Maria, C.A.B., Trugo. L.C., Neto, F.R.A., Moreira, R.F.A. and Alviano, C.S. (1996). Composition of green coffee water-soluble fractions and identification of volatiles formed during roasting. *Food Chemistry*, 55, 203-7.

De Maria, C.A.B., Trugo, L.C., Moreira, R.F.A. and Petracco, M. (1995) Simultaneous determination of total chlorogenic acids, trigonelline and caffeine in green coffee samples by high performance gel filtration chromatography, *Food Chemistry* 52, 447–449.

De Maria, C.A.B., Trugo, L.C., Moreira, R.F.A. and Werneck, C.C. (1994) Composition of green coffee fractions and their contribution to the volatile profile formed during roasting. *Food Chemistry*, 50, 141-145.

Dutra, E.R., Oliveira, L.S., Franca, A.S., Ferraz, V.P. and Afonso, R.J.C. (2001). A preliminary study on the feasibility of using the composition of coffee roasting exhaust gas for the determination of the degree of roast. *Journal of Food Engineering*, 47, 241–246.

Farah, A., Monteiro, M.C., Calado, V., Franca, A.S. and Trugo, L.C. (2006). Correlation between cup quality and chemical attributes of Brazilian coffee. *Food chemistry,* 98, 373-380.

Farah, A., De Paulis, T., Trugo, L.C. and Martin, P.R. (2005). Effect of roasting on the formation and degradation of chlorogenic acid lactones in roasted coffee, *Journal of Agricultural and Food Chemistry*, 53,1505–1513.

Farah, A. (2004). Distribuição nos grãos, importância na qualidade da bebida e biodisponibilidade dos ácidos clorogênicos do café. (Distribution in coffee beans, importance in beverage quality and biodisponibility of chlorogenic acids in coffee) Ph.D. Thesis, UFRJ (in Portuguese).

Fernandes, J. O. and Ferreira, M. A. (2000) Combined ion-pair extraction and gas chromatography-mass spectrometry for the simultaneous determination of diamines, polyamines and aromatic amines in Port wine and grape juice, *Journal of Chromatography A*, 886, 183-195.

Ferreira, L.A.B., Fragoso, M.A.C., Peratta, M.F., Silvo, M.C.C. and Rebeto, M.C. (1971) Constituintes minerais dos cafés de Angola. (Mineral constituents of Angola coffees). Proc. 5th International Scientific Colloquium on Green and Roasted Coffee Chemistry, 159-173.

Folstar, P. (1985) Lipids. In R.J. Clarke and R. Macrae (Eds.), *Coffee Vol. 1: Chemistry* (pp. 203–222), London: Elsevier Applied Science.

Franca, A.S., Oliveira, L.S., Mendonça, J.C.F. and Silva, X.A. (2005a) Physical and chemical attributes of defective crude and roasted coffee beans, *Food Chemistry,* 90, 84–89.

Franca, A.S., Mendonca, J.C.F. and Oliveira, S.D. (2005b) Composition of green and roasted coffees of different cup qualities, *LWT - Food Science and Technology*, 38, 709-715.

Freitas, M.L.G. 2001. A última impressão é a que fica - Introdução à classificação e degustação de café (The last impression stays... Introduction to coffee classification and cupping) Sindicafé MG, 74 p. (in Portuguese).

Ginz, M., Balzer, H.H., Bradbury, A.G.W. and Maier, H.G. (2000) Formation of aliphatic acids by carbohydrate degradation during roasting of coffee. *European Food Research and Technology,* 211, 404-410.

Gokmen, V. and Senyuva, H.Z. (2006). Study of colour and acrylamide formation in coffee, wheat flour and potato chips during heating, *Food Chemistry*, 99, 238-243.

Goodrum, J.W. and Geller, D.P. (2002). Rapid thermogravimetric measurements of boiling points and vapor pressure of saturated medium- and long-chain triglycerides. *Bioresource Technology*, 84, 75–80.

Grosch, W. (2001). Chemistry III: Volatile compounds. In: Clarke, R.J. and Vitzthum, O.Z. *Coffee: Recent Developments*, (pp. 68-89), Oxford: Blackwell Science.

Halász, A., Baráth, A., Simon-Sarkadi, L. and Holzapfel, W. (1994) Biogenic amines and their production by microorganisms in food, *Trends in Food Science and Technology,* 5, 42–49.

Homma, S. (2001) Chemistry II: Non-volatile compounds, Part II. In R.J.Clarke e O.G.Vitzthum (Eds.), *Coffee Recent Developments* (pp.50-67), London: Elsevier Applied Science.

Illy, E. (2002) The complexity of coffee, Scientific American, June, 86-91.

Kalač, P. and Krausová, P. (2005) A review of dietary polyamines: formation, implications for growth and health and occurrence in foods, *Food Chemistry,* 90, 219–230.

Lago, R.C.A. (2001) Lipídios em grãos de café (Lipids in coffee beans), *B. CEPPA* (Centro de Pesquisa e Processamento de Alimentos), 19, 319–341 (in portuguese).

Macrae, R. (1985) Nitrogenous compounds. In R.J. Clarke and R. Macrae (Eds.), *Coffee Vol. 1: Chemistry* (pp. 115–152) London: Elsevier Applied Science.

Mancha Agresti, P.D.C., Franca, A.S., Oliveira, L.S. and Augusti, R. (2008) Discrimination between defective and non-defective Brazilian coffee beans by their volatile profile, Food Chemistry, 106, 787-796.

Marcone, M.F. (2004) Composition and properties of Indonesian palm civet coffee (Kopi Luwak) and Ethiopian civet coffee, *Food Research International*, 37, 901-912].

Martín, M.J., Pablos, F. and Gonzalez, A.G. (1998) Discrimination between arabica and robusta green coffee varieties according to their chemical composition, Talanta, 46, 1259-1264.

Martin, M.J., Pablos, F. and Gonzalez, A.G. (1999) Characterization of Arabica and Robusta varieties and misture resolution according to their metal content. *Food Chemistry*, 66, 365-370.

Mazzafera, P. (1999) Chemical composition of defective coffee beans, *Food Chemistry*, 64, 547–554.

Mendes, L.C., Menezes, H.C., Aparecida, M. and Silva, A.P. (2001) Optimization of the roasting of robusta coffee (C. canephora conillon) using acceptability tests and RSM, *Food Quality and Preference*, 12, 153-162.

Mendonça, J.C.F.(2006) Avaliação do perfil de carboidratos em grãos de café defeituosos e sadios das espécies Coffea arabica e Coffea canephora (Evaluation of the carbohydrate profiles of defective and non-defective coffees of Coffea arabica and Coffea canephora species). Doctoral Proposal, Universidade Federal de Minas Gerais, Belo Horizonte, MG, Brazil, 114 pp. (in Portuguese).

Mendonça, J.C.F., Franca, A. S. and Oliveira, L.S. (2007) A comparative evaluation of methodologies for water content determination in green coffee, *LWT - Food Science and Technology*, 40, 1300-1303.

Mondello, L., Casilli, A., Tranchida, P.Q., Dugo, P., Costa, R., Festa , S. and Dugo, G. (2004). Comprehensive multidimensional GC for the characterization of roasted coffee beans, *Journal of Separation Science*, 27, 442-450.

Murkovic, M. and Derler, K. (2006). Analysis of amino acids and carbohydrates in green coffee, Journal of Biochemical and Biophysical Methods, 69, 25-32.

Nikolova-Damyanova, B., Velikova, R. and Gulab, N. J. (1998). Lipid classes, fatty acid composition and triacylglycerol molecular species in crude coffee beans harvested in Brazil, *Food Research International,* 31, 479–486.

Oliveira, L.S., Franca, A.S., Camargos, R.R.S. and Ferraz, V.P. (2008) Coffee oil as a potential feedstock for biodiesel production, Bioresource Technology, 99, 3244-3250.

Oliveira, L.S., Franca, A. S., Mendonça, J.C.F. and Barros-Júnior, M.C. (2006). Proximate composition and fatty acids profile of green and roasted defective coffee beans, *LWT - Food Science and Technology*, 39, 235–239.

Oliveira, S.D., Franca, A. S., Gloria , M.B.A. and Borges, M.L.A. (2005). The effect of roasting on the presence of bioactive amines in coffees of different qualities, *Food Chemistry,* 90, 287-291.

Oosterveld, A., Voragen, A.G.J. and Schols, H.A. (2003). Effect of roasting on the carbohydrate composition of coffea arabica beans, *Carbohydrate Polymers,* 54, 183-192.

Perrone, D., Farah, A., Donangelo, C.M., Tomas De Paulis, T. and Martin, P.R. (2008) Comprehensive analysis of major and minor chlorogenic acids and lactones in economically relevant Brazilian coffee cultivars, *Food Chemistry*, 106, 859-867.

Ramalakshmi, K., Kubra, I.R. and Rao, L.J.M. (2007). Physicochemical Characteristics of Green Coffee:Comparison of Graded and Defective Beans, *Journal of Food Science*, 72, S333-S337.

Ravindranath, R., Yousuf Ali Khan, R. and Reddy, O.T. (1972) Composition and characteristics of Indian coffee bean, spent grounds and oil. *Journal of Food and Agriculture Science*, 23, 307–310.

Reh, C.T., Gerber, A., Prodolliet, J. and Vuataz, G. (2006) Water content determination in green coffee - Method comparison to study specificity and accuracy, Food Chemistry, 96, Issue 3 423-430.

Rocha, S., Maeztu, L., Barros, A., Cid, C. and Coimbra, M.A. (2003). Screening and distinction of coffee brews based on headspace solid phase microextraction / gas chromatography / principal component analysis, *Journal of the Science of Food and Agriculture*, 84, 43-51.

Rodrigues, M.A.A., Borges, M. L. A., Franca, A. S. , Oliveira, L.S. and Correa, P.C. (2003) Evaluation of physical properties of coffee during roasting. *E-journal. International Commission of Agricultural Engineering*, 5, Manuscript FP 03004, 12 p.

Rossell, J. B., and Pritchard, J. L. R. (1991). Analysis of oilseeds, fats and fatty foods. London: Elsevier Applied Science.

Ryan, D., Shellie, R., Tranchida, P., Casilli, A., Mondello, L. and Marriott, P. (2004). Analysis of roasted coffee bean volatiles by using comprehensive two-dimensional gas chromatography-time-of-flight mass spectrometry, *Journal of Chromatography A*, 1054, 57-65.

Santos, M.H.S. (1996). Biogenic amines: their importance in foods, *International Journal of Food Microbiology*, 29, 213–231.

Santos, E.J. and Oliveira, E. (2001). Determination of mineral nutrients and toxic elements in brazilian soluble coffee by ICP-AES, *Journal of Food Composition and Analysis*, 14, 523-531.

Sanz, C., Ansorena, D., Bello, J. and Cid, C. (2001). Optimizing headspace temperature and time sampling for identification of volatile compounds in ground roasted Arabica coffee, *Journal of Agricultural and Food Chemistry*, 49,1364-1369.

Sivetz, M. and Desrosier, N.W. (1979). *Coffee Technology*. Westport ,CO: Avi Publishing Co.

Speer, K. and Kölling-Speer, I. (2001). Non-volatile compounds – lipids. In R.J. Clarke and O.G. Vitzhum (Eds.), *Coffee: Recent Developments* (pp. 33–49), Oxford: Blackwell Science.

Spiz, R.R., Jablonka, F.H. and Pereira, D.A. (1989). Composição em ácidos graxos: Triacilgliceróis, monoésteres de diterpenos e óleo de grãos de café. Congresso Brasileiro de Ciência e Tecnologia de Alimentos (p. 151). Resumos, Rio de Janeiro: SBCTA (in portuguese).

Stich, H. F., Rosin, M. P. and Bryson, L. (1982) Inhibition of mutagenicity of a model nitrosation reaction by naturally occurring phenolics, coffee and tea. *Mutation Research, 95*, 119-128.

Summa, C.A., De la Calle, B., Brohee, M., Stadler, R.H. and Anklam, E. (2007) Impact of the roasting degree of coffee on the in vitro radical scavenging capacity and content of acrylamide, *LWT - Food Science and Technology*, 40, 1849-1854.

Trugo, L.C. (1985) Carbohydrates In R.J. Clarke and R. Macrae (Eds.), *Coffee Vol. 1: Chemistry* (pp. 83-114), London: Elsevier Applied Science.

Turatti, J. M. (2001). Extração e caracterização de óleo de café (Extraction and characterization of coffee oil), Proceedings of Simpósio de Pesquisa dos Cafés do Brasil, Vitória, Brazil, 2, 1533–1539 (in portuguese).

Van Dam, R.M. (2006). Coffee and type 2 diabetes: From beans to beta-cells, *Nutrition, Metabolism and Cardiovascular Diseases*, 16, 69-77.

Vasconcelos, A.L. 2005. Caracterização de grãos defeituosos de café quanto a aspectos físico-químicos e teores de aminas, para diversos graus de torração (Characterization of defective coffee beans with respect to physical and chemical attributes and amine leves, for several roasting degrees) *M.Sc. Thesis*, Universidade Federal de Minas Gerais, Belo Horizonte, MG, Brazil, 101 pp. (in Portuguese).

Vasconcelos, A.L.S., Franca, A.S., Glória, M.B.A. and Mendonça, J.C.F. (2007) A comparative study of chemical attributes and levels of amines in defective green and roasted coffee beans. *Food Chemistry*, 101, 26-32.

Vega-Carrillo, H.R., Iskander, F.Y. and Manzanares-Acuña, E.(2002). Elemental content in ground and soluble/instant coffee, J*ournal of Radioanalytical and Nuclear Chemistry,* 252,75-80.

Vila, M.A., Andueza, S., de Peña, M.P. and Cid, C. (2005). Fatty acid evolution during the storage of ground, roasted coffees, JAOCS, 82, 639-646.

Vincent, J.C. (1987) Green Coffee Processing. In R.J. Clarke and R. Macrae (Eds.), *Coffee Vol. 2*: *Technology* (pp. 1 -58), London: Elsevier Applied Science.

Woodman, J.S. (1985) Carboxylic Acids In R.J. Clarke and R. Macrae (Eds.), *Coffee Vol. 1: Chemistry* (pp. 266-289), London: Elsevier Applied Science.

Yeretzian, C., Jordan, A. and Lindinger, W. (2003). Analysing the headspace of coffee by proton-transfer-reaction mass-spectrometry,*International Journal of Mass Spectrometry*, 223-224,115-139.

Zambonin, C.G., Balest, L., De Benedetto, G.E. and Palmisano, F. (2005). Solid-phase microextraction-gas chromatography mass spectrometry and multivariate analysis for the characterization of roasted coffees, *Talanta,* 66, 261-265.

In: Progress in Food Chemistry
Editor: E. N. Koeffer, pp. 139-166

ISBN: 978-1-60456-303-0

Chapter 5

STABILITY OF TOMATO CAROTENOIDS DURING PROCESSING AND STORAGE

***B. Stephen Inbara*[*1] *and B. H. Chen*[2,]**
Department of Food Science, Fu Jen University, Taipei 242, Taiwan

ABSTRACT

Carotenoids are an important class of micronutrients in tomato and tomato-based products, which are widely studied due to their beneficial effects in the prevention of chronic diseases such as cardiovascular disease and various types of cancers. However, carotenoids are susceptible to isomerization and/or oxidative degradation during processing and storage. The degradation of carotenoids and change in their isomeric forms has been reported to cause variation in biological activity. This chapter intends to review the recent studies dealing with the stability of tomato carotenoids during processing and storage. Typical thermal processing condition of boiling in water for a short period of time increased the yield of lycopene due to disruption of tomato cell matrix. However, high temperature along with long duration treatment caused detrimental effect on carotenoids. Lycopene, γ-carotene and δ-carotene were relatively stable to isomerization, while lutein and β-carotene were more prone to isomerization, which may be accounted for by the difference in the structural characteristics of carotenoids and their localization/accumulation in tomatoes. The lycopene loss under various house-hold cooking conditions followed the order: frying > baking > boiling > microwaving, and soaking tomato slices in vinegar retained more lycopene than in oil or oil/vinegar mixture. The stability of dehydrated tomato products was affected by various factors such as temperature, oxygen permeability, water activity and sample texture (fine or coarse). Dehydration to intermediate moisture content (20-40%) with a water activity at 0.69-0.86 and storage temperature at $\leq 18^{\circ}$ could minimize carotenoid loss in tomato products. Complete inactivation of natural enzymes by blanching may prevent carotenoid degradation in tomatoes during frozen storage. The higher the storage temperature, the faster the degradation rate, and the lycopene degradation under different storage conditions followed the order: air and light > air and dark > vacuum and dark. From the commercial point of view, the post-harvest life span of tomatoes could be extended under

* Tel.:886-2-29053626,Fax:886-2-29053415

controlled-atmosphere storage of high CO_2 and low O_2 level. Treating tomatoes with osmotic solution (sucrose or high dextrose equivalent maltodextrin) prior to processing or storage minimized the carotenoid loss. By subjecting the tomato sample to high hydrostatic pressure before storage, carotenoid degradation might be minimized by complete inactivation of enzymes.

1. INTRODUCTION

Tomato fruit (*Lycopersicon esculentum*) is a rich source of several micronutrients including carotenoids, polyphenols, vitamins and folate, among which carotenoids are frequently studied as the epidemiological evidence has demonstrated the relationship between dietary intake of the major tomato carotenoid lycopene and prevention of chronic disease such as cardiovascular disease and prostate cancer [1,2]. Of the various carotenoids, lycopene was reported to exhibit the highest antioxidant activity in terms of singlet oxygen quenching and inhibition of proliferation of human epithelial cancer cell lines [3-5]. Tomato and tomato-based products contribute to about 9 out of 14 carotenoids found in human serum and are a predominant source of approximately half of carotenoids [6]. Of late consumption of raw tomatoes has considerably reduced, instead, over 80% of tomatoes produced are consumed as processed products like tomato paste, juice, puree, catsup, sauce and salsa [7]. Annually, the American consumes an average of 17.9 pounds of fresh tomatoes and 68.7 pounds of processed tomato products [8]. Tonucci et al. [9] reported the level of individual carotenoids in tomato products to exceed their corresponding concentrations in whole tomatoes, with lycopene being present at the largest concentration, followed by γ-carotene, phytoene, neurosporene, phytofluene, β-carotene, ζ-carotene, lycopene-5,6-diol and lutein (table 1). Mechanical and/or thermal treatments during processing have been shown to enhance release of carotenoids from the tomato matrix. But, the various processing and storage conditions may change the composition of carotenoids, resulting in a reduction of nutritional value of tomatoes [7].

Carotenoids are sensitive to heat, light, oxygen, water activity, acids and metal ions due to the presence of long-chain conjugated double bonds. Consequently, a decrease in the contents of carotenoids may occur in processed tomato products, which should be mainly caused by isomerization and degradation. Changes in both carotenoid content and distribution of cis/trans isomers may significantly affect the biological activity of tomatoes [7,10]. Thus, the stability change of carotenoids during processing and storage is an important issue which needs to be addressed. This chapter aims to review the recent developments in stability of tomato carotenoids as affected by processing and storage conditions.

Table 1. Carotenoid content (mg/100 g) in whole tomatoes and tomato products

8	β-carotene	γ-carotene	ζ-carotene	Lutein	Lycopene	Neurosporene	Phytoene	Phytofluene	Lycopene-5,6-diol
Whole tomatoes	0.23 ± 0.04[a]	1.50 ± 0.28	0.21 ± 0.05	0.08 ± 0.02	9.27 ± 1.02	1.11 ± 0.13	1.86 ± 0.29	0.82 ± 0.14	0.11 ± 0.01
Tomato paste	1.27 ± 0.24	9.98 ± 1.15	0.84 ± 0.08	0.34 ± 0.11	55.45 ± 0.90	6.95 ± 0.84	8.36 ± 0.80	3.63 ± 0.38	0.44 ± 0.08
Tomato puree	0..41	2.94	0.25	0.09	16.67	2.11	2.40	1.08	0.17
Tomato sauce	0.45 ± 0.13	3.17 ± 0.64	0.29 ± 0.03	tr[b]	17.98 ± 1.47	2.48 ± 0.54	2.95 ± 0.43	1.27 ± 0.20	0.16 ± 0.02
Tomato juice	0.27 ± 0.04	1.74 ± 0.20	0.18 ± 0.03	0.06 ± 0.02	10.77 ± 1.07	1.23 ± 0.27	1.90 ± 0.19	0.83 ± 0.14	0.11 ± 0.03
Tomato soup	0.23 ± 0.05	1.95 ± 0.41	0.17 ± 0.02	0.09 ± 0.02	10.92 ± 2.92	1.53 ± 0.20	1.72 ± 0.17	0.72 ± 0.18	0.11 ± 0.03
Catsup	0.59 ± 0.12	3.03 ± 1.25	0.33 ± 0.05	nd[c]	17.23 ± 2.18	2.63 ± 0.73	3.39 ± 0.38	1.54 ± 0.18	0.18 ± 0.05
Spaghetti sauce	0.44 ± 0.07	3.02 ± 0.42	0.34 ± 0.07	0.16 ± 0.04	15.99 ± 0.90	3.15 ± 0.90	2.77 ± 0.66	1.56 ± 0.53	0.17 ± 0.03

[a] Source: Tonucci et al. 1995.
mean ± standard deviation (number of observations: 4 to 9); [b] traces (below 0.005 mg/100 g); [c] not detected.

2. Physical and Chemical Properties of Tomato Carotenoids

The structural characteristics of tomato carotenoids are presented in table 2. The color, photochemical and biological properties of carotenoids are mainly associated with the presence of extended conjugated double bond system. Carotenoids can readily undergo isomerization around each carbon-carbon double bond and theoretically a large number of stereoisomers are possible [11]. However, only a few exist because of the steric hindrance effect caused by cis double bonds, making the cis-isomers thermodynamically less stable than their corresponding all-trans forms [11]. In tomatoes, carotenoids are naturally present in all-trans form, which may undergo isomerization and/or oxidative degradation during processing or storage. The predominant all-trans-lycopene in tomatoes undergoes isomerization to form various cis-lycopene isomers including 5-cis-, 9-cis-, 13-cis- and 15-cis-lycopene (figure 1), which were reported to be present in both tomato products and human serum [12-15]. Compared to all-trans forms, the cis-isomers have a lesser tendency to aggregate or crystallize and hence may be more readily solubilized in chylomicrons, absorbed and transported in biological system [10,16]. Thus, the cis-isomers are more bioavailable than their all-trans counterparts. In addition, cis-isomers of lycopene, α-carotene and β-carotene were reported to possess a higher Trolox equivalent antioxidant capacity than their all-trans forms [17].

Table 2. Structural characteristics of tomato carotenoids

Carotenoid	Semisystematic name	Conjugated double bonds	Absorption spectrum (λ_{max})	Extinction coefficient ($\varepsilon^{1\%}_{1cm}$)
Lycopene	ψ,ψ-carotene	11	444, 470, 502	3450[a]
β-Carotene	β,β-carotene	11 (2 in ring)	425, 450, 477	2592[b]
α-Carotene	β,ε-carotene	10 (1 in ring)	422, 445, 473	2800[a]
γ-Carotene	β,ψ-carotene	11 (1 in ring)	437, 462, 494	2760[b]
ζ-Carotene	7,8,7′8′-tetrahydro-ψ,ψ-carotene	7	378, 400, 425	2555[b]
δ-Carotene	ε,ψ-carotene	10	431, 456, 489	3290[a]
Phytoene	7,8,11,12,7′,8′,11′12′-octahydro-ψ,ψ-carotene	3	276, 286, 297	1250[b]
Phytofluene	7,8,11,12,7′,8′-hexahydro-ψ,ψ-carotene	5	331, 348, 367	1577[b]
Lutein	β,ε-carotene-3,3′-diol	10 (1 in ring)	422, 445, 474	2550[c]
β-cryptoxanthin	β,β-caroten-3-ol	11 (2 in ring)	425, 449, 476	2386[a]

λ_{max}: Absorption wavelength maximum; $\varepsilon^{1\%}_{1cm}$: Specific extinction coefficient of a 1% carotenoid solution measured in a 1 cm light-path spectrophotometer cuvette; a-c: $\varepsilon^{1\%}_{1cm}$ measured with carotenoid dissolved in [a] petroleum ether, [b] hexane or [c] ethanol solvents.

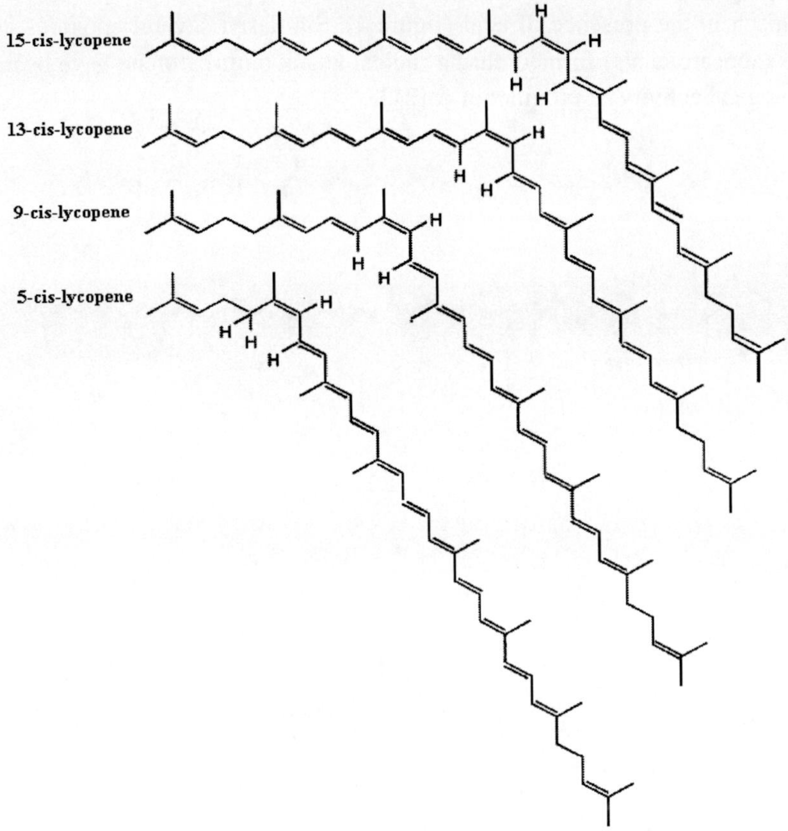

Figure 1. Major cis-isomers of lycopene in tomato products and human serum.

The antioxidant activity of tomato carotenoids is mainly derived from lycopene because of its acyclic structure consisting of 11 conjugated double bonds arranged in a linearly manner [3,18]. However, lycopene lacks provitamin A activity due to the absence of a β-ionone ring, while some other carotenoids such as β-carotene, α-carotene and γ-carotene do show provitamin A activity as each contains one or two β-ionone rings. Theoretically, β-carotene possesses 100% provitamin A activity, whereas α-carotene, γ-carotene, 9-cis-β-carotene, 13-cis-β-carotene, 9-cis-α-carotene and 13-cis-α-carotene were shown to be 53, 42-50, 38, 53, 13 and 16%, respectively [19]. The vitamin A value of commercial tomatoes is 200 μg retinol equivalents/kg [19].

The degradation of lycopene could result in formation of 2-methyl-2-hepten-6-one, apo-6′-lycopenal and some other reaction products during production and storage of tomato powder (figure 2) [20]. Also, the possible oxidative degradation products of lycopene generated during heating, as suggested by Kanasawud and Crouzet [21], are illustrated in figure 3. Hydroxylated derivatives of lycopene were detected in both tomato products and human serum. Khachik et al. [22,23] have proposed that lycopene may undergo oxidation during tomato processing or *in vivo* metabolism to form lycopene 5,6- and lycopene 1,2-epoxides, which may be in turn rearranged to 2,6,cyclolycopene-1,5-epoxides and subsequently hydrolyzed to their corresponding diols in tomatoes catalyzed by enzymes and human stomach in the presence of acid (figure 4). Similarly, several epoxides and carbonyl compounds (apocarotenals) formed during radical attack on β-carotene have been reported to possess biological activity as provitamin A [24].

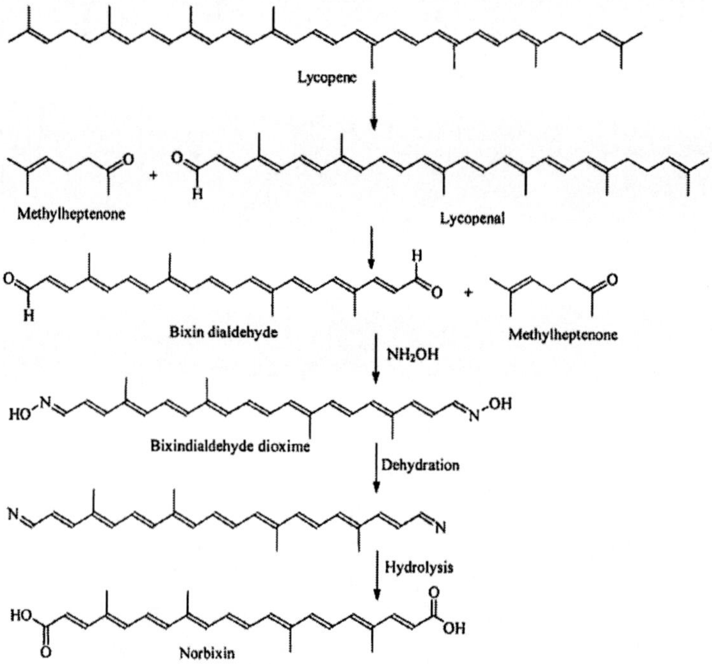

Source: Gould 1992.

Figure 2. Degradation pathway of lycopene during production of tomato powder and storage.

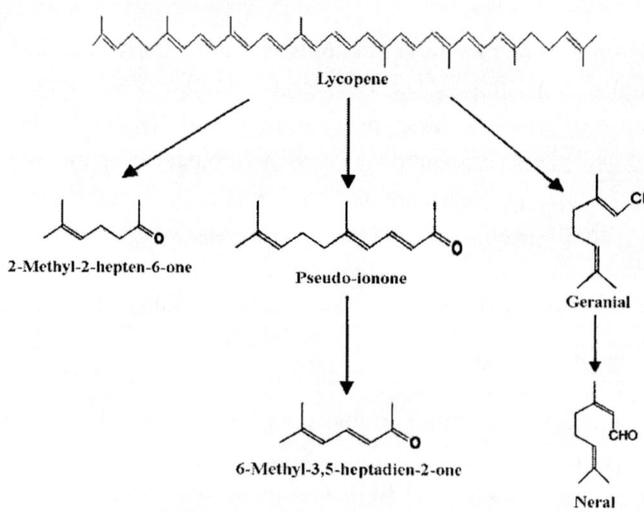

Source: Kanasawud and Crouzet 1990.

Figure 3. Oxidation products of lycopene during heating.

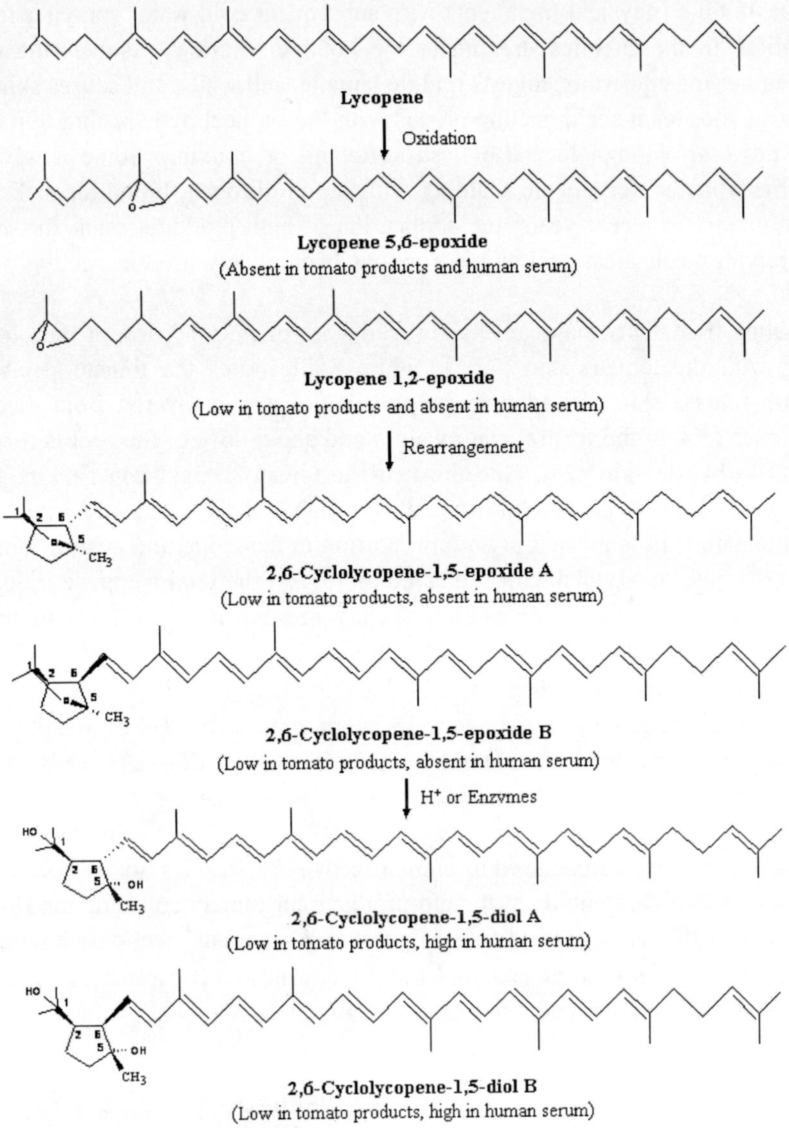

Source: Khachik et al. 1998; 2002.

Figure 4. Reaction pathways for the formation of oxidation and acid-catalyzed rearrangement products of lycopene in tomato products and human serum.

3. Carotenoid Loss during Peeling Treatment

Processing of tomatoes involves an initial peeling treatment before passing through mechanical peel eliminators. Tomatoes are peeled by one of the two commonly used procedures [20]: one uses a NaOH solution (lye solution) at a concentration of 160-200 g/l and at approximately 90° to soak tomatoes for 45-60 s (chemical treatment), followed by spraying with cold water to allow separation of peel, while the other uses only live steam on tomatoes for 45-60 s (physical treatment) with subsequent cold water spraying for complete peel separation. In the chemical treatment, the hot lye solution dissolves the epicuticular waxes, penetrates the epidermis, digests middle lamella, cell walls, and causes skin separation [20]. Likewise, the steam-scald peeling process can loosen peel by exposing tomatoes to live steam, but not long enough to cause flesh softening or cooking. Some newly developed peeling methods include cryogenic scalding with liquid nitrogen, liquid air or Freon 12 and infrared irradiation. In recent years, the application of high pressure steam for short time in combination with mechanical peel eliminators has been widely used in peeling procedure in the industry.

The peeling treatments may cause significant loss of pulp portion of the outer pericarp layer along with the tomato skin [7,25]. figure 5 illustrates the tomato peel component diagram with tomato skin and adhered pulp. Tomato pulp recovered from discarded peel amounts to over 15% of the fresh tomato weight and about 96% of the peel is recoverable as pulp and 4% as waste skin [25]. One third of the tomato weight can be lost as waste in processing plants [25]. It is well-known that the major and biologically-potent carotenoid lycopene in tomato fruit is located in high proportion in the epidermal area of tomatoes (skin and outer pericarp tissue), which constitutes 80 to 90% of the total lycopene in tomatoes [7]. In addition to lycopene, the other carotenoids are present at a low level in tomato skin. Knoblich et al. [26] recently reported the carotenoid contents in dried tomato peel removed by chemical treatment to be 734.0, 29.3, 14.5, 11.7 and 3.7 μg/g for lycopene, β-carotene, lutein, cis-β-carotene and zeaxanthin, respectively. In another study, a level of about 1180 μg/g of lycopene was extracted from tomato skin by supercritical fluid CO_2 [27]. Thus, it is apparent that a significant loss of tomato carotenoids can occur during peeling treatment.

The recovered pulp from tomato peel was reported to meet USDA Grade A Standards for color and flavor, and also can be used as animal feeds [25]. Besides, tomato peel was used to enrich the amounts of carotenoids in tomato products for human consumption. Reboul et al. [28] demonstrated that compared to tomato paste, a 6% tomato peel enrichment of tomato paste resulted in an increase of 58 and 99% more lycopene and β-carotene, respectively, with a higher bioavailability in human by intake of the latter.

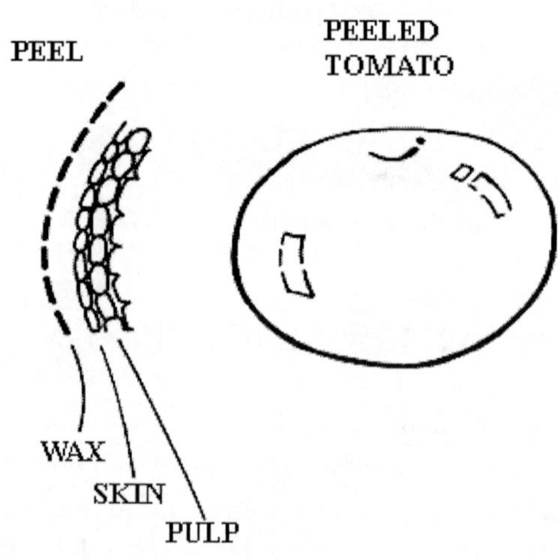

Figure 5. Tomato peel component diagram.

4. Stability of Carotenoids in Model Systems

Stability in a model system is of considerable importance as it represents a real isomerization/degradation pattern devoid of interference from the tomato matrix. The actual thermal stability of carotenoids may be misinterpreted in a system using raw tomatoes or tomato products that potentially contain heat-induced carotenoid precursors. Factors involved in food processing, such as enzymes in raw tomatoes, heating temperature, and additives could also affect the stability of tomato carotenoids. Hence, using pure authentic standards under simulated conditions would give a better understanding of actual carotenoid stability. However, stability studies of only a few selected carotenoid standards are currently available in the literature.

Lycopene, on either heating (50, 100, and 150°) or illumination (2000-3000 lux at 25°), underwent both isomerization and degradation simultaneously and the dominant reaction depended on heating temperature, illumination intensity and presence of catalyst [29]. The degradation dominated over isomerization following an increase of both temperature and heating or illumination time. The first order degradation rate of lycopene was 0.0075, 0.0124 and 0.1651 min^{-1} at 50, 100 and 150°, respectively, with an activation energy of 61.0 kJ/mol, indicating the lycopene degradation may proceed rapidly during heating at 150° and above (figure 6A). The oxidative degradation occurred at a temperature of ≤ 25°, while the isomerization accelerated at a temperature >75° [30-32]. On the other hand, lycopene undergoing illumination for 144 h degraded at a rate of 0.0003 min^{-1}, accompanied by a 13.1% loss of all-trans-lycopene, whereas a rise of 1.47, 0.92, 5.28 and 0.44% was shown for 5-cis-, 9-cis-, 13-cis- and 15-cis-lycopene, respectively (figure 6B) [29]. In another study, Shi et al. [33] reported that the illumination treatment of lycopene caused a greater loss in total lycopene than the heating treatment at 25, 100 and 180°, with the trans-isomer degradation rate proceeding faster than the cis-isomer formation rate.

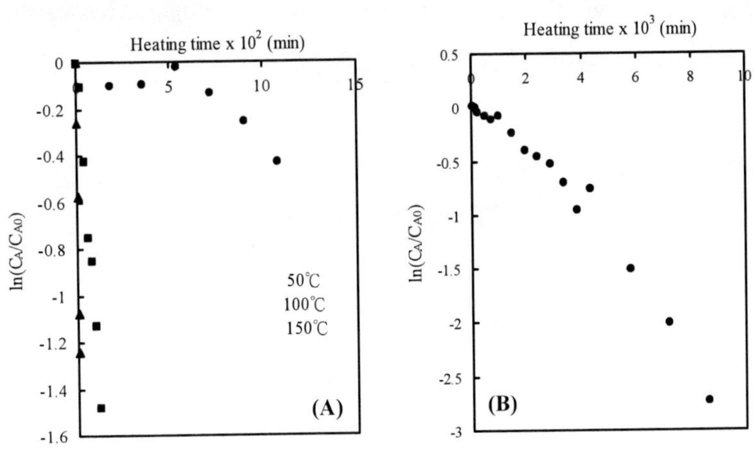

Source: Lee and Chen 2002.

Figure 6. First order kinetic plots for degradation of total lycopene during (A) heating at different temperatures and (B) illumination at 25° for 144 h. C_A: the total amount of lycopene after heating; C_{A0}: the initial amount of lycopene.

During the initial stage of heating or illumination, the isomerization of lycopene yielded 4 mono-cis-isomers in the following order: 13-cis > 5-cis > 9-cis > 15-cis-isomer. As the activation energy required to isomerize the central double bond is lower than the other positions [34], 13-cis-lycopene was more readily formed than the other cis-isomers. In addition, several di-cis-isomers formed during illumination or heating followed an increased trend initially during heating or illumination and then declined afterwards [29]. This can be attributed to instability of di-cis-isomer resulting in degradation after prolonged heating/illumination or conversion to the corresponding mono-cis-isomer.

All-trans-β-carotene crystals heated at 50, 100, 125 and 150° in an oven underwent degradation at a rate of 0.001, 0.007, 0.018 and 0.026 min^{-1}, respectively, with an activation energy of 39.0 kJ/mol, implying the higher the temperature, the faster the degradation rate (figure 7A) [35]. No significant formation of cis isomers occurred during oven heating at 50 and 100°. However, a large amount of both 13,15-di-cis- and 13-cis-isomers were produced at 125 and 150°. Conversely, the reflux heating treatment may accelerate the degradation rate through different mechanisms, generating several mono-cis-isomers at 70° in the following order: 13-cis > 9-cis > 15-cis. In comparison with oven heating, the isomerization is favored by reflux heating due to the low temperature (70°) employed and the non-polar solvent (hexane) used to dissolve β-carotene, which may promote isomerization. During illumination (2000 lux) at -5.4° in the presence or absence of iodine as catalyst, all-trans-β-carotene resulted in a large formation of 13,15-di-cis-isomer, followed by 13-cis-, 9-cis- and 15-cis-isomers, with 13,15-di-cis and 13-cis isomers being more readily formed in the presence of iodine [35]. Obviously, the isomerization was favored in iodine-catalyzed illumination, while the degradation dominated in non-iodine-catalyzed illumination. The total β-carotene degraded at a rate of 0.024 day^{-1} on illumination at -5.4° for 20 h (figure 7B) [35]. On the contrary, a higher degradation rate of 0.040 day^{-1} was observed for photodegradation of β-carotene when exposed to a 250 ft. candle light at 28° for 30 days, which may be due to the difference in illumination conditions as a high temperature for a long exposure time was used [36].

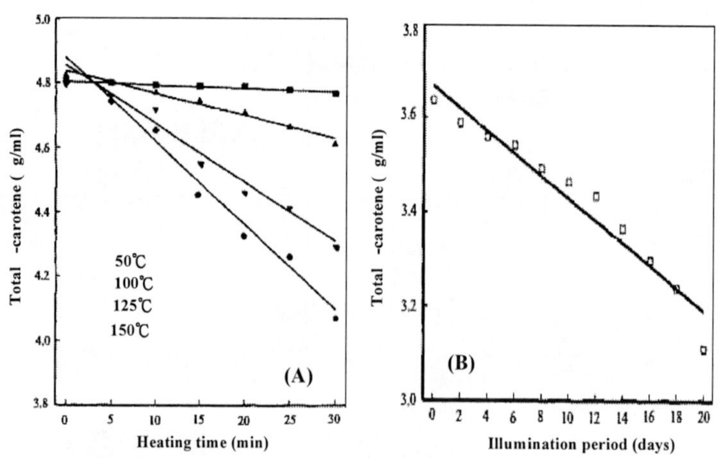

Source: Chen and Huang 1998

Figure 7. Kinetic plots for degradation of β-carotene during (A) oven heating at various temperatures and (B) illumination at -5.4° for 20 h.

It has been well established that among the mono-cis-β-carotene isomers, 13-cis-β-carotene was the major isomer formed in the dark, while 9-cis-β-carotene was kinetically favored under light [36-38]. In addition, a mono-cis isomer can be converted to another cis isomer only through the intermediate all-trans form and the formation of 13,15-di-cis isomer may occur through 13-cis or 15-cis isomer [34,37]. Also, the geometric configuration did not seem to affect the stability, as no significant difference in degradation rate was observed between 9-cis- and all-trans-β-carotene when heated in safflower seed oil (table 3) [39].

When all-trans-α-carotene was subjected to oven heating at 150 or illumination (2000 lux) for 30 min, a larger amount of 13-cis-α-carotene was generated, whereas both 9- and 15-cis isomers were not significantly affected [37]. By comparison, 13-cis-α-carotene was formed at a higher level than 13-cis-β-carotene, indicating that all-trans-β-carotene may be more stable to thermal isomerization than all-trans-α-carotene.

Heating of lycopene, all-trans-β-carotene, 9-cis-β-carotene and lutein in safflower seed oil at 75, 85 and 95^0 caused degradation to occur through a first order kinetics with the thermal stability following the order: lutein > β-carotene > lycopene (table 3) [39]. When exposed to light at 4600 lux and 25^0 or 2000 lux and 4^0 during storage, lutein underwent degradation loss at 8.0 and 2.8% per day, respectively [40,41]. The difference in degradation rate may be accounted for by the difference in illumination intensity and storage temperature. The degradation rate increased following a rise in storage temperature, but storage at freezing temperatures retained most of lutein, demonstrating that a storage temperature from -12 to 20° could prevent lutein loss.

Table 3. Reaction rate constants and activation energies for degradation of lycopene, β-carotene, 9-cis-β-carotene and lutein during heating in safflower seed oil

Carotenoid[a]	Temperature (^{0})	Rate constant (min^{-1})[b]	R^2	Activation energy (kJ/mol)[c]
Lycopene[A]	75	0.0018	0.945	
	85	0.0036	0.973	82.84 ± 9.83
	95	0.0086	0.990	
β-Carotene[B]	75	0.0007	0.991	
	85	0.0020	0.959	109.62 ± 1.72
	95	0.0054	0.944	
9-Cis-β-carotene[B]	75	0.0008	0.945	
	85	0.0018	0.924	105.02 ± 20.38
	95	0.0059	0.973	
Lutein[C]	75	0.0006	0.964	
	85	0.0022	0.957	104.18 ± 20.50
	95	0.0045	0.960	

Source: Henry et al. 1998.

[a] Data for carotenoid with same capital letters in the first column are not significantly different (P < 0.01).

[b] Mean ± standard deviation for two replicates.

[c] Values obtained from the slope of Arhenius plot.

5. Stability of Tomato Carotenoids during Processing

5.1. Processing at Different Temperatures

Thermal processing condition in a typical food preparation like cooking in water at 80-100^0 for a short time (≤ 30 min) did not show significant degradation of carotenoids in tomatoes [42]. Nevertheless, they are susceptible to thermal isomerization to varying degree depending on their structural characteristics and cellular localization in tomatoes [43]. Cooking of homogeneous tomato slurry at 88° for 2, 15 and 30 min raised total all-trans lycopene and antioxidant activity by 54.4 and 27.9%, 171.1 and 33.9%, and 164.3 and 62.1%, respectively, accompanied by a simultaneous increase in total cis-lycopene by 5.8, 17.4 and 34.9%. This may explain why a higher bioavailability can occur for heat-processed tomatoes compared to fresh ones.

In an attempt to study the effect of heating treatment on the isomeric ratio of lycopene, Schierle et al. [14] heated tomato paste in water or olive oil at 75° for varied length of time and observed a decline in the percentage of all-trans-lycopene with a concomitant increase in the level of cis-lycopene isomers, but the total carotenoid remained unchanged (table 4). Furthermore, heating in oil could have a greater impact on isomerization than heating in water, especially for both 9-cis- and 5-cis-lycopene. Thus, both heating condition and heating medium can affect lycopene isomerization significantly.

Table 4. Effect of heating on lycopene isomerization in aqueous and oily dispersions of tomato paste[a]

Duration of heat treatment (min)	Isomers of lycopene (%)				
	All-trans	5-cis	9-cis	13-cis + 15-cis	Other-cis
10	92.6	4.5	0.9	1.6	0.5
15	92.3	4.4	0.9	1.6	0.5
30	88.1	5.1	2.1	2.3	2.5
60	87.1	5.2	2.2	2.7	3.0
120	86.2	5.5	2.7	2.6	3.1
180	83.4	6.1	3.6	3.2	3.8
0	87.4	4.8	4.3	3.0	0.5
30	85.2	5.8	5.5	2.9	0.5
90	83.5	6.2	5.9	3.3	1.2
120	80.3	7.0	6.9	3.2	2.6
180	76.7	8.1	8.8	3.1	3.3

Source: Schierle et al. 1997.

[a] Tomato paste dispersed in demineralised water or in cold-pressed olive oil in a ratio of 1 g/10 ml and heated for 3 h in a water bath (75°).

Nguyen et al. [43] depicted that during heating in boiling water for 30 min, tomato carotenoids like lutein and β-carotene were isomerized to a greater extent, while lycopene, γ-carotene and δ-carotene were relatively stable to isomerization, with the total carotenoid content remaining the same (figure 8). Similarly, in contrast to lycopene, a significant amount of cis-β-carotene was formed when different commercial tomato products were heated in a retort [43,44] (figure 9). This phenomenon was also observed by several authors [45,46]. Two main factors responsible for the difference in thermal stability of tomato carotenoids are: (i) variation in molecular size, shape and structure of carotenoids that determine hydrophobicity, solubility, crystalline state and ease of crystal formation and (ii) different locations of synthesis and accumulation in the cell, that is, lycopene is accumulated as crystals within the lumina of thylakoids where they remain enveloped inside a membrane, whereas β-carotene is dissolved in lipid material of the globules in a plastoglobulin-type structure [43, 47–53]. Figures 10a and 10b show the electron micrograph of chloroplast from green tomato tissue during ripening and lycopene crystalloids in mature red tomato chromoplast, respectively, both of which illustrate lycopene and β-carotene to be associated with different cellular organelles.

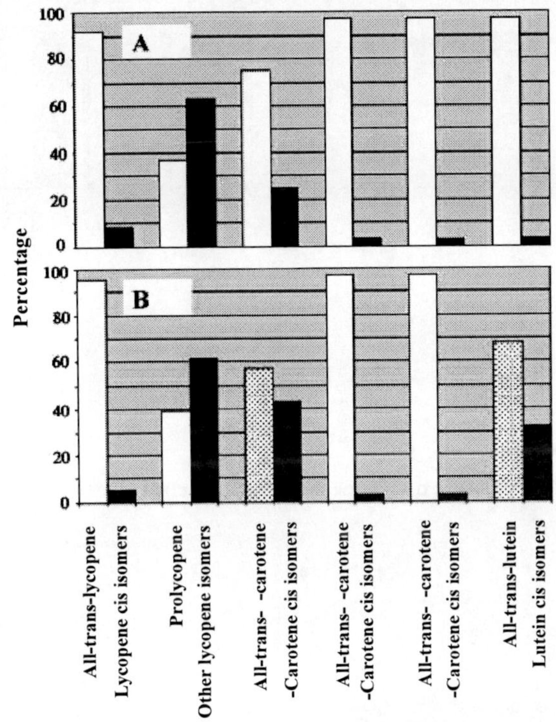

Source: Nguyen et al. 2001.

Figure 8. Distribution of carotenoids and their isomers in (A) fresh tomatoes and (B) thermally treated samples (boiling in water for 30 min).

Thermal processing at high temperatures for long duration can result in degradation of cis-isomers. Heating of tomato pulp at 100° for 120 min under atmospheric pressure caused lycopene degradation to occur following a pseudo first order reaction at a rate of 0.0023 min^{-1} [54]. Likewise, the lycopene level in tomato juice during heating at 90-100° for 7 min dropped by 1-2%, respectively, while a higher loss of 17% occurred at 130° [55]. The high-temperature-short-time treatment (121° for 4 s) of tomato juice could enhance leaching of lycopene from the cell matrix with minimum degradation [12]. However, a high lycopene loss (25%) was observed for tomato pulp heated at 100° for 2 h in the presence of oxygen, but a low loss of 5-8% in the presence of CO_2 [56]. Thermal processing of tomatoes into paste also resulted in a decrease in lycopene concentration by 9-28%, which may be associated with a long processing time required to achieve the final solid content [57]. It was also shown that lycopene in tomatoes were relatively resistant to degradation compared to pure lycopene in model systems, which should be due to the protection provided by some other functional components including tocopherol, ascorbic acid and phenolic compounds. The other processing methods like extraction, homogenization, sterilization and pasteurization also caused considerable isomerization of lycopene and β-carotene, with the homogenization step and/or subsequent heat treatment significantly decreasing the contents of all-trans forms of lycopene and β-carotene (table 5) [46].

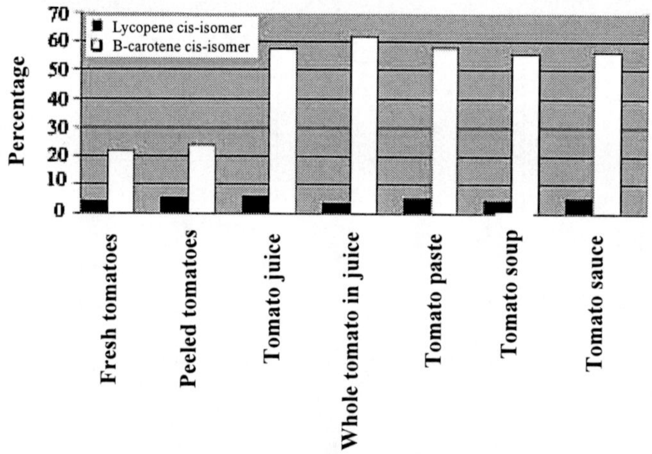

Source: Nguyen et al. 2001.

Figure 9. Effect of thermal processing on lycopene and β-carotene cis-isomer percentages.

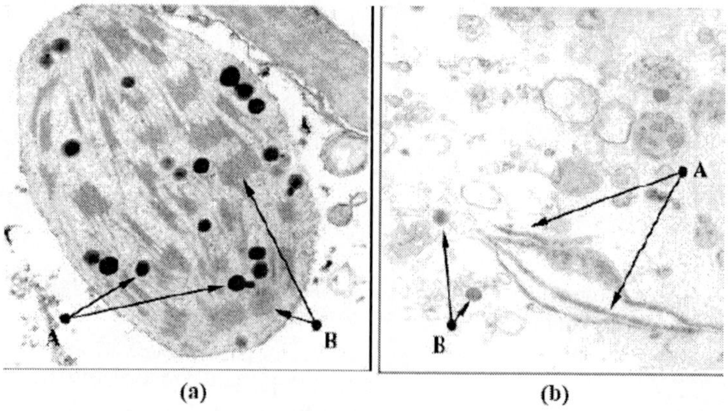

Source: Nguyen et al. 2001.

Figure 10. Electron micrographs of (a) chloroplast from green tomato tissue undergoing ripening. A: plastoglobulin-type structure; B: thylakoids and (b) lycopene crystalloids in mature red tomato chromoplast. A: lycopene crystalloids; B: plastoglobulin-type sacs in which β-carotene reportedly accumulates.

Table 5. Changes in contents of all-trans-lycopene and all-trans-β-carotene during production of tomato juice

Sample	All-trans-lycopene[a,b] (mg/100 g)	All-trans-β-carotene[a,b] (mg/100 g)
Wet weight basis		
After extraction	8.91 ± 0.55[A]	0.24 ± 0.02[A]
After homogenization	6.70 ± 0.11[B]	0.21 ± 0.01[A,B]
After sterilization	7.66 ± 0.22[C]	0.19 ± 0.00[B]
After pasteurization	7.49 ± 0.24[B,C]	0.19 ± 0.01[B]
Dry weight basis		
After extraction	214.1 ± 13.3[A]	5.77 ± 0.46[A]
After homogenization	133.6 ± 4.3[B]	4.22 ± 0.12[B]
After sterilization	159.4 ± 4.6[C]	4.03 ± 0.04[B]
After pasteurization	150.7 ± 4.9[B,C]	3.76 ± 0.30[B]

Source: Seybold et al. 2004.

[a] mean ± standard deviation.

[b] values within columns with the same letter are not significantly different ($P > 0.05$).

5.2. Processing under Domestic Cooking Conditions

Mayeaux et al. [32] made a critical comparison of house-hold cooking conditions like microwaving, baking and frying of tomato samples on lycopene content, and the lycopene loss followed the order: frying > baking > microwaving (figure 11). The hydroperoxide free radicals produced during frying at high temperatures may be responsible for the accelerated degradation. Approximately a 35% loss of lycopene occurred during microwaving at 1000 w for 60 s, whereas during baking at 177 and 218° for 15, 30 and 45 min, a decline of 35.9 and 48.5%, 54.4 and 58.7%, and 62.7 and 74.9% of lycopene was shown, respectively. But, lycopene was severely degraded with a loss of 70 and 75%, respectively, when fried in sunflower oil at 145 and 165° for 2 min. A similar trend was observed by Sahlin et al. [58], who reported a decrease in lycopene content and antioxidant activity by 6.5 and 10.0%, 10.0 and 17.8%, and 48.2 and 36.2%, respectively, during boiling (15 min), baking (18 min) and frying (in olive oil for 4 min) of tomato samples. A high lycopene loss shown in both studies may be caused by severe cooking condition. In addition, the domestic processing practices generally include soaking of tomato slices for a short period of time in a marinade containing oil and vinegar. Soaking tomato pieces in vinegar for 20 min at 20° retained more lycopene and possessed higher antioxidant activity than soaking in oil or oil/vinegar mixture, which further demonstrated the detrimental effect of oil on lycopene [58].

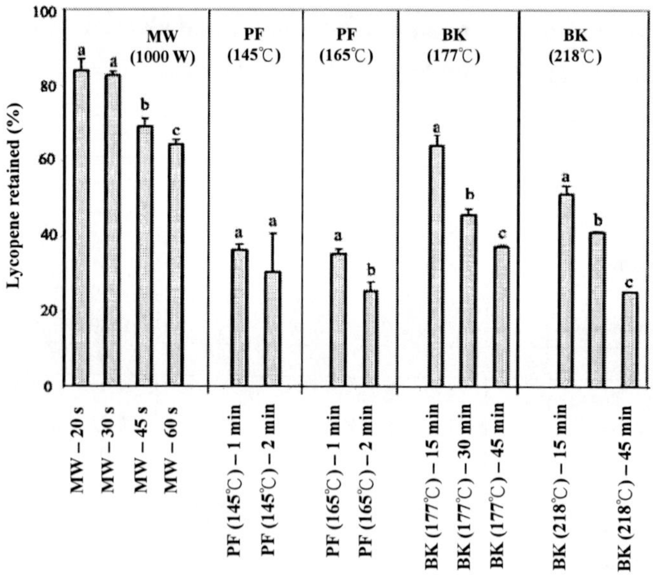

Source: Mayeaux et al. 2006.

Figure 11. Percentage of lycopene retained after microwaving, pan-frying and baking of tomato samples. MW: Microwaving; PF: Pan-frying; BK: Baking; Significant difference ($P < 0.05$) between 2 columns in the same cooking conditions is expressed by different letters.

5.3. Processing by Dehydration

Dehydration is one of the important processing methods to dry tomato halves, slices, quarters and powder for enhancement of shelf-life stability for subsequent incorporation into pizza and various vegetable dishes [59]. Temperature, oxygen permeability, moisture content and texture (fine or coarse) of the tomato sample are the factors determining the stability of dried tomato products. Industrial processing of tomatoes to a final moisture content of <15% often require high temperatures (60-110°) with air flow rate at 0.5-2.0 m/s over a period of 2-10 h in the presence of oxygen, resulting in carotenoid degradation [60]. Although many studies have indicated a little or no degradation of lycopene during drying, isomerization did occur in dehydrated products. Shi et al. [61] reported a formation of 16.6% of cis-lycopene isomers in air-dried tomato pulp, with a total lycopene loss of only 3.9%. Similarly, a maximum formation of 6.25% cis-isomers of lycopene was reported for drum-dried tomato powder [62]. Drying of tomato halves at 80^{0} with air flow at 1.5 m/s to a final moisture content of 10% did not cause any significant loss of lycopene, but a large loss (12%) occurred at 110° for the moisture content reduced to <12% (table 6) [60]. Thus, freeze-drying is preferred over air-drying as the latter can lead to progressive carotenoid degradation because of long exposure to oxygen and heat. It was also suggested that low temperature treatment, reduction of tomato thickness by using tomato slices or quarters, and drying to intermediate moisture content (20-40%), all of which could prevent lycopene loss during air-drying [60]. Intermediate moisture content may decrease the oxygen permeability during drying, inactivate the prooxidant trace metal ions, delay the propagation reaction in lipid autoxidation by forming hydrogen bond with hydroperoxide and compete with oxygen for the active absorption sites [63].

Table 6. Lycopene content of fresh and dried tomato halves during air drying at 80° and 110° for different time duration

Air Drying at 80°			Air Drying at 110°		
Time (min)	Moisture (%)	Lycopene content[a] (mg/g TS[b])	Time (min)	Moisture (%)	Lycopene content[a] (mg/g TS[b])
0	94.1	0.88	0	94.6	0.94
190	75.4	0.91	110	77.0	0.90
270	52.7	0.87	150	56.9	0.93
320	45.8	0.86	160	51.9	0.94
350	29.6	0.94	170	47.6	0.93
390	23.2	0.90	190	26.7	0.94
410	11.7	0.88	200	12.7	0.84
430	8.6	0.90	230	10.0	0.83

Source: Zanoni et al. 1999.

[a] Data are mean of two replicates with three determinations per replicate.

[b] TS: total solids.

Protection against lycopene loss can also be achieved by subjecting the tomato samples to osmotic pretreatment (soaking in sucrose solution) prior to drying, as demonstrated by Shi et al. [61] (table 7). Possibly, the presence of osmotic solution on tomato surface may prevent oxygen from penetrating into the tomato matrix.

Table 7. Changes in contents of all-trans- and cis-isomers of lycopene during different drying treatment of tomato samples

Sample	Total lycopene[a,b] (μg/g dry basis)	Lycopene loss (%)	All-trans-isomers (%)	Cis-isomers (%)
Fresh tomato	75.5^{A}	0	100	0
Osmotic treatment[c]	75.5^{A}	0	100	0
Osmotic treatment + vacuum dried	73.7^{B}	2.4	93.5	6.5
Vacuum dried	73.1^{C}	3.2	89.9	10.1
Air dried	72.6^{D}	3.9	84.4	16.6

Source: Shi et al. 1999.

[a] Data presented as means of triplicate determinations.

[b] Values within columns with the same letter are not significantly different ($p < 0.01$).

c Soaking in 65°Brix sucrose solution at 25° for 4 h.

6. Stability of Tomato Carotenoids during Storage

6.1. Post-Harvest Storage

The synthesis of carotenoids in tomato fruits continues to proceed even after harvest, and vine-ripened tomatoes were reported to produce more carotenoids than those ripened on storage. Nevertheless, maintaining appropriate post-harvest conditions are necessary to increase the amount of carotenoids in tomatoes [64]. Following a rise in ripening index (a/b), both lycopene and β-carotene contents increased linearly in vine-ripened tomatoes, whereas an exponential trend was observed for detached mature-green tomatoes when washed with 125 mg/L chlorine and allowed to ripen in a well-ventilated room at 20° [64]. The concentrations of lycopene and β-carotene in post-harvest-ripened tomatoes were almost twice as high as those in vine-ripened tomatoes. With storage temperature at 7°, tomatoes of Tradiro cultivar variety showed a 2-fold increase in lycopene content compared to those stored at 15 and 25° for 10 days [65]. Thus, by maintaining an appropriate post-harvest storage condition, the level of carotenoids in tomatoes could be greatly enhanced.

Controlled-atmosphere storage (CAS) has been proved effective in delaying ripening to extend the post-harvest life span of fruits and vegetables. During CAS, the harvested tomato fruits are exposed to inert gases to maintain quality and retard senescence. A high level of CO_2 and low O_2 were reported to suppress the chlorophyll degradation and ethylene synthesis, leading to prevention of total carotenoid and lycopene accumulation (figure 12) [66]. Besides, CAS may suppress fungal spoilage, inhibit activities of α- and β-galactosidase, polygalacturonase cellulose and NAD-cytochrome c oxidase as well as reduce levels of pectic substance, organic acids, sugars and amino acids, thereby preventing or delaying physiological disorders that might soften the tomato fruit [66,67]. Approximately, 3-5% O_2 and/or 0-3% CO_2 was efficient for storage of mature green tomatoes [66]. However, after prolonged storage under high concentration of CO_2, a decrease in a/b ratio may occur because of CO_2 injury (figure 13A) [67]. In addition, the maturation time could be extended on exposure to high CO_2 levels (figure 13B), which should be an advantage from the commercial point of view.

6.2. Frozen Storage with or without Blanching

Carotenoids in tomato and tomato products can undergo chemical or enzymatic degradation even when stored at freezing temperatures, especially in the amorphous portion of the food matrix, where a rise in oxygen solubility is possible following a drop in temperature [68]. Blanching is a commonly used pretreatment for vegetable/fruit products prior to storage to inactivate oxidative enzymes [69]. During storage of unblanched tomato products, carotenoids can undergo enzymatic oxidation in addition to chemical and autocatalytic reactions [70]. Also, inadequate blanching due to underestimation of time and temperature parameters can be responsible for residual enzyme activities [69,71,72]. The activity of oxidative enzymes like peroxidase and lipoxygenase was reduced progressively with storage time at freezing temperatures (figure 14), which is mainly due to changes in solute concentration, ionic strength, pH, oxygen solubility, water activity, viscosity and residual volume of the concentrated phase, all of which may result in aggregation and/or conformational modification of enzyme molecules [70,73,74].

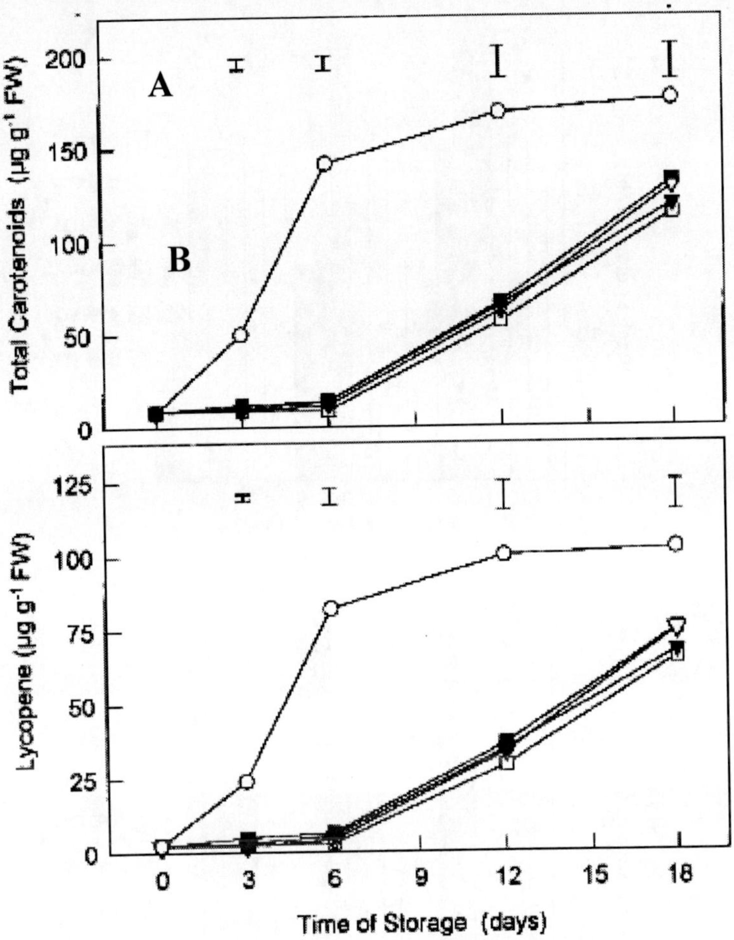

Source: Sozzi et al. 1999.

Figure 12. Effect of controlled atmosphere storage on (A) carotenoid and (B) lycopene biosyntheses in tomato fruit. (○) Control; (▽) 3% O_2; (▼) 3% O_2 + 100 mg/l C_2H_4; (□) 20% CO_2; (■) 20% CO_2 + 100 mg/l C_2H_4; FW: fresh weight.

Several authors observed a progressive color loss accompanied by a reduction of carotenoid content during frozen storage of tomatoes [70,72,73,75]. Most studies attributed the carotenoid loss to oxidative reactions, but the mechanism involved in color changes has not been completely elucidated, as both enzyme-mediated and oxidative reactions can occur at a significant rate in partially blanched and frozen tomatoes as well as unblanched tomato samples during storage [76,77]. Calligaris et al. [70] reported a sharp loss in red color of unblanched tomato puree compared to the blanched ones during storage at -7° and -18°, which may be due to simultaneous enzymatic co-oxidation and chemical oxidation for the former and chemical oxidation for the latter. A contrasting phenomenon was shown by Dermesonlouoglou et al. [72], who demonstrated blanched tomatoes to undergo a larger lycopene loss (0.250 mg/100 g per day) for blanched tomatoes than for untreated samples (0.182 mg/100 g) when stored at -15°.

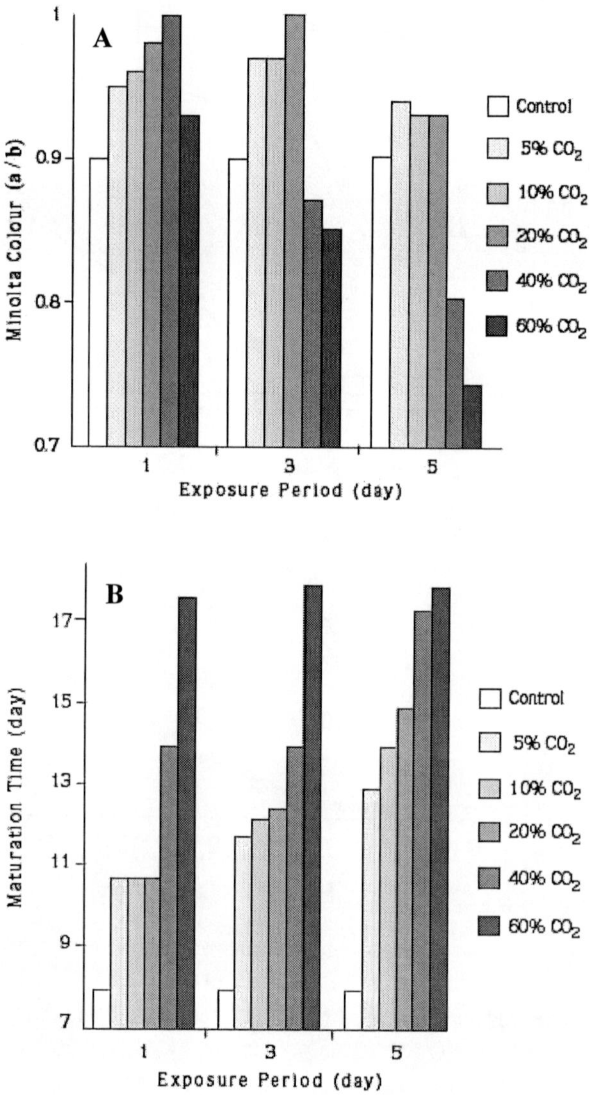

Source: Batu and Thompson 1998.

Figure 13. Effect of mature-green-tomato-fruit exposure to various levels of CO2 for 1, 3 and 5 days with fixed 5.5% O2 supply on (A) Minolta color values (a/b), representing the carotenoid accumulation and (B) maturation time in days.

This is probably because of the difference in blanching condition as a temperature of 100° for 20 min was used for the former, while a mild condition of 80° for 80 s for the latter should have caused residual enzyme activity leading to carotenoid degradation.

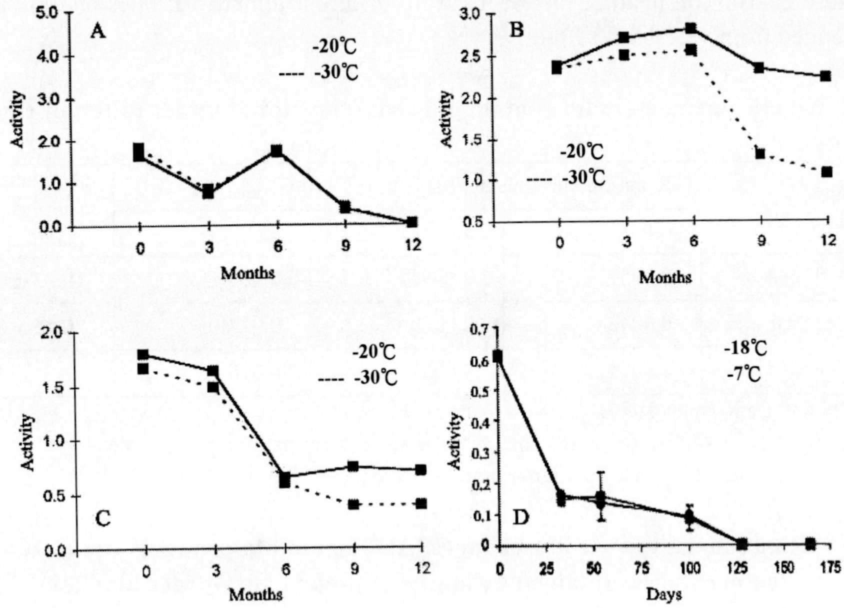

Source: Lisiewska and Kmiecik 2000; Calligaris et al. 2002.

Figure 14. Decrease in enzyme activity with storage time. A: Peroxidase; B: Catalase; C: Lipase; D: Lipoxygenase.

Thus, freezing does not prevent the degradation of carotenoids and the activity of naturally-occurring oxidative enzymes in tomato should play a major role for a reduction in the sensory properties and nutrients, despite the fact that the biochemical activity of enzymes declined rapidly in tomatoes on frozen storage [70,73]. Nevertheless, freezing of tomato samples can still prevent carotenoid degradation under the condition of complete enzyme inactivation.

6.3. Effect of Temperature, Time, Light and Oxygen during Storage

With storage of tomato pulp at -20, 5 and 25° for 60 days, Sharma and Le Maguer [54] noticed an increased lycopene degradation following a rise in temperature under three different storage conditions, which followed the order: air and light > air and dark > vacuum and dark (table 8). The lycopene degradation was shown to fit a pseudo first order kinetics and the activation energy ranged from 19.9-27.7 kJ/mol. A maximum lycopene loss of 77.6% occurred when stored under air and light at 25°, whereas a 16.2% loss was found even when stored at -20° under vacuum and dark over a period of 60 days, which should be due to an autocatalytic reaction. Likewise, a rise in storage temperature from -30 to -20° lowered lycopene and β-carotene contents in tomato cubes by 24 and 17%, respectively, after 12-month storage[73]. A similar trend was shown for different tomato products during storage at 30, 40 and 50° for 90 days, with the degradation rate increasing along with a raise in temperature (table 9) and the activation energy was 71.70 and 108.55 kJ/mol for tomato pulp and paste, respectively [78]. Hackett et al. [30] also reported an increased degradation rate for temperature 25-100° on heating oleoresins from different tomato varieties and the activation energy ranged from 48.1-62.8 kJ/mol.

Table 8. Kinetic parameters for tomato pulp samples stored under different conditions[a]

Storage condition	Reaction rate constant (day^{-1})			Activation energy[b] (kJ/mol)
	-20°	5°	25°	
Air and light	0.0057	0.0092	0.0250	19.87 ± 6.38[A]
Dark and air	0.0048	0.0078	0.0220	20.45 ± 6.70[A]
Vacuum and dark	0.0024	0.0067	0.0180	27.74 ± 2.76[A]

Source: Shi and Le Maguer 1996.

[a] Data are the mean of duplicate measurements with two determinations per sample.

[b] Values with the same letter are not significantly different ($p < 0.01$).

Table 9. Rate constants for color changes (ΔE^a) in tomato products stored at various temperatures, obtained by applying pseudo-zero-order kinetics

	Rate constant (day^{-1})[b]
Pulp at 30°	0.0094
Pulp at 40°	0.0188
Pulp at 50°	0.0580
Over-heated pulp at 40°	0.0090
Puree at 40°	0.0092
Paste at 30°	0.0117
Paste at 40°	0.0440
Paste at 50°	0.1689

Source: Giovanelli and Lavelli 2002.

[a] $\Delta E = [(a-a_0)^2 + (b-b_0)^2 + (L-L_0)^2]^{0.5}$, where a_0, b_0 and L_0 are the color indices at the beginning of storage.

[b] Data are mean of duplicate analyses.

Storage of tomato juice at room temperature for 6 months did not show significant lycopene change, but dropped by 2 % when exposed to sunlight for 6 months [79]. Tomato juice processed by hot-breaking of tomatoes at 82°, screening and heating at 121° for 40 s, and subjected to storage under light or dark at 4, 25 and 35° for 12 weeks, the degradation loss rose following an increase in temperature and time, and was higher under light than under dark [80]. However, the degradation of carotenoids in canned juice stored under dark or light was low, as the contact between juice and light or oxygen was minimized. Also, all-trans-lycopene showed the highest degradation loss, followed by all-trans-β-carotene and all-trans-lutein. More cis-isomers were formed from lycopene than lutein or β-carotene during storage and the dominant isomers were 13-cis and 9-cis for lutein and β-carotene, while the major lycopene isomers formed were 5-cis, 9-cis, 13-cis and 15-cis [80]. Thus, light, oxygen, temperature and time are the major factors responsible for the stability of carotenoids in tomato and tomato products during storage.

6.4. Storage after Dehydration

The stability of carotenoids also depends on the dehydration conditions to which the tomato samples were subjected before storage. Though several studies affirm that carotenoids are substantially stable during industrial drying [59-61], a significant oxidative loss does occur during storage of dehydrated tomato / tomato products, which can be attributed to exposure of a large surface area to air. Freeze-dried and oven-dried tomato pulps did not show any lycopene loss during drying, but when stored at room temperature for 4 months in a closed container, a 97 and 73.3-78.9% loss of lycopene did occur, respectively [54]. Perhaps, the voluminous and fluffy nature of freeze-dried samples may account for a high lycopene loss compared to a thin crust of sheets in oven-dried samples. With tomato halves (10% moisture content) air-dried at 80 and 110° and subjected to storage for 90 days in the air under darkness at 37°, a lycopene loss over 70% was found for both temperatures (table 10) [60]. Anguelova and Warthesen [81] also reported a loss of 30-40% and 60% of total lycopene for spray-dried commercial tomato powders stored at 6 and 45° for 6 weeks, respectively, with lycopene-5,6-diol and 5,5′-di-cis-lycopene being the main oxidation and isomerization products.

Zanoni et al. [82] optimized storage conditions of dried tomato halves by factorial design using several variables like moisture content (10-60%), temperature (5-30°) and storage time (1-38 days). The optimum moisture content to minimize color change over a 30-day storage period under vacuum in the dark was determined to be 20-40%, corresponding to a water activity (a_w) of 0.69-0.86 at a storage temperature of ≤ 18°. Both temperature and moisture content were claimed to be the critical factors in carotenoid degradation during storage of dried tomato products. Theoretically, the moisture content has to be reduced during drying to lower water activity so that the oxidation rate can be terminated and growth of spoilage microorganisms can be inhibited [82]. However, drying to a very low moisture level (≤12%) can promote oxidation, as evidenced in a previous study regarding the effect of water activity on rate of lipid oxidation [83]. Boskovich [84] proposed that a low storage temperature in combination with an extremely low moisture content or water activity may exhibit a pro-oxidant effect. Therefore, drying to an intermediate moisture level, instead of complete dehydration, should be an interesting alternative to increase shelf-life of tomato and tomato products during storage.

Literature data regarding the stability of lycopene in dehydrated tomato products do not lead to univocal conclusions. Giovanelli and Paradiso [85] found the tomato pulp dried to an intermediate moisture content (23%) to be more sensitive to lycopene degradation than to a low moisture level (9%). This contradictory result was justified as the prevailing solvent effect of water facilitating mobility of reaction substrates and cosubstrates. Furthermore, the lycopene degradation of tomato pulp with an intermediate moisture content showed an inversed relationship with storage temperature, amounting to 75, 38 and 28% at 4, 20 and 37°, respectively. Likewise, Lovric et al. [63] noticed a different trend with maximum color retention in tomato powder stored at 20° than at -10, 2 or 37° under air and dark. This was postulated that all-trans-lycopene may be converted to its corresponding cis isomers during drying and the reisomerization from cis to all-trans form is favored at 20° than at other temperatures. Since cis isomers are more susceptible to oxidation than all-trans isomers, lycopene oxidation during storage occurred faster at low temperatures (-10 and 2°), facilitating formation of a high ratio of cis isomers.

Table 10. Lycopene content of dried tomato halves during storage in air and darkness at 37^0

Time (days)	Residual lycopene (%)[a]	
	Sample dried at 80^0	Sample dried at 110
0	100	100
30	46	38
40	44	35
50	39	31
60	34	27
90	26	19

Source: Zanoni et al. 1999.

[a] Data are mean of two replicates with three determinations per replicate.

The carotenoid (particularly lycopene) loss during storage can be reduced by 5-35% in osmodehydrating tomatoes in high dextrose equivalent maltodextrin (HDEM) solution (56.5 %) under an optimized condition of 1:5 ratio of tomato to HDEM syrup at 35° for 1 h [72]. The lycopene loss can be reduced by 5-35% compared to the other freezing methods (blanched and unblanched), with isomerization being the main reaction to proceed during osmotic treatment (figure 15).

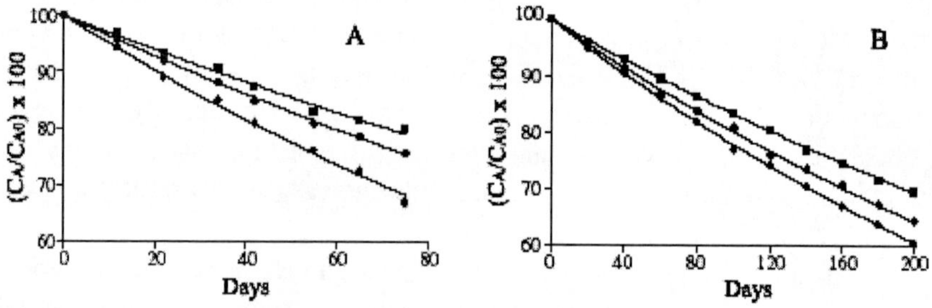

Source: Dermesonlouoglou et al. 2007.

Figure 15. Total lycopene loss in frozen tomatoes, untreated, blanched and osmotically pretreated (HDEM) at storage temperatures. A: -5°; B: -15°; (◆): untreated; (•): blanched; (■): HDEM (high dextrose equivalent maltodextrin); CA: the total amount of lycopene on storage; CA0: the initial amount of lycopene.

A recent study revealed a high hydrostatic pressure applied to tomato samples before storage could offer a sterilization effect to inactivate enzymes and reduce lycopene degradation [86]. On storage (4 or 24°) of lycopene standard and tomato purees pressurized in a thermostated (20°) hydraulic reactor to different isostatic pressures (100-600 MPa) showed better protection of lycopene than untreated samples, with a minimum loss at 400 and 500 MPa, respectively.

7. Conclusion

Carotenoids in a model system are more prone to isomerization and/or oxidative degradation than in tomato matrix. Carotenoids in tomato/tomato products are largely influenced by processing or storage conditions of high temperature treatment for long duration. Thus, processing or storage of tomato samples at elevated temperature and in the presence of light and oxygen should be avoided. Tomato samples should also be dried to intermediate moisture content to minimize carotenoid degradation. There is still a need to develop a novel technology to prevent carotenoid loss during processing and storage of tomatoes. The stability of tomato carotenoids other than lycopene and β-carotene also needs to be investigated in more detail, as a synergistic effect in biological activity may be possible.

References

[1] Giovannucci, E. *J. Natl. Can. Inst.* 1999, *91*, 317-331.

[2] Giovannucci, E.; Rimm, E. B.; Liu, Y.; Stampfer, M. J.; Willett, W. C. *J. Natl. Can. Inst.* 2002, *94*, 391-398.

[3] Miller, N. J.; Sampson, J.; Candeias, L. P.; Bramley, P. M.; Rice-Evans, C. A. *FEBS lett.* 1996, *384*, 240-242.

[4] Levy, J.; Bosin, E.; Feldman, B.; Giat, Y.; Miinster, A.; Danilenko, M.; Sharoni, Y. *Nutr. Cancer* 1995, *24*, 257-266.

[5] Gärtner, C.; Stahl, W.; Sies, H. *Am. J. Clin. Nutr.* 1997, *66*, 116-122.

[6] Khachik, F.; Beecher, G.; Smith, J. C. *J. Cell Biochem. Suppl.* 1995, *22*, 236-246.

[7] Shi, J.; Le Maguer, M. *Crit. Rev. Food Sci. Nutr.* 2000, *40*, 1-42.

[8] Canene-Adams, K.; Campbell, J. K.; Zaripheh, S.; Jeffery, E. H.; Erdman, Jr., J.W. *J. Nutr.* 2005, *135*, 1226-1230.

[9] Tonucci, L. H.; Holden, J. M.; Beecher, G. R.; Khachik, F.; Davis, C. S.; Mulokozi, G. *J. Agric. Food Chem.* 1995, *43*, 579-586.

[10] Boileau, A. C.; Merchen, N. R.; Wasson, K.; Atkinson, C. A.; Erdman, J. W. *J. Nutr.* 1999, *129*, 1176-1181.

[11] Zechmeister, L. Cis-trans Isomeric Carotenoids, Vitamin A and Arylpolyenes; Academic Press: NY, 1962.

[12] Lin, C. H.; Chen, B. H. *Eur. Food Res. Technol.* 2005, *221*, 274-280.

[13] Rajendran, V.; Pu, Y. S.; Chen, B. H. *J. Chromatogr. B* 2005, *824*, 99-106.

[14] Schierle, J.; Bretzel, W.; Bühler, I.; Faccin, N.; Hess, D.; Steiner, K.; Schüep, W. *Food Chem.* 1997, *59*, 459-465.
[15] Wang, C. Y.; Chen, B. H. *Eur. Food Res. Technol.* 2006, *222*, 347-353.
[16] Britton, G. *FASEB J.* 1995, *9*, 1551-1558.
[17] Bohm, V.; Puspitasari-Nienaber, N. L.; Ferruzzi, M. G.; Schwartz, S. J. *J. Agric. Food Chem.* 2002, *50*, 221-226.
[18] Stahl, W.; Sies, H. *Arch. Biochem. Biophys.* 1996, *336*, 1-9.
[19] Gross, J. *Pigments in Vegetables;* van Nordsrand Reinhold: NY, 1991.
[20] Gould, W. A. *Tomato Production, Processing, and Technology;* CTI Publications: Baltimore, MD, 1992.
[21] Kanasawud, P.; Crouzet, J. C. *J. Agric. Food Chem.* 1990, *38*, 1238-1242.
[22] Khachik, F.; Pfander, H.; Traber, B. *J. Agric Food Chem.* 1998, *46*, 4885-4890.
[23] Khachik, F.; Carvalho, L.; Bernstein, P. S.; Muir, G. J.; Zhao, D. Y.; Katz, N. B. *Exp. Biol. Med.* 2002, *227*, 845-851.
[24] Krinsky, N.I.; Yeum, K. J. *Biochem. Biphys. Res. Comm.* 2003, *305*, 754-760.
[25] United States Environmental Protection Agency (USEPA). *Commercial Feasibility Of Recovering Tomato Processing Residuals For Food Use;* USEPA Environmental Protection Technology Series and EPA-60012-78-202, National Technical Information Service: Springfield, VA, 1978; pp 4.
[26] Knoblich, M.; Anderson, B.; Latshaw, D. *J. Sci. Food Agric.* 2005, *85*, 1166-1170.
[27] Topal, U.; Sasaki, M.; Goto, M.; Hayakawa, K. *J. Agric. Food Chem.* 2006, *54*, 5604-5610.
[28] Reboul, E.; Borel, P.; Mikail, C.; Abou, L.; Charbonnier, M.; Caris-Veyrat, C.; Goupy, P.; Portugal, H.; Lairon, D.; Amiot, M. J. *J. Nutr.* 2005, *135*, 790-794.
[29] Lee, M. T.; Chen, B. H. *Food Chem.* 2002, *78*, 425-432.
[30] Hackett, M. M.; Lee, J. H.; Francis, D.; Schwartz, S. J. *J. Food Sci. – Food Chemistry and Toxicology* 2004, *69*, 536-541.
[31] Mayer-Melbach, E.; Schuchmann, H. P.; Regler, M.; Behsnilian, D. *Food Res. Int.* 2005, *38*, 1103-1108.
[32] Mayeaux, M.; Xu, Z.; King, J. M.; Prinyawiwatkul, W. *J. Food Sci.* 2006, *71*, 461-464.
[33] Shi, J.; Wu, Y.; Bryan, M.; Le Maguer, M. *Nutraceutical and Food* 2002, *7*, 179-183.
[34] Zechmeister, L. *Chem. Rev.* 1944, *34*, 267-322.
[35] Chen, B. H.; Huang, J. H. *Food Chem.* 1998, *62*, 299-307.
[36] Pesek, C. A.; Warthesen, J. J. *J. Agric. Food Chem.* 1990, *38*, 1313-1315.
[37] Chen, B. H.; Chen, T. M.; Chien, J. T. *J. Agric. Food Chem.* 1994, *42*, 2391-2397.
[38] Pesek, C. A.; Warthesen, J. J.; Taoukis, P. S. *J. Agric. Food Chem.* 1990, *38*, 41-45.
[39] Henry, L. K.; Catignani, G.L.; Schwartz, S.J. *JAOCS* 1998, *75*, 823-829.
[40] Shi, X. M.; Chen, F. *Nahrung* 1997, *41*, 38-41.
[41] Kopas-Lane, L. M.; Warthesen, J. J. *J. Food Sci.* 1995, *60*, 773-776.
[42] Dewanto, V.; Wu, X.; Adom, K. K.; Liu, R. H. *J. Agric. Food Chem.* 2002, *50*, 3010-3014.
[43] Nguyen, M. L.; Francis, D.; Schwartz, S. J. *J. Sci. Food Agric.* 2001, *81*, 910-917.
[44] Nguyen, M. L.; Schwartz, S. J. *Proc. Soc. Exp. Biol. Med.* 1998, *218*, 101-105.
[45] Abushita, A. A.; Daood, H. G.; Biacs, P. A. *J. Agric. Food Chem.* 2000, *48*, 2075-2081.
[46] Seybold, C.; Fröhlich, K.; Bitsch, R.; Otto, K.; Böhm, V. *J. Agric. Food Chem.* 2004, *52*, 7005-7010.

[47] Ray, K.; Misra, T. N. *J. Photochem. Photobiol A: Chem*. 1997, *107*, 201-205.
[48] Bartley, G. E.; Scolnik, P. A.; Beyer, P. Eur. *J. Biochem*. 1999, 259, 396-403.
[49] Bonk, M.; Hoffmann, B.; Von Lintig, J.; Schleds, M.; Al-Babili, S.; Hobeika, E.; Klenning, H.; Bayer, P. *Eur. J. Biochem.* 1997, *247*, 942-950.
[50] Ljubesic, N.; Wrischer, M.; Devide, Z. *Int. J. Develop. Biol.* 1991, *35*, 251-258.
[51] Bathgate, B.; Purton, M. E.; Grierson, D.; Goodenough, P. W. *Planta* 1985, *165*, 197-204.
[52] Mohr, W. P. *Ann. Bot.* 1979, *44*, 427-434.
[53] Rosso, S. W. *J. Ultrastruct. Res.* 1968, *25*, 307-322.
[54] Sharma, S. K.; Le Maguer, M. *Food Res. Int.* 1996, *29*, 309-315.
[55] Miki, N.; Akatsu, K. *Nippon Shokuhin Kogyo Gakkaishi* 1970, *17*, 175-181.
[56] Cole, E. R.; Kapur, N. S. *J. Sci. Food Agric.* 1957, *8*, 366-368.
[57] Takeoka, G. R.; Dao, L.; Flessa, S.; Gillespie, D. M.; Jewell, W. T.; Huebner, B.; Bertow, D.; Ebeler, S. E. *J. Agric. Food Chem.* 2001, *49*, 3713-3717.
[58] Sahlin, E.; Savage, G. P; Lister, C. E. *J. Food Comp. Anal.* 2004, *17*, 635-647.
[59] Giovanelli, G.; Zanoni, B.; Lavelli, V.; Nani, R. *J. Food Engg.* 2002, *52*, 135-141.
[60] Zanoni, B.; Peri, C.; Nani, R.; Lavelli, V. *Food Res. Int.* 1999, *31*, 395-401.
[61] Shi, J.; Le Maguer, M.; Kakuda, Y.; Liptay, A.; Niekamp, F. *Food. Res. Int.* 1999, *32*, 15-21.
[62] Nguyen, M. L.; Schwartz, S. *J. Food Technol.*. 1999, *53*, 38-45.
[63] Lovric, T.; Sablek, Z.; Boskovic, M. *J. Sci. Food Agric.* 1970, *21*, 641-647.
[64] Giovanelli, G.; Lavelli, V.; Peri, C.; Nobili, S. 1999, *79*, 1583-1588.
[65] Toor, R. K.; Savage, G. P.; Heeb, A. *J. Food Comp. Anal.* 2006, *19*, 20-27.
[66] Sozzi, G. O., Trinchero, G. D.; Fraschina, A. A. *J. Sci. Food Agri.* 1999, *79*, 1065-1070.
[67] Batu, A.; Thompson, A. K. *Tr. J. Agric. Fores.* 1998, *22*, 405-410.
[68] Kristott, J. In *The Stability and Shelf-life of Food;* Kilcast, D.; Subramaniam, P.; Ed.; Woodhear Publishing Limited: Cambridge, 2000; pp 25-32.
[69] Fellows, P. J. In *Food Processing Technology – Principles and Practice;* Fellows, P. J.; Ed.; Woodhead Publishing Limited: Cambridge, 2000; pp 233-240.
[70] Calligaris, S.; Falcone, P.; Anese, M. *J. Food Sci. – Sensory and Nutritive Qualities of Food* 2002, *67*, 2432-2435.
[71] Barrett, D. M.; Theerakulkait, C. *Food Technol.* 1995, *49*, 62-65.
[72] Dermesonlouoglou, E. K.; Giannakourou, M. C.; Taoukis, P. S. *Food Chem.* 2007, *103*, 985-993.
[73] Lisiewska, Z.; Kmiecik, W. *Food Chem.* 2000, *70*, 167-173.
[74] Fennema, O. R. In *Principles of Food Science Part 2: Physical Principles of Food Preservation;* Karel, M.; Fennema, O. R.; Lund, D. B.; Ed.; Marcel Dekker Inc.: NY, 1975; pp 173-215.
[75] Biacs, P.; Wissgott, U. *Nahrung* 1997, *5*, 306-310.
[76] Manzocco, L.; Nicoli, M. C.; Anese, M.; Pitotti, A.; Maltini, E. *Food Res. Int.* 1999, *31*, 363-370.
[77] Velasco, P. J.; Lim, M. H.; Pangborn, R. M.; Whitaker, J. R. *Biotechnol. Appl.* Biochem. 1989, *11*, 118-127.
[78] Giovanelli, G.; Lavelli, V. *J. Sci. Food Agric.* 2002, *82*, 1263-1267.
[79] Miki, N.; Akatsu, K. *Nippon Shokuhin Kogyo Gakkaishi* 1971, *17*, 309-312.
[80] Lin, C. H.; Chen, B. H. *Food Chem.* 2005, *90*, 837-846.

[81] Anguelova, T.; Warthesen, J. J. Food Sci. – Food Chemistry and Toxicology 2000, 65, 67-70.
[82] Zanoni, B.; Pagliarini, E.; Foschino, R. *J. Sci. Food Agric.* 2000, *80*, 2203-2208.
[83] Labuza, T. P. *CRC Crit. Rev. Food Technol.* 1971, *2*, 355-405.
[84] Boskovic, M. A. *J. Food Sci.* 1979, *44*, 84-86.
[85] Giovanelli, G.; Paradiso, A. *J. Agric. Food Chem.* 2002, *50*, 7277-7281.
[86] Qiu, W.; Jiang, H.; Wang, H.; Gao, Y. *Food Chem.* 2006, *97*, 516-523.

In: Progress in Food Chemistry
Editor: E. N. Koeffer, pp. 167-181
ISBN: 978-1-60456-303-0

Chapter 6

AN OVERVIEW OF SIMULATION STUDIES ON MICROWAVE PROCESSING OF FOOD PRODUCTS

Adriana S. Franca* and Leandro S. Oliveira
Programa de Pós-Graduação em Ciência de Alimentos/UFMG
Av. Antônio Carlos, 6627 – 31270-901 – Belo Horizonte, MG – Brasil

ABSTRACT

Microwaves have been employed as a heat source since the 1940s, with applications in the food and chemical processing industries. The inherent complexity of microwave heating itself, associated to the coupled transport phenomena that occur as a result of microwave application, has led several researchers to develop models and present simulation studies describing heat and mass transfer occurring during microwave processing of food products. The discretization techniques employed for model solution include finite differences (FD), finite volume (FV) and the finite element method (FEM). Even though with model complexity and simulation results accuracy increasing over the past years, there are still issues to be addressed in terms of modeling and simulation applied to microwave processing. In view of the above, the objective of the present study was to present an overview of the mathematical models that describe transport phenomena occurring during microwave treatment of food products and comment on the discretization techniques that have been employed to solve such models, in order to pinpoint the modeling and simulation issues that need to be addressed in future studies.

1. INTRODUCTION

Microwaves have been employed as a heat source since the 1940s, with applications in the food and chemical engineering industries. The food industry is the largest consumer of microwave energy, where it is employed for cooking, thawing, tempering, drying, freeze-drying, pasteurization, sterilization, baking, heating and re-heating (Oliveira and Franca,

* E-mail:adrianafranca@pesquisador.cnpq.br.Tel:+55-31-34096910.Fax:+55-31-34096989

2002). Furthermore, the industrial and domestic use of microwaves has increased dramatically over the past few decades. Recent improvements in the design of high-powered microwave ovens, reduced equipment manufacturing costs and trends in electrical energy costs offer a significant potential for developing new and improved industrial microwave processes (Vadivambal and Jayas, 2007).

Conventional thermal treatments usually involve exposure of food to high temperatures for long periods of time, which can result in depreciation of flavor, color and nutrient content. In view of such problems, microwave has gained popularity as an alternative thermal processing method in association with improved thermal efficiency, shorter processing time and improved product quality. However, microwave processing also presents its drawbacks. Besides cost issues, an inherent problem associated with microwave processing of foods is the non-uniformity in heating and the consequent uneven temperature distribution throughout the material, i.e., presence of hot (high temperature) and cold (low temperature) spots (Pandit et al., 2007). To reduce such problem, the product is kept in movement (rotation) within the microwave cavity, so that different parts of the product receive an average of electromagnetic field intensity over a period of time. Intermittent heating (turning the power on and off) has also been successfully employed to reduce hot spots and temperature gradients tend to diminish with increasing the on-off frequency (Oliveira and Franca, 2002). The factors that affect the uniformity of heating can be divided into two general categories: cavity effects and product interaction (Vadivambal and Jayas, 2007). Cavity effects are associated to design limitations, location of the microwave inlet point, shape of the cavity, microwave reflections, etc. Factors related to product interactions include food dielectric properties, penetration depth, thickness, shape, size, rotation and others, and will obviously vary from product to product (Kelen et al., 2006).

Conventional heating of a solid food product takes place by convection at the surface, followed by conduction within the material. Microwave heating, on the other hand, is associated to a volumetrically distributed heat source inside the material, due to molecular friction resulting from dipolar rotation of polar solvents and from the conductive migration of dissolved ions. The dipolar rotation is caused by variations of the electrical and magnetic fields in the product (Alton, 1998). Water, the major constituent of most food products, is the main source for microwave interactions due to its dipolar nature. Heat is thus generated within the material, leading to faster heating rates and shorter processing times compared to conventional heating. The material properties that are the most important in microwave heating are the complex relative permittivity and the loss tangent, or dielectric loss. The real part of the permittivity is called the dielectric constant and determines how much of the incident energy is reflected at the sample surface and how much enters the sample. The most important property in microwave processing is the dielectric loss, which predicts the ability of the material to convert the incoming energy into heat (Ku et al., 2002). A comprehensive review on dielectric properties of agricultural and food products is presented by Venkatesh and Raghavan (2004). Recent review papers on microwave processing of food products are also available (Ohlsson and Bengtsson, 2001; Sumnu and Sahin, 2005; Zhang et al., 2006; Vadivambal and Jayas, 2007).

Modeling of microwave heating involves coupling the models for microwave power absorption and temperature and water content distributions inside the product. This requires solution of mass and energy balances, with the microwave effects incorporated as a source term in the energy equation. Due to the inherent complexity of the models, analytical solutions can not be obtained and simulation techniques must me employed. Even though the number of experimental studies available has been increasing considerably over the past decade, they are still restricted to specific conditions and do not encompass all situations that are of interest. Furthermore, microwave heating is quite complex and far from being fully understood, so several issues remain unresolved. In that regard, as computer simulation tools become more sophisticated and accurate, the models that describe microwave processing can be more complex and realistic, thus providing a better description and understanding of the physical phenomena. In view of the above, the objective of the present study was to present an overview of the mathematical models that describe transport phenomena occurring during microwave treatment of food products and of the discretization techniques that have been employed to solve such models, in order to establish trends for future simulation studies.

2. Model Development

In this section, a brief description of the mathematical models that have been employed to describe the transport phenomena that take place when a food product is submitted to microwave radiation is presented. Such review is based on literature published over the last ten years restricted to food applications and does not represent a comprehensive review on the subject.

2.1. Heat Generation Due to Microwave Irradiation

Microwave energy penetrates a given material and produces a volumetrically distributed heat source, due to molecular friction resulting from dipolar rotation of polar solvents and from the conductive migration of dissolved ions. Dipolar rotation results from variations of the electrical and magnetic fields, and energy generation due to microwaves (Q) can be modeled according to the following equation:

$$Q = \frac{1}{2}\omega\varepsilon_0 k''\overline{E}.E^* \qquad (1)$$

where ω is the wave frequency, ε_o is the free space permittivity, k'' is the relative dielectric loss and E* is the complex conjugate of the electric field intensity (E). The intensity of the electric field varies throughout the material and can be evaluated by solving Maxwell's equations:

$$\begin{aligned} \nabla^2 E^R + E^R\psi^E - E^I\chi^E &= 0 \\ \nabla^2 E^I + E^I\psi^E - E^R\chi^E &= 0 \end{aligned} \qquad (2)$$

where ψ^E and χ^E are dimensionless parameters based on dielectric properties, E^R is the dimensionless real electric field component and E^I corresponds to the dimensionless imaginary electric field component. Solution of this system of equations requires a restriction of the simulation domain because the electromagnetic field is distributed in both the sample and the surrounding medium. Therefore, appropriate boundary conditions must be applied at the restricted area (Givoli and Keller, 1989; Oliveira and Franca, 2002). Considering that (i) the simulation domain is defined as a cylindrical region involving the irradiated product (see dashed line in figure 1), (ii) that the irradiated material is large enough along the *z*-axis and that (iii) the electric field of the incident wave is polarized along the *z*-axis and varies in both *x* and *y* directions, the problem can be solved for either radial or lateral (x-axis) irradiation (see figure 1). The corresponding boundary conditions for radial irradiation are (Balanis, 1989):

$$\frac{\partial E^R}{\partial r} + c_1 E^R + c_2 E^I = -c_3 \tag{3}$$

$$\frac{\partial E^I}{\partial r} + c_1 E^I - c_2 E^R = -c_4 \tag{4}$$

with

$$c_1 = R\alpha_0 \frac{J_1(\alpha_0 R) J_0(\alpha_0 R) + Y_1(\alpha_0 R) Y_0(\alpha_0 R)}{J_0(\alpha_0 R)^2 + Y_0(\alpha_0 R)^2} \tag{5}$$

$$c_2 = -\frac{1}{\pi} \frac{2}{J_0(\alpha_0 R)^2 + Y_0(\alpha_0 R)^2} \tag{6}$$

$$c_3 = -\frac{4}{\pi} \frac{Y_0(\alpha_0 R)}{J_0(\alpha_0 R)^2 + Y_0(\alpha_0 R)^2} \tag{7}$$

$$c_4 = -\frac{4}{\pi} \frac{J_0(\alpha_0 R)}{J_0(\alpha_0 R)^2 + Y_0(\alpha_0 R)^2} \tag{8}$$

where J_n and Y_n correspond to nth order Bessel functions of the 1st and 2nd kind, respectively, R is the boundary radius and α_0 is the free space wave number.

The corresponding boundary conditions for lateral irradiation are (Givoli and Keller, 1989; Ayappa et al., 1992):

$$\frac{\partial E^R}{\partial r} = \sum_n \mathrm{Re}(C_n)\cos(n\phi) + \sum_n \mathrm{Re}(C_n)\int_0^{2\pi} E^R(1,\phi)\cos n(\phi-\phi')d\phi' - \sum_n \mathrm{Im}(D_n)\int_0^{2\pi} E^I(1,\phi)\cos n(\phi-\phi')d\phi' \tag{9}$$

$$\frac{\partial E^I}{\partial r} = \sum_n \text{Im}(C_n)\cos(n\phi) + \sum_n \text{Re}(C_n)\int_0^{2\pi} E^R(1,\phi)\cos n(\phi-\phi')d\phi' + \sum_n \text{Im}(D_n)\int_0^{2\pi} E^I(1,\phi)\cos n(\phi-\phi')d\phi' \quad (10)$$

with

$$C_n = \xi_n i^n k_2\left[J_n'(k_2) - J_n(k_2)\frac{H_n^{(1)'}(k_2)}{H_n^{(1)}(k_2)}\right] \qquad \xi_n = \begin{cases}1, & n=0\\ 2 & \forall n>0\end{cases} \quad (11)$$

$$D_n = \frac{\delta_n k_2 H_n^{(1)'}(k_2)}{H_n^{(1)}(k_2)} \qquad \delta_n = \begin{cases}1/2, & n=0\\ 1 & \forall n>0\end{cases} \quad (12)$$

where r and ϕ correspond to the radial and angular coordinates, respectively, Re and Im refer to real and imaginary terms, respectively, H_n is the nth order Hankel function of the first kind, J_n is the nth order Bessel function of the first kind and k_2 is the wave propagation constant in region 2.

Rotation of the sample can be also simulated, by changing the direction of radiation incidence around the sample employing the following equation (Oliveira and Franca, 2002):

$$\varphi = \varphi_0 + \omega t \quad (13)$$

where φ represents the location of the sample at time t, φ_0 corresponds to the location of the sample when irradiation begins, ω is the source (or sample) angular velocity and t is the time.

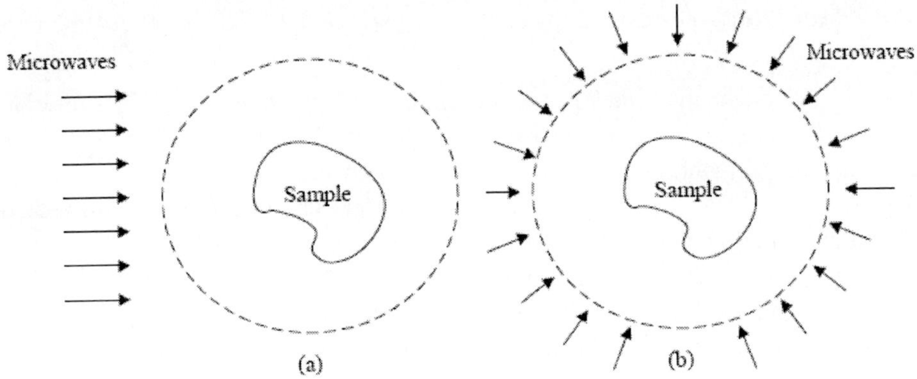

Figure 1. Definition of the simulation domain (inside the dashed lines) for (a) lateral and (b) radial irradiation.

Solution of Maxwell´s equations, although complex, allows for evaluation of the heat generated by microwaves based on the knowledge of dielectric properties alone (Oliveira and Franca, 2002) and has been widely employed in simulation studies dealing with the effect of microwave application on heat and mass transfer in food/biological products (Clemens and Saltiel, 1996; Burfoot et al., 1996; Zhao and Turner, 2000; Zhang et al., 2000; Oliveira and Franca, 2000, 2002; Bhattacharya et al., 2002; Ratanadecho et al., 2002; Basak and Ayappa,

2002; Oliveira et al., 2003; Dinčov et al., 2004; Yang and Gunasekaran, 2004; Campañone and Zaritzky, 2005; Akkari et al., 2005; Rattanadecho, 2006; Basak and Meenakshi, 2006; Vegh and Turner, 2006; Basak, 2007; Zhu et al., 2007; Geedipalli et al., 2007).

As energy is absorbed within the material, the electric field intensity decreases as a function of the distance from the surface of the material. Several simulation studies have modeled the heat generation by microwaves assuming that the microwave power decreases exponentially as a function of penetration into the sample. This type of approach is known as Lambert's law and can be expressed as:

$$Q = Q_0 e^{-d/\delta} \tag{14}$$

where Q_0 is the transmitted power flux at the surface, d is the sample characteristic lenght and δ is the microwave penetration depth, defined as the distance from the sample surface where the absorbed power is 1/*e* of the absorbed power at the surface. Beyond this depth, volumetric heating due to microwave energy is negligible. It is noteworthy to mention that most studies that employed Lambert´s approximation only considered microwave penetration in one direction (Franca and Haghighi, 1996; Oliveira and Franca, 2000, 2002; Pandit and Prasad, 2003; Yang and Gunasekaran, 2004; Campañone and Zaritzky, 2005; Mao et al., 2005; Chatterjee et al., 2007; Datta, 2007) and only a few recent studies have considered microwave penetration in two directions (Sanga et al., 2002; Pandit and Prasad, 2003; Romano et al., 2005; Cuccurullo et al., 2007). In this case, Lambert´s law is represented in cartesian and cylindrical coordinates for two-dimensional samples as (Pandit and Prasad, 2003):

$$Q = 2\alpha P_S''[\exp(-2\alpha(L_1/2 - x)) + \exp(-2\alpha(L_2/2 - y))] + 2\alpha P_S''[\exp(-2\alpha(L_1/2 + x)) + \exp(-2\alpha(L_2/2 + y))] \tag{15}$$

$$Q = 2\alpha P_C''/r[\exp(-2\alpha(R - r)) + \exp(-2\alpha(R + r))] + 2\alpha P_C''[\exp(-2\alpha(L/2 - z)) + \exp(-2\alpha(L/2 + z))] \tag{16}$$

where α is the attenuation factor, L_1 and L_2 are sample dimensions in Cartesian (x,y) coordinates, R and L are sample dimensions in cylindrical (r,z) coordinates, and P''_s and P''_c correspond to the incident power per unit area at the slab and cylinder surfaces, respectively.

This type of approach, although simple, is dependent on the knowledge of the amount of radiation transmitted at the sample surface. Furthermore, it can only be employed above a minimum value of the characteristic sample dimension. Such critical sample dimension has been evaluated and correlations with respect to the microwave penetration depth are available for both slabs (Ayappa et al., 1991) and cylinders (Oliveira and Franca, 2002).

A few studies have considered that the heat generation by microwaves is constant throughout the material. Wu et al. (2004) and Tao et al. (2005) employed such approximation for modeling heat and mass transfer in porous materials subjected to microwaves. The authors justified that the microwave power distribution could be assumed constant since the sample size was much smaller than the microwave penetration depth. A recent study by Zhang and Datta (2006) also assumed uniform heat generation, based on domestic oven power levels and applied it to simulate microwave baking of bread dough.

2.2. Heat and Mass Transfer

Heat transfer resulting from microwave incidence over a solid material can be described by the transient heat equation:

$$\rho c_p \frac{\partial T}{\partial t} = \nabla.(k(\nabla T)) + Q \tag{17}$$

where T is the temperature, c_p is the specific heat capacity, k is the thermal conductivity, ρ is the density and Q is the heat generation term that can be evaluated according to the models discussed in the previous section, depending on the problem being analyzed. This equation has been widely employed to describe microwave heating of solids, especially food products (Zhao and Turner, 2000; Oliveira and Franca, 2000, 2002; Oliveira, Franca and Oliveira, 2003; Pandit and Prasad, 2003; Mao et al., 2005; Romano et al., 2005; Rattanadecho, 2006; Basak and Meenakshi, 2006; Basak, 2007; Cuccurullo et al., 2007; Geedipalli et al., 2007).

Some studies have dealt with sample thawing, for which phase change must be taken into account (Basak and Ayappa, 2002; Ratanadecho et al., 2001a; Rattanadecho, 2004). Heat is considered to be transmitted through both the liquid and solid phases by conduction alone, and the effect of phase change is incorporated into the heat conduction equation through variations of thermal properties with temperature. The moving boundary between the frozen and unfrozen layers is evaluated according to the Stefan equation (Ratanadecho et al., 2001a; Rattanadecho, 2004):

$$\frac{\partial R}{\partial t} = \frac{1}{\rho_1 L}\left(\lambda_1 \left.\frac{\partial T_1}{\partial x}\right|_{x=R} - \lambda_i \left.\frac{\partial T_i}{\partial x}\right|_{x=R} \right) \tag{18}$$

where R corresponds to the thawing front position, L is the latent heat, T is the temperature, λ is the effective thermal conductivity and subscripts i and l correspond to ice and liquid water, respectively. The model presented by Basak and Ayappa (2002) considers the presence of a mushy zone between the liquid and solid phases, in which thermal and dielectric properties are functions of the liquid volume fraction, which in turn depends on temperature.

Most of the modeling and simulation studies applied to microwave heating have focused on solid products and, in the last ten years, only a few studies have focused on microwave induced natural convection (Franca and Haghighi, 1996; Zhang et al., 2000; Ratanadecho et al., 2002; Chatterjee et al., 2007) or microwave heating of flowing liquids (Zhu et al., 2007). Evaluation of microwave heating of liquid samples is quite complex, since it requires solution of the continuity, momentum and energy balances. The resulting equations, considering an incompressible Newtonian fluid, are:

Continuity:

$$\nabla.\vec{v} = 0 \tag{19}$$

Momentum:

$$\rho\left[\frac{\partial \vec{v}}{\partial t}+\vec{v}.\nabla\vec{v}\right]=\vec{B}-\nabla P+\mu\left(\nabla^2\vec{v}\right) \tag{20}$$

Energy:

$$\rho c_p\left[\frac{\partial T}{\partial t}+\vec{v}.\nabla T\right]=k\left(\nabla^2 T\right)+Q \tag{21}$$

where $\vec{v}$ is the velocity, ρ is the density, P is pressure, μ is viscosity, $\vec{B}$ represent body forces (in most applications mainly the gravity field), T is the temperature, c_p is the specific heat capacity, k is the thermal conductivity, ρ is the density and Q is the heat generation term due to microwaves. In the case of natural convection, Boussinesq approximation is usually employed. The flow is treated as incompressible, with the natural convection effect being considered only in the buoyance force term. A detailed description of the development of heat and mass transfer equations is available in textbooks (Burmeister, 1993; Incropera, 2006).

The microwave effect on heating of liquids has been evaluated by either solving Maxwell´s equations or by employing Lambert´s law. Lambert´s approximation was employed by Franca and Haghighi (1996) and Chatterjee et al. (2007), whereas Zhang et al. (2000), Ratanadecho et al. (2002) and Zhu et al. (2007) solved Maxwell´s equations, with different levels of simplification.

The models discussed previously allow for a detailed description of heat transfer due to microwaves. However, as the sample heats, moisture is transferred towards its surface, due to internal evaporation and pressure-driven flow. Moisture accumulation at the food surface constitutes a well-known problem in microwave heating, preventing occurrence of the usually desired surface crispiness that is attained with conventional heating (Datta and Ni, 2002) and causing the food to become soggy. Furthermore, microwave has been employed as an alternative to conventional drying of food products, either alone or combined with other techniques (Zhang et al., 2006; Ressing et al., 2007). In that regard, several models that account for coupled heat and mass transfer during microwave heating have been presented (Ni et al., 1999; Ratanadecho et al., 2001b; Sanga et al., 2002; Dinčov et al., 2004; Wu et al., 2004; Tao et al., 2005; Zhang and Datta, 2006). A brief discussion of such models is presented as follows. Readers are referred to the specific articles for details of the mathematical models and the respective equations.

The simplest model that allows for a description of heat and mass transfer occurring due to the action of microwaves consists on solution of the heat and mass transfer diffusion equations. This model was employed by Sanga and co-workers (2002) to evaluate heat and mass transfer occurring during microwave drying of shrinking materials. Microwave heat generation was evaluated based on Lambert´s approximation. Coupling between heat and mass was taken into account through the evaluation of moisture diffusivity dependence of temperature and moisture by an empirical model. Sample shrinkage was taken into account, but the specific details of how it was evaluated were not discussed in the paper.

A few studies have incorporated the effect of sample porosity (Ni et al., 1999; Ratanadecho et al., 2001b; Datta and Ni, 2002; Dinčov et al. 2004). Ni and co-workers (1999) presented a model for microwave heating of hygroscopic porous materials. The model consisted of the mass conservation equations for vapor, liquid water and air coupled to the energy equation. Mass conservation consisted on both diffusive and convective (Darcy) flows inside a porous media. An exponential drop of the absorbed energy with the penetration depth of the microwaves was assumed (Lambert´s approximation). Later, the same authors (Datta and Ni, 2002) modified their model by adding the effects of infrared and hot air assisted heating, in order to provide alternatives for surface moisture removal.

Ratanadecho et al. (2001b) presented an experimental and numerical study on heat and mass transfer in unsaturated porous materials submitted to microwave drying, coupled to Lambert´s approach for microwave heat generation. The proposed one-dimensional model was based on the solution of mass and energy conservation equations for the liquid and vapor phases, with fluid velocities evaluated according to Darcy´s law. Dinčov et al. (2004) also presented a two-phase heat and mass transfer model for microwave heating considering the effect of material porosity. Heat transfer was evaluated based on two equations, one representing both the solid and liquid and thus including the effect of microwave heating, and the other representing the gas phase, with material properties being averaged for each equation. Fluid velocities (liquid and gas) were evaluated based on Darcy´s law. Mass transfer equations were solved for both liquid and gas phases, with the interface mass transfer being determined from a heat balance between the phases. The effect of microwaves was assessed by solution of Maxwell equations using Finite Differences Time Domain (FDTD), whereas the coupled heat and mass balances were evaluated using a commercial computational fluid dynamics (CFD) software. A recent study (Ressing et al., 2007) presented a model to simulate the puffing of a dough ball being dehydrated under vacuum with microwave energy. Microwave heat generation was based on Lambert´s approximation and the thermal model was based on the transient heat conduction equation. The effect of drying was taken into account by employing "wet" and "dry" dough elements, being randomly distributed according to the mass ratio of water in the dough. Puffing was simulated by a solid mechanics model. "Wet" and "dry" dough elements presented distinct thermal behaviors as a consequence of the effect of water on thermal properties. However, it was assumed that the structural behavior would not be affected by the presence of water. Model solution was based on a commercial FEM code. A few studies have presented models to evaluate microwave freeze-drying, incorporating the effect of phase change to the coupled heat and mass transfer models (Wang and Shi, 1998; Wu et al., 2004; Tao et al., 2005; Wang and Chen, 2005) with the heat due to microwaves considered constant.

3. MODEL SOLUTION

An evaluation of the models previously presented indicates that, given the inherent complexity of the microwave heating phenomena, numerical methods are needed in order to solve even the more simplified versions of the models. An evaluation of the simulation studies published over the last decade indicates that the majority of the simulations have employed finite differences (FD), finite or control volumes (CV) and finite element discretization techniques (FEM). The Finite Differences Time Domain (FDTD) technique has been specifically employed for the solution of Maxwell´s equations (Zhang et al., 2000; Rattanadecho, 2006; Zhu et al., 2007), with one of the previously mentioned discretization methods being employed for the solution of the heat, momentum and mass transfer models.

Finite differences is a simple and intuitive discretization method. Detailed description of the discretization procedure applied to heat conduction problems is available even in heat transfer textbooks (Incropera, 2006). It has been employed to describe transport phenomena during microwave processing for one (Lu et al., 1998; Ni et al., 1999; Chen et al., 2001; Datta and Ni, 2002; Wang and Chen, 2005), two (Yang and Gunasekaran, 2004; Akkari et al., 2005; Rattanadecho, 2006) and three-dimensional (Burfoot et al., 1996; Campañone and Zaritzky, 2005) simulation studies over the last decade.

The finite element method has been widely applied to simulate transport phenomena associated to microwave irradiation. Some of the advantages of the FEM include the ability to handle complex geometries and boundary conditions, spatial and temporal properties variations, and the fact that FEM-based computer codes are generic and can be applied to solve a wide range of problems (Oliveira and Franca, 2002). This technique has been extensively applied to simulation of microwave processing in the food industry, with the majority of the studies focusing on microwave heating of solid foods (Oliveira and Franca, 2000, 2002; Oliveira et al., 2003; Pandit and Prasad, 2003; Mao et al., 2005; Romano et al., 2005) and fewer works on coupled heat and mass transfer (Zhou et al., 1995; Sanga et al., 2002), microwave heating of liquids (Franca and Haghighi, 1996), phase change associated with thawing (Basak and Ayappa, 2002; Battacharya et al, 2002), heat and mass transfer during baking (Zhang and Datta, 2006) and vacuum microwave drying (Ressing et al., 2007).

Application of the finite or control volume (FV or CV) discretization technique to transport phenomena associated to microwave processing is quite recent compared to FD and FEM and has been applied to microwave heating of solids (Zhao and Turner, 2000) and liquids (Zhang et al., 2000; Ratanadecho et al., 2001, 2002; Chatterjee et. al., 2007) and heat and mass transfer in porous media without (Dinčov et al., 2004; Tao et al., 2005) and with phase change (Wu et al., 2004).

4. Conclusion

An evaluation of the models proposed and implemented to describe heat and mass transfer due to the effect of microwaves indicates that at this point a more comprehensive model can be built, as a combination of the models already available in the literature. Such model would comprise the coupled heat and mass balances in fluids or porous solid foods, including the effects of temperature and moisture variations on thermal and dielectric properties. Phase change should also be taken into account. Heat generation due to microwave should be taken into account by solving Maxwell´s equations in order to ensure a more generic approach. However, given the simplicity of Lambert´s approximation, it should still be employed if sample size allows it. Combined heating and drying mechanisms such as hot air, vacuum, infrared heating and others (Zhang et al., 2006) could also be considered. However, the question about whether or not such a complete a model can be solved, and if so, which technique should be employed, still remains.

An evaluation of the studies employing FD indicates that this technique is adequate for solution of models describing heat and mass transfer due to microwaves, taking into account material porosity and phase change, as shown by several 1D studies. However, employment of FD discretization for 2 and 3D problems is still restricted to regularly shaped objects and this technique is not appropriate for complex geometries. The FEM method is a powerful discretization technique and does have the necessary features to handle a complex model in 2 or 3D, either for microwave heating alone or including coupled heat and mass transfer equations. An evaluation of the available studies on natural convection caused by microwaves indicates that the finite volume method is the more appropriate technique nowadays, given the availability of a majority of FV-based commercial CFD softwares. The employment of such commercial codes becomes a necessity, as the models become more complex. However, FV simulations available in the literature are still restricted to regular geometries.

Modeling and simulation of microwave processing of food products is a complex research subject and a lot of work still has to be done. With the natural evolution of models and softwares allowing for more realistic descriptions, care must me taken with software accuracy. Unstructured meshes or adaptive procedures can be employed in order to ensure that regions presenting high temperature and moisture gradients (hot spots, thawing or sublimation fronts, etc.) are tracked and such techniques could be applied to either FEM (Franca et al., 1995; Franca and Haghighi, 1996) or FV (Martins et al., 2002, 2004) based codes. Furthermore, boundary conditions must be also re-evaluated. A recent study by Verboven et al. (2003) evaluated airflow patterns and the resulting heat transfer coefficients in a standard household microwave cavity with a cylindrical food inside. Simulation results showed significant variations in the heat transfer coefficient (h) along the surface of a cylindrical food material, indicating that the commonly employed assumption of constant heat and mass transfer coefficients along the food surface could also contribute to simulation errors. It is common knowledge that food geometry will affect air flow and heat/mass transfer coefficients. The more irregular the geometry, more variations in h values should be expected and should be taken into account, either as boundary conditions or by means of conjugate analysis (Martins and Oliveira, 2005). Researchers must also keep in mind that simulation and experiments must be conducted together, ensuring that models and softwares are properly validated and verified. Finally, as already pointed out almost 10 years ago (Palombizio and Yakovlev, 1999), there is still need to improve the interface between simulation studies and industry needs and applications.

ACKNOWLEDGEMENTS

The authors gratefully acknowledge financial support from the following Brazilian Government Agencies: CNPq and FAPEMIG.

REFERENCES

Alton, W. J. (1998). Microwave pasteurization of liquids, Society of Manufacturing Engineers, *Paper No*. EM98-211.

Ayappa, K. G., Davis, H. T., Davis, E.A. and Gordon, J. (1992) Two-dimensional finite element analysis of microwave heating, *AIChe Journal*, 38, 1577–1592.

Ayappa, K. G., Davis, H. T., Crapiste, G., Davis, E. A. and Gordon, J. (1991). Microwave heating: an evaluation of power formulations, *Chemical Engineering Science*, 46, 1005-1016.

Akkari, E., Chevallier, S. and Boillereaux, L. (2005). A 2D non-linear "grey-box" model dedicated to microwave thawing: Theoretical and experimental investigation, Computers and *Chemical Engineering*, 30, 321-328.

Balanis, C.A. (1989) Advanced Engineering Electromagnetics, *Wiley*: New York.

Basak, T. (2007). Role of lateral and radial irradiations on efficient microwave processing of food cylinders, *Chemical Engineering Science*, 62, 3185-3196.

Basak, T. and Meenakshi, A. (2006) A theoretical analysis on microwave heating of food slabs attached with ceramic plates: Role of distributed microwave incidence, *Food Research International,* 39, 932-944.

Basak, T. and Ayappa, K. G. (2002). Role of length scales on microwave thawing dynamics in 2D cylinders, International *Journal of Heat and Mass Transfer*, 45, 4543-4559.

Bhattacharya, M., Basak, T. and Ayappa, K. G. (2002). A fixed-grid finite element based enthalpy formulation for generalized phase change problems: role of superficial mushy region, International *Journal of Heat and Mass Transfer*, 45, 4881-4898.

Burfoot, D., Railton, C. J., Foster, A.M. and Reavell, S. R. (1996). Modelling the pasteurisation of prepared meals with microwaves at 896 MHz, *Journal of Food Engineering,* 30, 117-133.

Burmeister, L.C. (1993). Convective Heat Transfer, 2nd ed., *Wiley:* New York.

Campañone, L.A. and Zaritzky, N.E. (2005). Mathematical analysis of microwave heating process, *Journal of Food Engineering*, 69, 359-368.

Chatterjee, S., Basak, T. and Das, S.K. (2007). Microwave driven convection in a rotating cylindrical cavity: A numerical study, *Journal of Food Engineering*, 79, 1269-1279.

Chen, G., Wang, W. and Mujumdar, A.S. (2001). Theoretical study of microwave heating patterns on batch fluidized bed drying of porous material, *Chemical Engineering Science*, 56, 6823-6835.

Clemens, J. and Saltiel, C. (1996). Numerical modeling of materials processing in microwave furnaces, International *Journal of Heat and Mass Transfer*, 39, 1665-1675.

Cuccurullo, G., Cinquanta, L. and Sorrentino, G. (2007) A procedure to achieve fine control in MW processing of foods, *Infrared Physics and Technology*, 49, 292-296.

Datta, A.K. (2007) Porous media approaches to studying simultaneous heat and mass transfer in food processes. II: Property data and representative results, *Journal of Food Engineering,* 80, 96-110.

Datta, A.K. and Ni, H. (2002). Infrared and hot-air-assisted microwave heating of foods for control of surface moisture, *Journal of Food Engineering*, 51, 355-364.

Dinčov, D.D., Parrott K. A. and Pericleous, K. A. (2004). Heat and mass transfer in two-phase porous materials under intensive microwave heating, *Journal of Food Engineering*, 65, 403-412.

Franca, A.S. and Haghighi, K. (1996). Adaptive finite element analysis of microwave driven convection, *International Communications in Heat and Mass Transfer*, 23, 177-186.

Franca, A.S., Oliveira, L.S., Haghighi, K. and Krutz, G. (1995) The application of adaptive finite element analysis to heat and mass transfer problems, *Journal of Agricultural and Engineering Research*, 62, 49-60.

Geedipalli, S.S.R., Rakesh, V. and Datta, A.K. (2007) Modeling the heating uniformity contributed by a rotating turntable in microwave ovens, *Journal of Food Engineering*, 82, 359-368.

Givoli, D. and Keller, J.B. (1989) Exact non-reflecting boundary conditions. *Journal of Computational Physics,* **82,** 172–192.

Incropera, F.P. (2006). Fundamentals of Heat and Mass Transfer, 6th edition, *Wiley*: New York.

Kelen, A., Ress, S. Nagy, T., Pallai, E. and Pintye-Hodi, K. (2006) Mapping of temperature distribution in pharmaceutical microwave vacuum drying, *Powder Technology* , 162 , 133–137.

Ku, H. S., Siores, E., Taube, A. and Ball, J. A. R. (2002) Productivity improvement through the use of industrial microwave technologies, *Computers and Industrial Engineering*, 42, 281-290.

Lu, L., Tang, J. and Liang, L. (1998). Moisture distribution in spherical foods in microwave drying. *Drying Technology*, 16, 503-524.

Mao, W., Watanabe, M. and Sakai, N. (2005) Analysis of temperature distributions in Kamaboko during microwave heating, *Journal of Food Engineering*, 71, 187-192.

Martins, M.A. and Oliveira, L.S. (2005). Cooling of Apples as a Conjugate Heat Transfer Problem, ASAE Paper no. 056065, *St Joseph*, MI.

Martins, M.A., Oliveira, L.S. and Valle, R.M. (2004). Adaptivity for finite volume on unstructured triangular meshes: a study of thermal injury in teeth, *International Journal for Numerical Methods in Engineering,* 61, 1625-1643.

Martins, M.A., Oliveira, L.S., Valle, R.M. and Burgarelli, D. (2002). Error estimation and adaptivity for finite-volume methods on unstructured triangular meshes: elliptic heat transfer problems, *Numerical Heat Transfer*, Part B, 42, 461-483.

Ni, H., Datta, A.K. and Torrance, K. (1999). Moisture transport in intensive microwave heating of biomaterials: a multiphase porous media model, *International Journal of Heat and Mass Transfer,* 42, 1501-1512.

Oliveira, M.E.C. and Franca, A.S. (2000). Finite element analysis of microwave heating of solid products, *International Communications in Heat and Mass Transfer*, 27, 527-536.

Oliveira, M.E.C. and Franca, A.S. (2002). Microwave heating of foodstuffs, *Journal of Food Engineering,* 53, 347-359.

Oliveira, M.E.C., Franca, A.S. and Oliveira, L.S. (2003). Numerical analysis of the use of microwaves in the treatment of malignant tumors. Ciencia y Engenharia/ *Science and Engineering Journal,* 12, 79-83.

Palombizio, A. and Yakovlev, V.V. (1999). Parallel worlds of microwave modeling & industry: a time to cross?, *Microwave World,* 20, 14-19.

Pandit, R.B. and Prasad, S. (2003). Finite element analysis of microwave heating of potato - transient temperature profiles, *Journal of Food Engineering*, 60, 193-202.

Pandit, R.B., Tang, J., Liu, F. and Mikhaylenko, G. (2007) A computer vision method to locate cold spots in foods in microwave sterilization processes, *Pattern Recognition*, 40, 3667-3676.

Rattanadecho, P. (2006). The simulation of microwave heating of wood using a rectangular wave guide: Influence of frequency and sample size, *Chemical Engineering Science*, 61, 4798-4811.

Rattanadecho, P. (2004). Theoretical and experimental investigation of microwave thawing of frozen layer using a microwave oven (effects of layered configurations and layer thickness), *International Journal of Heat and Mass Transfer*, 47, 937-945.

Ratanadecho, P., Aoki, K. and Akahori, M. (2002). A numerical and experimental investigation of the modeling of microwave heating for liquid layers using a rectangular wave guide (effects of natural convection and dielectric properties), Applied *Mathematical Modelling*, 26, 449-472.

Ratanadecho, P., Aoki, K. and Akahori, M. (2001a) A numerical and experimental investigation of the modelling of microwave melting of frozen packed beds using a rectangular wave guide, *International Communications in Heat and Mass Transfer*, 28, 751-762.

Ratanadecho, P., Aoki, K. and Akahori, M. (2001b) Experimental and numerical study of microwave drying in unsaturated porous material, *International Communications in Heat and Mass Transfer,* 28, 605-616.

Ressing, H., Ressing, M. and Durance, T. (2007) Modeling the mechanisms of dough puffing during vacuum microwave drying using the finite element method, *Journal of Food Engineering,* 82, 498-508.

Romano, V.R., Marra, F. and Tammaro, U. (2005). Modelling of microwave heating of foodstuff: study on the influence of sample dimensions with a FEM approach, *Journal of Food Engineering,* 71, 233-241.

Sanga, E. C. M., Mujumdar, A. S. and Raghavan, G. S. V. (2002). Simulation of convection-microwave drying for a shrinking material, *Chemical Engineering and Processing*, 41, 487-499.

Sumnu, G. and Sahin, S. (2005) Recent Developments in Microwave Heating. In. Da-Wen Sun (Ed.) Emerging Technologies for Food Processing (pp. 419-444), London: *Academic Press.*

Tao, Z., Wu, H., Chen, G. and Deng, H. (2005). Numerical simulation of conjugate heat and mass transfer process within cylindrical porous media with cylindrical dielectric cores in microwave freeze-drying, *International Journal of Heat and Mass Transfer*, 48, 561-572.

Ohlsson, T. and Bengtsson, N. (2001). Microwave Technology and Foods. In S. L. Taylor (Ed.) Advances in Food and Nutrition Research (pp. 65-140), London: *Academic Press.*

Vadivambal, R. and Jayas, D.S. (2007). Changes in quality of microwave-treated agricultural products-a review, *Biosystems Engineering*, 98, 1-16.

Vegh, V. and Turner, I.W. (2006). A hybrid technique for computing the power distribution generated in a lossy medium during microwave heating, *Journal of Computational and Applied Mathematics*, 197, 122-140.

Venkatesh, M.S. and Raghavan, G.S.V. (2004). An overview of microwave processing and dielectric properties of agri-food materials, *Biosystems Engineering*, 88, 1-18.

Verboven, V., Datta, A.K., Anh, N.T., Scheerlinck, N. and Nicolaï, B.M. (2003). Computation of airflow effects on heat and mass transfer in a microwave oven, *Journal of Food Engineering,* 59, 181-190.

Wang, Z.H. and Shi, M.H. (1998). Numerical study on sublimation-condensation phenomena during microwave freeze drying, *Chemical Engineering Science*, 53, 3189-3197.

Wang, W. and Chen, G. (2005). Heat and mass transfer model of dielectric-material-assisted microwave freeze-drying of skim milk with hygroscopic effect, *Chemical Engineering Science,* 60, 6542-6550.

Wu, H., Tao, Z., Chen, G., Deng, H., Xu, G. and Ding, S. (2004). Conjugate heat and mass transfer process within porous media with dielectric cores in microwave freeze drying, *Chemical Engineering Science*, 59, 2921-2928.

Yang, H.W. and Gunasekaran, S. (2004). Comparison of temperature distribution in model food cylinders based on Maxwell's equations and Lambert's law during pulsed microwave heating, *Journal of Food Engineering*, 64, 445-453.

Zhang, M., Tang, J., Mujumdar, A.S. and Wang, S. (2006). Trends in microwave-related drying of fruits and vegetables, *Trends in Food Science and Technology*, 17, 524-534.

Zhang, J. and Datta, A.K. (2006). Mathematical modeling of bread baking process, *Journal of Food Engineering,* 75, 78-89.

Zhang, Q., Jackson, T.H. and Ungan, A. (2000). Numerical modeling of microwave induced natural convection, *International Journal of Heat and Mass Transfer*, 43, 2141-2154.

Zhao, H. and Turner, I.W. (2000). The use of a coupled computational model for studying the microwave heating of wood, *Applied Mathematical Modelling*, 24, 183-197.

Zhou L., Puri V.M., Anantheswaran R.C. and Yeh G. (1995). Finite Element Modeling of Heat and Mass Transfer in Food Materials During Microwave Heating - Model Development and Validation, *Journal of Food Engineering*, 25, 509-529.

Zhu, J., Kuznetsov, A.V. and Sandeep, K.P. (2007). Mathematical modeling of continuous flow microwave heating of liquids (effects of dielectric properties and design parameters), *International Journal of Thermal Sciences*, 46, 328-341.

In: Progress in Food Chemistry
Editor: E. N. Koeffer, pp. 183-199
ISBN: 978-1-60456-303-0

Chapter 7

LOW MOLECULAR WEIGHT OXIDANT-STABLE PROTEASE FROM THE INTESTINE OF SMOOTH HOUND (*MUSTELUS MUSTELUS*) — PURIFICATION AND CHARACTERIZATION

Ali Bougatef, Kemel Jellouli, Rafik Balti, Yosra Ellouz-Triki, Ahmed Barkia and Moncef Nasri*

Laboratoire de Génie Enzymatique et de Microbiologie - Ecole Nationale d' Ingénieurs de Sfax, B.P. "W" 3038 Sfax, Tunisia

ABSTRACT

An extracellular low molecular weight (LMW) protease from the intestine of smooth hound (*Mustelus mustelus*) was purified and characterized. The enzyme was purified to homogeneity by fractionation with ammonium sulphate, Sephadex G-100 gel filtration and DEAE-cellulose anion exchange chromatography with a 10.7-fold increase in specific activity and 22.6% recovery. The molecular weight of the purified enzyme was estimated to be 14,800 Da by SDS-PAGE and gel filtration. *Mustelus mustelus* protease appeared as a single band in native-PAGE. The optimum pH and temperature for the enzyme activity were pH 8.0 and 60 °C, respectively. The relative activity at pH 9.0 was 80.5% and the enzyme showed high pH stability between 6.0 and 9.0.

The enzyme showed extreme stability towards oxidizing agents, retaining more than 80% of its initial activity after 1 h incubation at 30 °C in the presence of 1% H_2O_2 and 2% sodium perborate. Furthermore, the purified enzyme showed relative stability and compatibility with commercial liquid detergents. The enzyme retained more than 75 and 61% of its initial activity after preincubation 60 min at 30 °C in the presence of Dixan and Ariel.

The purified enzyme was strongly inhibited by soybean trypsin inhibitor (SBTI) and phenylmethylsulphonyl fluoride (PMSF) a serine-protease inhibitor. The kinetic protease

* Corresponding author: Tel.: 216 74-274-088; fax: 216 74-275-595; E-mail address: mon_nasri@yahoo.fr; moncef.nasri@enis.rnu.tn.

constants K_m and k_{cat} of the purified enzyme for casein were 0.313 mM and 0.088 s^{-1}, respectively, while the catalytic efficiency k_{cat}/K_m was 0.281 s^{-1} mM^{-1}.

Keywords: Low molecular weight protease; Purification; Biochemical characterization; Smooth hound (Mustelus mustelus); Detergents compatibility.

INTRODUCTION

Proteases constitute the most important group of industrial enzymes used in the world today, accounting for about 50% of the total industrial enzyme market (Rao et al., 1998). They have diverse applications in a wide variety of industries such as detergent, food, agrochemical and pharmaceutical industries (Gupta et al., 2002; Zukowski, 1992). Proteases are mainly derived from animal, plant and microbial sources.

Today, there is an increasing demand for fish proteolytic enzymes in food processing. Viscera, one of the most important by-products of fishing industry, have wide biotechnological potential as a source of digestive enzymes, especially proteases that have high activity over a wide range of pH and temperature conditions (Gildberg, 1992; Cancre et al., 1999; Shahidi and Kamil, 2001) and exhibit high catalytic activity at relatively low concentration (Haard, 1998). These characteristics of fish proteases have made them suitable for different applications in many food-processing operations. In addition, fish enzymes could be utilized to produce bioactive peptides from fish proteins. Considering the specific characteristics of these enzymes, fish processing by-products are currently used for enzyme extraction.

A variety of digestive proteolytic enzymes has been isolated from the internal organs of fish such as sardine (*Sardina pilchardus*) (Bougatef et al., 2007); smooth hound (*Mustelus mustelus*) (Bougatef et al., 2007), true sardine (*Sardinops melanostictus*) and arabesque greenling (*Pleuroprammus azonus*) (Kishimura et al., 2006), yellowfin tuna (*Thunnus albacores*) (Klomklao et al., 2006), shark (*Centroscymunus coelolepis*) (Nguyen et al., 1998), sea bream (*Sparus latus* Houttuyn) (Zhou et al., 2007) and African coelacanth (*Latimeria chalumnae*) (Tanji et al., 2007).

The most important digestive enzymes from fish viscera are the aspartic protease pepsin, and serine proteases trypsin, chymotrypsin, elastase and collagenase. Acidic proteases from fish stomachs display high activity between pH 2.0 and 4.0, while alkaline digestive proteases, such as trypsin, are most active between pH 8.0 and 10.0.

During fish processing, large quantities of waste, including heads and viscera, are generated and discarded. They can represent about 30% of the original raw material. These wastes, which represent an environmental problem to the fishing industry, constitute an important source of proteolytic enzymes and protein. Traditionally, these materials have been converted to powdered fish flour used as animal feed (Strom and Eggum, 1981), but the abundance of proteolytic enzymes and proteins in fish viscera open the possibility of further utilisations.

One alternative to convert the fish processing wastes into more marketable and acceptable products is to produce fish powders or fish protein hydrolysates that may be used as carbon and/or nitrogen source for biomass and metabolites production. In a previous paper, we have shown that protease synthesis was strongly induced when *Bacillus subtilis* strain was grown in media containing only sardinelle (*Sardinella aurita*) heads and viscera powder (Ellouz et al, 2001). Moreover, several studies revealed that fish protein hydrolysates performed effectively as a nitrogenous source in microbial growth and enzyme production (Clausen et al., 1985; Gildberg et al., 1989; Dufossé et al., 2001; Triki-Ellouz et al., 2003; Ghorbel et al., 2005).

An interesting alternative is to isolate and purify proteolytic enzymes which can be used in the food industry or in fish protein hydrolysate preparation. The recovery of proteolytic enzymes from fish viscera might be a solution to the pollution generated by fish processing industries.

The present paper describes the purification procedure and some biochemical characterization of low molecular weight protease from smooth hound (*Mustelus mustelus*).

Materials and Methods

Reagents

Casein sodium salt from bovine milk, ethylenediaminetetraacetic acid (EDTA), soybean trypsin inhibitor (SBTI), phenylmethylsulfonyl fluoride (PMSF), benzamidine, trichloroacetic acid, glycine, ammonium sulphate, bovine serum albumin and markers for molecular weights 14,000-66,000 Da were purchased from Sigma Chemical Co. (St. Louis MO, USA). Sodium dodecyl sulphate (SDS), acrylamide, ammonium persulphate, N,N,N',N'-tetramethyl ethylenediamine (TEMED), Coomassie Brilliant Blue R-250 were from Bio-Rad Laboratories (Mexico). Sephadex G-100 and diethylaminoethyl (DEAE)-cellulose were from Pharmacia Biotech (Uppsala, Sweden). Tris (hydroxymethyl) aminomethane was procured from Panreac Quimica SA (Spain). All other reagents were of analytical grade.

Smooth Hound Viscera

Smooth hound (*M. mustelus*) was purchased from the local market at Sfax City, Tunisia. It was washed twice with water and intestine were separated, and then stored in sealed plastic bags at -20 °C until used for enzyme extraction.

Preparation of Enzyme Extract

Intestine from *M. mustelus* (150 g) were rinsed with distilled water, and homogenized for 60 sec with 300 ml extraction buffer A (10 mM Tris-HCl, pH 8.0). The mixture was centrifuged twice at 8,500g for 30 min at 4 °C. The pellet was discarded and the supernatant was collected and used as crude protease extract.

Enzyme Purification

Ammonium Sulphate Precipitation

The crude enzyme extract was subjected to ammonium sulphate fractionation 0-20%, 20-60% and 60-80%. The precipitates obtained after centrifugation at 13,000*g* for 30 min were suspended in buffer A and dialyzed 24 h at 4 °C against repeated changes in the same buffer.

Size-Exclusion Chromatography

The 20-60% ammonium sulphate precipitate was subjected to gel filtration on a Sephadex G-100 column (2.6 × 150 cm) pre-equilibrated with buffer B (25 mM Tris-HCl, pH 8.0 containing 0.5‰ Triton X-100). Enzyme fractions of 5 ml were eluted at a flow rate of 25 ml/h with the same buffer, and were analyzed for enzyme activity and protein content. Active enzyme fractions were pooled.

Anion Exchange Chromatography

The active fractions from the Sephadex G-100 were applied to a DEAE cellulose column (2 × 25 cm) previously equilibrated with buffer C (25 mM Tris-HCl, pH 8.0). After being washed with the same buffer, bound proteins were eluted with a linear gradient of sodium chloride in the range of 0-0.5 M in the equilibrating buffer. Fractions of 5 ml were collected at a flow rate of 85 ml/h. The fractions with high protease activities were pooled and stored at -20°C for further analyses. All the purification steps were conducted at temperatures not exceeding 4 °C.

Polyacrylamide Gel Electrophoresis

Sodium dodecyl sulphate-polyacrylamide gel electrophoresis (SDS-PAGE) was carried out for the determination of purity and molecular weight of the purified enzyme as described by Laemmli (1970), using a 5% (w/v) stacking and 15% (w/v) separating gels. Samples were prepared by mixing the purified enzyme at 1:5 (v/v) ratios with distilled water containing 10 mM Tris-HCl pH 8.0, 2.5% SDS, 10% glycerol, 5% β-mercaptoethanol and 0.002% bromophenol blue. Samples were heated at 100 °C for 5 min before electrophoresis. After electrophoresis, the gels were stained with 0.25% Coomassie Brilliant Blue R-250 in 45% ethanol-10% acetic acid and destained with 5% ethanol and 7.5% acetic acid. The molecular weight of the enzyme was estimated using a low molecular weight calibration kit as markers. The molecular mass markers used are: Bovine serum albumin (66,000 Da); ovalbumin (45,000 Da); glyceraldehyde-3-deshydrogenase (36,000 Da); carbonic anhydrase (29,000 Da); bovine trypsinogen (24,000 Da) and bovine α-lactoalbumin (14,200 Da).

Native PAGE and Zymography

Native-PAGE was performed according to the procedure of Laemmli (1970), except that the sample was not heated and SDS and reducing agent were left out.

Zymography was performed on native-PAGE. Briefly, after electrophoresis, the gel was submerged in 1% casein in 100 mM Tris HCl buffer, pH 8.0 and incubated at 37 °C for 90 min. After washing, the gel was stained with Coomassie Brilliant Blue R250 for zymography analysis. Clear zone on the blue background indicated the presence of proteinase.

Protein Concentration

Protein concentration was determined by the method of Bradford [1976] using bovine serum albumin as a standard, and during the course of enzyme purification by measuring the absorbance at 280 nm.

Determination of Protease Activity

Protease activity in the crude extract was measured by the method of Kembhavi et al. (1993) using casein as a substrate. A 0.5 ml aliquot of the enzyme, suitably diluted, was mixed with 0.5 ml 100 mM Tris-HCl (pH 8.0) containing 1% casein, and incubated for 10 min at 60 °C. The reaction was stopped by addition of 0.5 ml 20% (w/v) trichloroacetic acid. The mixture was allowed to stand at room temperature for 15 min and then centrifuged at 10,000*g* for 15 min to remove the precipitate. The acid soluble material was estimated spectrophotometrically at 280 nm. A standard curve was generated using solutions of 0-50 mg/l tyrosine. One unit of protease activity was defined as the amount of enzyme required to liberate 1 μg tyrosine per min under the experimental conditions used.

Biochemical Properties

Effect of pH on Activity and Stability of the Protease

The optimum pH of the purified enzyme was studied over a pH range of 5.0-12.0. For the measurement of pH stability, the enzyme was incubated at 30 °C for 30 min in different buffers at 100 mM and then the residual proteolytic activity was determined under standard assay conditions. The following buffer systems were used: sodium acetate, pH 5.0-6.0; phosphate buffer, pH 7.0; Tris-HCl buffer, pH 8.0; glycine-NaOH buffer, pH 9.0-12.0.

Optimum Temperature and Thermal Stability

The effect of temperature on protease activity was studied from 30 °C to 80 °C for 10 min at pH 8.0. Thermal stability of the purified protease was determined by incubating the enzyme 60 min at different temperatures, and residual enzyme activities were estimated at regular intervals under standard conditions. The non-heated enzyme was considered as control (100%).

Effects of Metals Ions, Enzyme Inhibitors and Denaturing Reagents

The effect of metal ions (5 mM) on enzyme activity was investigated by adding the monovalent (Na^+ and K^+) and divalent metal ions (Ca^{2+}, Mn^{2+}, Zn^{2+}, Co^{2+}, Cu^{2+}, Ba^{2+} and Mg^{2+}) to the reaction mixture. The activity was compared with that of the reaction that was free of the corresponding metal ions. The effects of various concentrations of $CaCl_2$ and NaCl on protease activity were also evaluated.

The effects of inhibitors on protease activity were studied using phenylmethylsulfonyl fluoride (PMSF), soybean trypsin inhibitor (SBTI), benzamidine, β-mercaptoethanol and ethylene-diaminetetraacetic acid (EDTA). The purified enzyme was preincubated with inhibitors for 30 min at 25 °C and then the remaining enzyme activity was estimated using casein as a substrate, and compared with the control activity obtained without inhibitors. The effect of some surfactants (Triton X-100, Tween 80 and SDS) and oxidizing agents (H_2O_2 and sodium perborate) on enzyme stability was studied by pre-incubating the enzyme for 1 h at 30 °C. The residual activity was measured at pH 8.0 and 60 °C. The activity of the enzyme (without any additive) was taken as 100%.

Stability in the Presence of Liquid Detergents

The compatibility of the LMW protease with commercial liquid laundry detergents was studied using Dixan (Henkel-Spain), Nadhif (Henkel-Alki-Tunisia) and Lav^{+} (Tunisia). The detergents were diluted 100-fold in tap water to simulate washing conditions. The enzyme was incubated in various detergents solutions for 1 h at 30 °C and the residual activity was determined. The enzyme activity of a control (without detergent), incubated under the similar conditions, was taken as 100%.

Kinetic Properties

The effect of casein concentration on protease activity was determined at 60 °C. The apparent Michaelis-Menton constant (K_m) and the substrate turnover number (V_{max}) were calculated from Lineweaver-Burk plots (Lineweaver and Burk, 1934). Value of turnover number (k_{cat}) was calculated from the following equation: $k_{cat} = V_{max}/[E]$, where [E] is the active enzyme concentration and V_{max} is the maximal velocity.

Results and Discussion

Purification of the Protease

The enzyme from the intestine of *M. mustelus* was purified by the three-step procedure described in Section 2. In the first step, the crude enzyme extract was fractionated with ammonium sulphate. The fraction F2 (20-60% (w/v) saturation) showed higher specific activity (1048 U/mg of protein) than F1 (0-20%; 79.78 U/mg of protein) and F3 (60-80%; 43.53 U/mg of protein). No activity was detected in final supernatant. The 20-60% ammonium sulphate precipitate, which gave the highest specific activity, was subjected to gel filtration on a Sephadex G-100 column. The elution profiles of protease activities and proteins from Sephadex G-100 are shown in figure 1. The elution resulted in two peaks of proteolytic activity. Fractions (from peak 2: P_2) containing protease activity were pooled and then loaded on DEAE-cellulose column pre-equilibrated with buffer C and eluted with a linear gradient 0-0.5 M NaCl in the same buffer (figure 2). Protease activity appeared in a single peak together with adsorbed fractions. The results of the purification procedure are summarized in table 1. After the final purification step, the protease was purified 10.7-fold with a recovery of 22.6% and a specific activity of 6952 U/mg of protein.

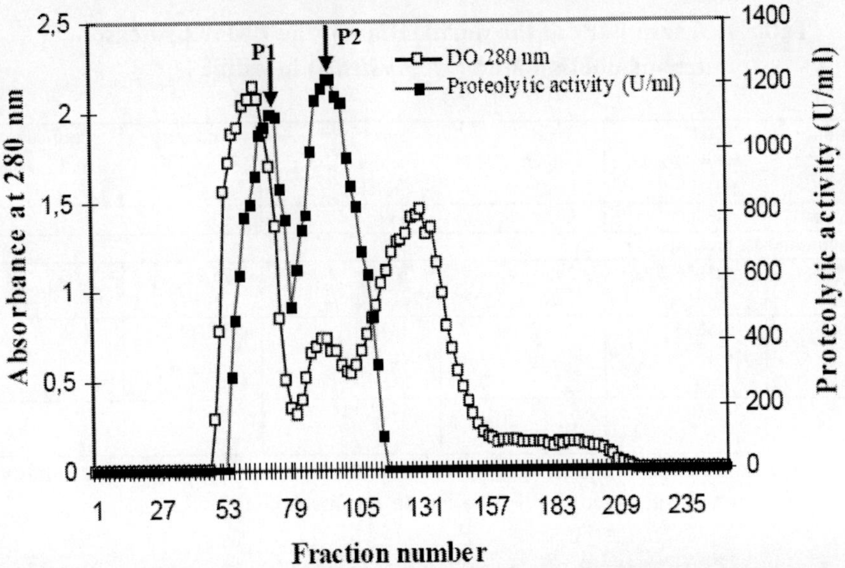

The enzyme preparation (20-60% saturation with ammonium sulphate) was applied to a 2.6 x 150 cm column, equilibrated and eluted with buffer B. Fractions (5 ml) collected from the column were assayed for proteins content at 280 nm and protease activity as described in Materials and Methods. Flow rate = 25 ml/h.

Figure 1. Purification profile of the LMW protease from smooth hound (*M. mustelus*) intestine by gel filtration on Sephadex G-100 column.

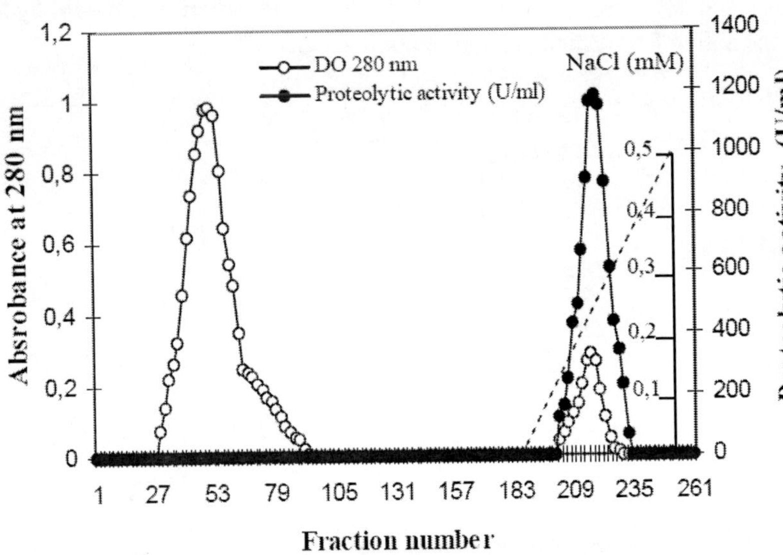

The adsorbed protein fractions were eluted with a linear gradient of sodium chloride in the range of 0-0.5 M in the equilibrating buffer C. Fractions (5 ml) collected from the column were assayed for proteins content at 280 nm and protease activity as described in Materials and Methods. The chromatography was carried out at a flow rate of 85 ml/h.

Figure 2. Purification profile of the LMW protease from smooth hound (*M. mustelus*) intestine by DEAE-cellulose column (2.5 × 25 cm) pre-equilibrated with buffer C.

Table 1. A summary of the purification of the LMW protease from smooth hound (*M. mustelus*) intestine

Purification steps	Total activity (U)	Total protein (mg)	Specific activity(U/mg protein)	Recovery (%)	Purification fold
Crude extract	403800	632	639	100	1
Ammonium sulphate precipitation					
(NH4)2SO4 (20-60%)	303926	290	1048	75.26	1.64
Sephadex G-100 gel filtration	148870	30.72	4846.02	36.86	7.58
DEAE-Cellulose	91420	13.15	6952.09	22.63	10.7

All operations were carried out at 4 °C. Only precipitate formed between 20-60% saturation with ammonium sulphate was subjected to gel-filtration on Sephadex G-100.

Biochemical Characterization

Molecular Weight

The homogeneity of the purified protease was checked by SDS-PAGE under reducing conditions. As shown in figure 3, the purified enzyme has a molecular weight of approximately 14,800 Da when analysed using SDS-PAGE, corresponding with that determined by gel filtration. Purity of the enzyme was also evaluated by using native gel electrophoresis and zymogram. As shown in figure 4, a clear band of casein hydrolysis was observed in the native-PAGE, indicating the homogeneity of the enzyme.

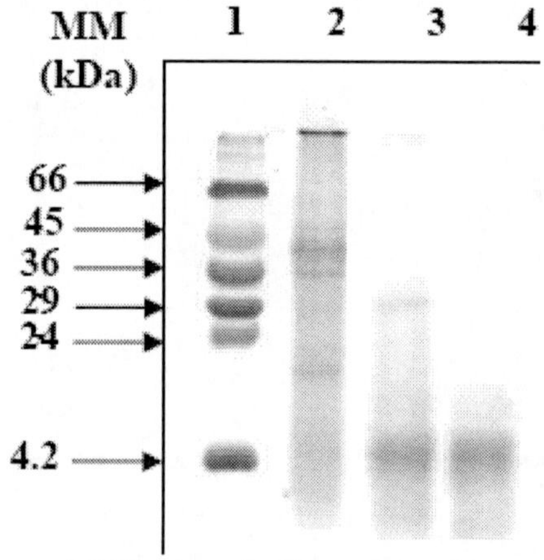

Lane 1: standard protein markers of different molecular weights; lane 2: crude extract; lane 3: after gel filtration; lane 4: purified protease.

Figure 3. SDS-polyacrylamide gel electro-phoresis of the purified protease from smooth hound (*M. mustelus*) intestine.

Figure 4. Native-PAGE (1) and zymogram (2) of the purified protease from smooth hound (*M. mustelus*) intestine.

Effect of pH on Activity and Stability

The effect of pH on protease activity was studied by using casein as a substrate at various pH values at 60 °C. The purified enzyme was highly active between pH 7.0 and 9.0, with an optimum around pH 8.0 (figure. 5a). The relative activities at pH 7.0 and 9.0 were about 80.5% of that at pH 8.0. As seen in figure 5a, protease activity decreased significantly above pH 9.0 and was only 44.5 and 21.5% of the maximum activity at pH 10.0 and 11.0, respectively. These findings are in accordance with several earlier reports showing optimum activity at pH 8.0 (Bougatef et al., 2007; Castillo-Yanez et al., 2005; Klimova at al., 1990). The optimum pH of *M. mustelus* protease was higher than that of the 14.8 kDa collagenase from the Mackerel *S. japonicus,* which had optimum activity around pH 7.5 (Park et al., 2002),.

The pH stability profile of the purified protease showed that the enzyme is very stable in a broad pH range, maintaining over 100% of its original activity between pH 7.0 and 8.0, after incubation 30 min at 30 °C, and more than 80% of its activity was retained at pH 6.0 and 9.0 (figure 5b).

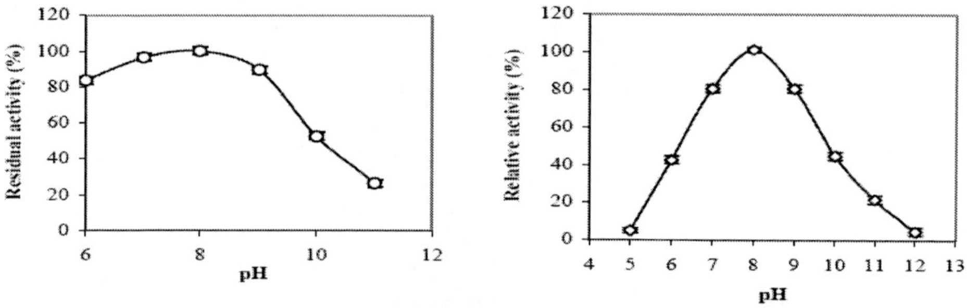

Proteolytic activity was assayed using casein as a substrate. The protease activity was evaluated in the pH range of 5.0-12.0 using buffers of different pH values at 60 °C. The maximum activity obtained at pH 8.0 was considered as 100% activity. The pH stability of the enzyme was determined by incubating the enzyme in different buffers for 30 min at 30 °C and the residual activity was measured at pH 8.0 and 60 °C. The activity of the enzyme before incubation was taken as 100%. Buffer solutions used for pH activity and stability are presented in Materials and Methods.

Figure 5. Effect of pH on activity (a) and stability (b) of the purified protease.

Effect of Temperature on Activity and Stability of the Enzyme

The effect of temperature on the activity of *M. mustelus* protease was examined at various temperatures (figure 6a). The LMW protease was active at temperatures from 30 to 70 °C with an optimum around 60 °C. The relative activities at 50 and 70 °C were about 81.8 and 59%, respectively, of that at 60 °C. The optimum temperature for *M. mustelus* protease was higher than that from Mackerel, *S. japonicus* (Park et al., 2002), which had optimum temperature at 55 °C.

The thermal stability profiles showed that the purified enzyme is completely stable at 40 °C. At 50 °C, the enzyme retained more than 84% of its initial activity after 1 h incubation, while 18% of the maximal activity remained within 15 min of incubation at 60 °C. However, the enzyme was completely inactivated after 15 min incubation at 70 °C.

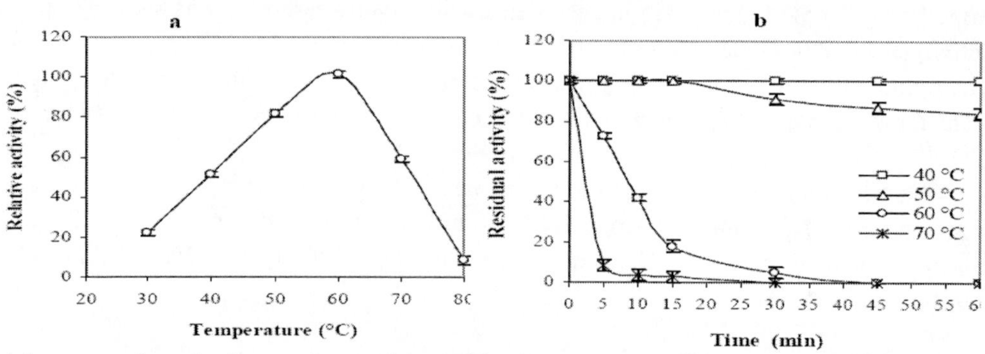

Activity was evaluated using casein as substrate. The temperature profile was determined by assaying protease activity at temperatures between 30 and 80 °C. The activity of the enzyme at 60 °C was taken as 100%. The temperature stability was determined by incubating purified enzyme at 40, 50, 60 and 70 °C from 0 to 60 min at pH 8.0 and residual enzyme activities were estimated at regular intervals under standard conditions. The non-heated enzyme was considered as control (100%).

Figure 6. Effect of temperature on activity (a) and stability (b) of the purified LMWprotease.

Effect of Enzyme Inhibitors on Protease Activity

Proteases can be classified by their sensitivity to various inhibitors (North, 1982). In order to determine the nature of the purified protease, the effect of a variety of enzyme inhibitors, such as chelating agent and a specific group reagent on enzyme activity was investigated (table 2). The enzyme was strongly inhibited by the serine-protease inhibitor (PMSF) and by soybean trypsin inhibotor (SBTI). Benzamidie (5 mM), a synthetic trypsin inhibitor, showed also strong inhibition, approximately 37%. Therefore, these results suggest that the enzyme is a member of the serine-protease family.

No inhibition was observed when the cystein type inhibitor, i.e, β-mercaptoethanol was used. Metalloenzyme inhibitor EDTA (5 mM) inhibited the protease activity by 20%, indicating the importance of Ca^{2+} in enzyme stabilization. Indeed, serine-proteases are known to contain two Ca^{2+} binding sites and the removal of Ca^{2+} from the strong binding site is associated with significant decrease in thermal stability (Lee and Jang, 2001).

Table 2. Effect of enzyme inhibitors on smooth hound (*M. mustelus*) protease

Inhibitors	Concentration (mM)	Residual enzyme activity (%)
None		100
PMSF	1	52
	5	12
EDTA	1	100
	5	80
Benzamidine	1	91
	5	63
β-mercaptoethanol	5	100
SBTI	1 mg/ml	0

Enzyme activity measured in the absence of any inhibitor was taken as 100%. The remaining protease activity was measured after preincubation of the purified enzyme with each inhibitor at 25 °C for 30 min. PMSF: phenylmethylsulfonyl fluoride; EDTA: ethylenediaminetetraacetic acid. SBTI: Soybean Trypsin Inhibitor.

Effect of Metal Ions

The effects of different metal ions (5 mM) on the activity of smooth hound protease were studied at pH 8.0 and 60 °C (table 3). The addition of $CaCl_2$ increased protease activity. Mg^{2+} and Ba^{2+} showed no influence on the enzyme activity. However, strong inhibition was observed with Co^{2+}, Cu^{2+}, Zn^{2+} and Mn^{2+}, which inhibited the enzyme activity by 87, 79, 72 and 68%, respectively. The enzyme activity was not affected by Na^{+} and slightly activated by K^{+}.

Table 3. Effect of various metal ions (5 mM) on enzyme activity

Ions	None	Ca^{2+}	Mg^{2+}	Zn^{2+}	Mn^{2+}	Cu^{2+}	Ba^{2+}	Co^{2+}	Na^{+}	K^{+}
Relative activity (%)	100	113	100	28	32	21	92	13	100	109

Since Ca^{2+} induce the activity, it is necessary to study the effect of its concentration on protease activity. As shown in table 4, maximum activity was obtained with 2 mM Ca^{2+}.

Beyond 2 mM Ca^{2+}, protease activity decreased. These results indicated that the enzyme require Ca^{2+} for its optimal activity.

Table 4. Effect of $CaCl_2$ concentration on the activity of *M. mustelus* protease

Concentration (mM)	1	2	3	5	7	10
Relative activity (%)	100	120	117	115	77.9	74

Effect of Calcium Ions on Enzyme Stability

To determine whether Ca^{2+} enhanced the stability of the *M. mustelus* protease during the inactivation, the stability was examined by incubating the enzyme for 6 h at 40 °C, in the absence or presence of 2 mM $CaCl_2$ or 2 mM EDTA, followed by measuring the residual activity under standard conditions. As shown in figure 7, in the absence of $CaCl_2$, no loss of activity was observed after 1 h incubation, then the activity decreased with increasing time, maintaining 77.2% of its original activity when incubated for 6 h. However, no loss of activity was observed when incubated with $CaCl_2$. The activity was considerably reduced in the presence of metalloenzyme inhibitor (EDTA). These findings are in line with several earlier reports showing that active site structure of serine proteases contains Ca^{2+} binding site(s) and the removal of Ca^{2+} from the strong binding site is associated to a significant reduction of thermal stability (Vieille and Zeikus, 2001).

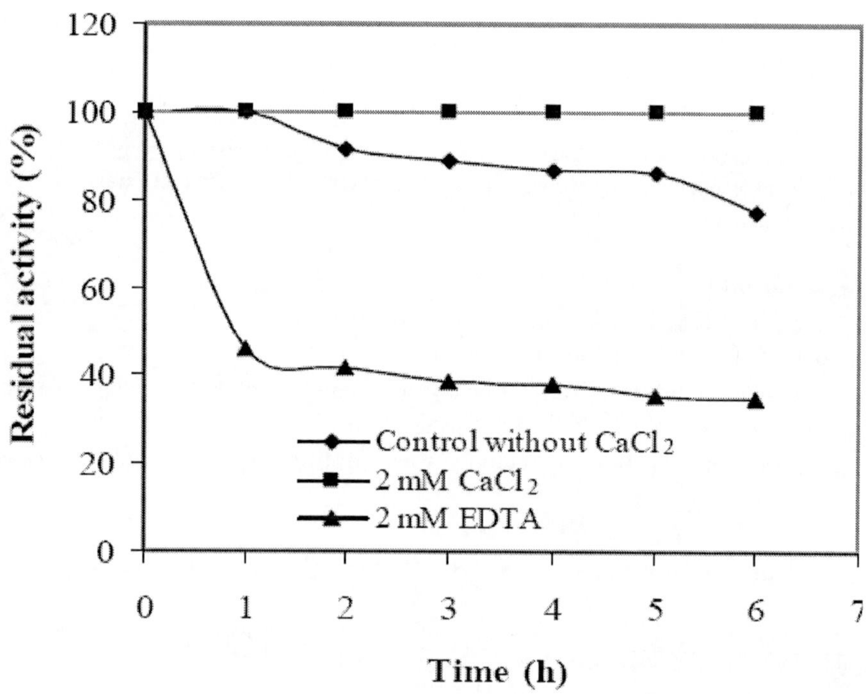

The enzyme was preincubated at 40 °C in the absence or presence of $CaCl_2$ or EDTA, and residual enzyme activity was determined from 0 to 6 hours at 1 hour interval. The non-incubated enzyme was considered as control.

Figure 7. Stability of the *M. mustelus* protease in the absence and presence of $CaCl_2$ or EDTA.

Effect of NaCl Concentration

The effect of NaCl on the activity of *M. mustelus* protease was studied at pH 8.0 and 60 °C by addition of NaCl to the reaction mixture. As shown in figure 8, the activity of the enzyme was not affected with NaCl concentration up to 7.5% (w/v). Beyond 7.5%, protease activity decreased with increasing NaCl concentration. The relative activity at 10 and 15% was 69.3 and 26.3%, respectively. The decrease in activity might be due to the denaturation of enzyme caused by the "salting out" effect with increasing NaCl concentration. Therefore, this enzyme can be used in hydrolysis of proteins in high salt fish products.

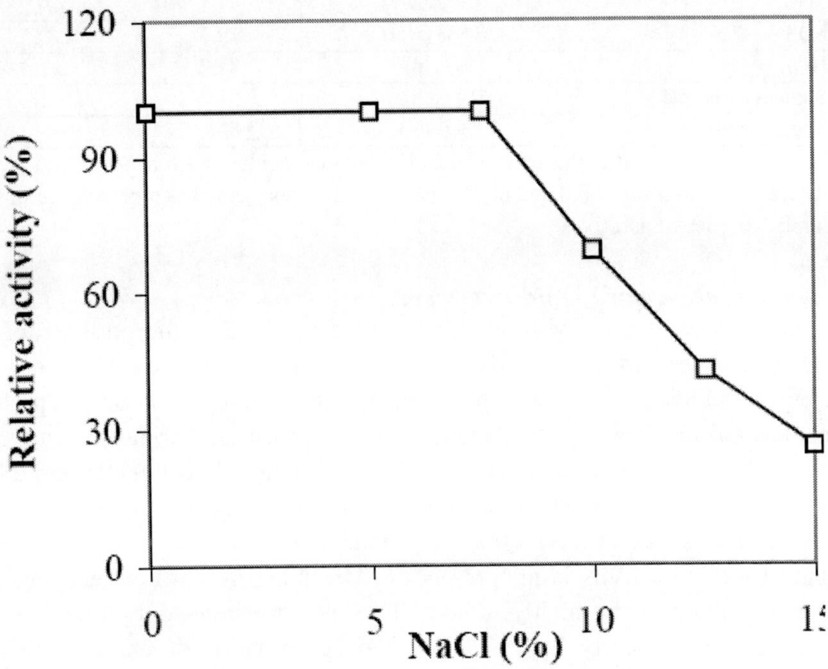

Figure 8. Effect of NaCl concentration on activity of *M. mustelus* protease.

Effect of Oxidizing Agents and Surfactants on Protease Stability

In order to be effective during washing, a good detergent protease must be compatible and stable with all commonly used detergent compounds such as surfactants, bleaches, oxidizing agents and other additives, which might be present in the formulation (Kumar and Takagi, 1999; Gupta et al., 1999).

As shown in table 5, the enzyme was highly stable in the presence of the non-ionic surfactants like Tween 80 and Triton X-100. In addition, the *M. mustelus* protease activity was little influenced by oxidizing agent, and retained 91, 80% of its activity after incubation 1 h at 30 °C in the presence of 1 and 2% sodium perborate and 81.7% in the presence of 1% hydrogen peroxide. This is a very important characteristic for its eventual use in detergent formulations.

Table 5. Stability of *M. mustelus* LMW protease in the presence of various surfactants and detergents

Additifs	Concentration	Residual activity (%)
None		100
Tween 80	1% (v/v)	91
	5%	76
Triton X-100	1% (v/v)	86.5
	5%	86
SDS	0,1% (w/v)	41.1
SDS	0,5% (w/v)	12.7
H_2O_2	1% (v/v)	81.7
Sodium perborate	1% (w/v)	91
Sodium perborate	2% (w/v)	80

The enzyme was pre-incubated with surfactants and oxidizing agents for 1 h at 30 °C and the remaining activity was measured at pH 8.0 and 60 °C. The activity is expressed as a percentage of the activity level in the absence of additives.

Stability in the Presence of Liquid Detergents

The high activity of the LMW weakly alkaline protease in the presence of chelating agents (EDTA) and its stability towards oxidizing agents were very useful for application as liquid detergent additive. To check the compatibility of *the M. mustelus* protease with detergents, the enzyme was preincubated in the presence of various commercial liquid laundry detergents for one hour at 30 °C and pH 9.0. The liquid detergents were diluted 100-fold in tap water to simulate washing conditions. The data presented in table 6 show that the enzyme is relatively stable in the presence of Dixan and Nadhif. The enzyme retained more than 75 and 61% of its activity in the presence of Dixan and Nadhif, respectively. However, the enzyme was found to be highly affected by Lav+, retaining only 17.8% of its initial activity. These results clearly indicated that the performance of enzymes in detergents depends on number of factors, including the detergents compounds since the proteolytic stability varied with each laundry detergent.

Table 6. Stability of the *M. mustelus* protease in the presence of various commercial liquid detergents

Commercial detergents	Remaining activity (%)
None	100
Dixan (Henkel-Spain)	75.5
Nadhif (Henkel-Alki-Tunisia)	61
Lav+ (Tunisia)	17.8

The enzyme was pre-incubated with commercial detergent diluted 100-fold in tap water for 1 h at 30 °C and the remaining activity was measured at pH 8.0 and 60°C. Enzyme activity of control sample without any detergent, incubated under the similar conditions, was taken as 100%.

Kinetic Properties

Kinetic constants K_m and k_{cat} of the purified enzyme were calculated using lineweaver-Burk plots. K_m and k_{cat} of the purified enzyme were 0.313 mM and 0.088 s^{-1}, respectively. The K_m of *M. mustelus* protease was lower than that of the collagenase (1.1 mM) of Mackerel,

S. japonicus, which had a same molecular weight (Park et al., 2002). The catalytic efficiency (k_{cat}/K_m) of *M. mustelus* protease was 0.281 s^{-1} mM^{-1}.

CONCLUSION

The purification to homogeneity of the LMW protease was achieved by ammonium sulphate precipitation (20-60% saturation), gel filtration through Sephadex G-100 and anion exchange chromatography on DEAE-cellulose. After the final purification step, the enzyme was purified 10.7-fold with a specific activity of 6952 U/mg and 22.6% recovery. The purified enzyme preparation was homogenous on SDS-PAGE and its molecular weight was estimated to be 14,800 Da. The enzyme was strongly inhibited by PMSF and SBTI and did not show esterase specific activity on *N*α-benzoyl-L-arginine ethyl ester hydrochloride.

The enzyme showed an optimum temperature at 60°C and optimum pH of 8.0. The enzyme was stable at a pH range of 6.0-10.0 and at temperatures in the range of 40-50 °C. The enzyme was compatible with some tested liquid detergents, retaining more than 75.5 and 61% of its initial activity with Dixan and Nadhif, respectively.

Further research is needed to determine properties of *M. mustelus* protease as a possible biotechnological tool in the fish processing and food industries.

ACKNOWLEDGEMENTS

This work was funded by the « Ministère de l'Enseignement Supérieur, de la Recherche Scientifique et de la Technologie».

REFERENCES

Bradford, M. (1976). A rapid and sensitive method for the quantification of microgram quantities of protein utilizing the principle of protein dye binding. *Analytical Biochemistry*, *72*, 248-254.

Bougatef, A., Souissi, N., Fakhfakh, N., Ellouz-Triki, Y., and Nasri, M. (2007). Purification and characterization of trypsin from the viscera of sardine (*Sardina pilchardus*). *Food Chemistry, 102*, 343-350.

Bougatef, A., Balti, R., Ben Zaied, S., Souissi, N., and Nasri, M. (in press). Pepsinogen and pepsin from the stomach of smooth hound (*Mustelus mustelus*): Purification, characterization and amino acid terminal sequences. *Food chemistry*, doi:10.1016/j.foodchem.2007.08.077.

Cancre, I., Ravallec, R., Van Wormhoudt, A. V., Stenberg, E., Gildberg, A., and Le Gal, Y. (1999). Secretagogues and growth factors in fish and crustacean protein hydrolysates. *Marine Biotechnology*, *1*, 489-494.

Castillo-Yanez, F.J., Pacheco-Aguilar, R., Garcıa-Carreno, F.L., and Navarrete-Del Toro, M.A. 2005, Isolation and characterization of trypsin from pyloric caeca of Monterey Sardine *Sardinops sagax caerulea*. Comp. Biochem. Physiol., 140B, 91-98.

Clausen, E., Gildberg, A., and Raa, J. (1985). Preparation and testing of an autolysate of fish viscera as growth substrate for bacteria. *Applied and Environmental Microbiology, 50*, 1556-1557.

Dufossé, L., De la Broise, D., and Guérard, F. (2001). Evaluation of nitrogenous substrates such as peptones from fish : A new method based on Gompertz modeling of microbial growth. *Current Microbiology*, *42*, 32-38.

Ellouz, Y., Bayoudh, A., Kammoun, S., Gharsallah, N., and Nasri, M. (2001). Production of protease by Bacillus subtilis grown on sardinelle heads and viscera flour. *Bioresource Technology*, 80- 49-51.

Ghorbel, S., Souissi, N., Triki-Ellouz, Y., Dufossé, L., Guérard, F., and Nasri, M. (2005). Preparation and testing of sardinella protein hydrolysates as nitrogen source for extracellular lipase production by *Rhizopus oryzae*. *World Journal of Microbiology and Biotechnology*, *21*, 33-38.

Gildberg, A. (1992). Recovery of proteinase and protein hydrolysate from fish viscera. *Bioresource Technology*, *39*, 271-276.

Gildberg, A., Batista, I., and Ström, E. (1989). Preparation and characterization of peptones obtained by two-step enzymatic hydrolysis of whole fish. *Biotechnology and Applied Biochemistry*, *11*, 413-423.

Gupta, R., Beg, Q. K., and Lorenz, P. (2002). Bacterial alkaline proteases: molecular approaches and industrial applications. *Applied Microbiology and Biotechnology*, *59*, 13-32.

Gupta, R., Gupta, K., Saxena, R. K., and Khan, S. (1999). Bleach-stable, alkaline protease from *Bacillus* sp. *Biotechnology Letters, 21*, 135-138.

Haard, N. F. (1998). Specialty enzymes from marine organisms. *Food Technology, 52*, 64-67.

Kembhavi, A. A., Kulkarni, A., and Pant, A. (1993). Salt-tolerant and thermostable alkaline protease from *Bacillus subtilis* NCIM No.64. *Applied Biochemistry and Biotechnology*, *38*, 83-92.

Kishimura, H., Hayashi, K., Miyashita, Y., and Nonami Y. (2006). Characteristics of trypsins from the viscera of true sardine (*Sardinops melanostictus*) and the pyloric ceca of arabesque greenling (*Pleuroprammus azonus*). *Food Chemistry, 97,* 65-70.

Klimova, O.A., Borukhov, S.I., Solovyeva, N.I., Balaevskaya, T.O., and Strogin, A.Y. (1990). The isolation and properties of collagenolytic proteases from crab hepatopancreas. *Biochemical and Biophysical research communications*., 166, 1411-1420.

Klomklao, S., Benjakul, S., Visessanguan, W., Kishimura, H., Simpson B. K., and Saeki, H. (2006). Trypsins from yellowfin tuna (Thunnus albacores) spleen: Purification and characterization, *Comparative Biochemistry and Physiology, Part B, 144,* 47-56.

Kumar, C. G., and Takagi, H. (1999). Microbial alkaline proteases from a bioindustrial viewpoint. *Biotechnology Advances, 17*, 561-594.

Laemmli, U. K. (1970). Cleavage of structural proteins during the assembly of the head of bacteriophage T4. *Nature*, *227*, 680-685.

Lee, S., and Jang, D. J. (2001). Progressive rearrangement of subtilisin Carlsberg into orderly and inflexible conformation with Ca^{2+} binding. *Biophysical Journal. 81*, 2972-2978.

Lineweaver, H., and Burk, D. (1934). The determination of enzyme dissociation constants. *Journal of the American Chemical Society, 56*, 665-666.

Nguyen, A., Nungaray, J., Martel, A., Le Goffic, F., Molle, D., and Leonil, J. (1998). Purification and characterization of the main pepsinogen from the shark, *Centroscymunus coelolepis*. *Journal of Biochemistry, 124*, 287-293

North, M. J. (1982). Comparative biochemistry of the proteinases of eukaryotic microorganisms. *Microbialogical Reviews, 46*, 308-340.

Park, P. J., Lee, S. H., Byun, H. G., Kim, S. H., and Kim, S. K. (2002). Purification and characterization of a collagenase from the Mackerel, *Scomber japonicus*. *Journal of Biochemistry and Molecular Biology, 35*, 576-582.

Rao, M. B., Tanksala, A. M., Ghatge, M. S., and Deshpande, V. V. (1998). Molecular and biotechnological aspects of microbial proteases. *Microbiology and Molecular Biology Reviews, 62*, 597-635.

Shahidi, F., and Kamil, J. Y. V. A. (2001). Enzymes from fish and aquatic invertebrates and their application in the food industry. *Trends in Food Science and Technology, 12*, 435-464.

Strom, T., and Eggum, B. O. (1981). Nutritional value of fish viscera silage. *Journal of the Science of Food and Agriculture, 32*, 115-120.

Tanji, M., Yakabe, E., Kageyama, T., Yokobori, S. I., Ichinose, M., Miki, K, Ito, H., and Takashi, K. (2007). Purification and characterization of pepsinogens from the gastric mucosa of African coelacanth, *Latimeria chalumnae* and properties of the major pepsins. *Comparative Biochemistry and Physiology, 146*, 412-420.

Triki-Ellouz, Y., Ghorbel, B., Souissi, N., Kammoun, S., and Nasri, M. (2003). Biosynthesis of protease by *Pseudomonas aeruginosa* MN7 grown on fish substrate. *World Journal of Microbiology and Biotechnology, 19*, 41-45.

Vieille, C., and Zeikus, J. G. (2001). Hyperthermophilic enzymes : sources, uses and molecular mechanisms for thermostability. *Microbiology and Molecular Biology Reviews, 65*, 1-43.

Zhou, Q., Fu, X. P., Zhang, L. J., Su, W. J., and Cao, M. J. (2007). Purification and characterization of sea bream (*Sparus latus* Houttuyn) pepsinogens and pepsins. *Food Chemistry, 103*, 795-801.

Zukowski, M. M. (1992). Production of commercially valuable products. In: Biology of Bacilli: Application to Industry (RH Doi and M Mc Gloughlin, eds), 311-337, *Butterworth-Heinemann*, London.

In: Progress in Food Chemistry
Editor: E. N. Koeffer, pp. 201-216

ISBN: 978-1-60456-303-0

Chapter 8

QSAR Analysis: A New Method in Food Research

Luciana Scotti[1], Marcus T. Scotti[2], Hamilton Ishiki[3], Marcelo J. P. Ferreira[2], Vicente P. Emerenciano[2] and Elizabeth I. Ferreira[1]

[1] Faculdade de Farmácia, Universidade de São Paulo,
Caixa Postal 05508-900, São Paulo, SP, Brazil.
[2] Instituto de Química, Universidade de São Paulo,
Caixa Postal 26077, 05513-970, São Paulo, SP, Brazil.
[3] Universidade do Oeste Paulista, Rua José Bongiovani 700, 19050-900,
Presidente Prudente, São Paulo, SP, Brazil

Abstract

Quantitative structure-activity relationships (QSAR) represent an attempt to correlate structural or property descriptors of compounds with several types of biological activities. These physicochemical descriptors, which include parameters, related with hydrophobicity, topology, electronic properties, and steric effects are determined empirically or, more recently, by computational methods. Activities used in QSAR studies (the dependent parameters) include chemical measurements and biological assays. QSAR software programs generate equations (models) by statistically identifying molecular descriptors and/or substructural molecular attributes that are correlated with dependent parameter. These programs are capable of identifying similar structural alerts associated with activity in a test compound and through a computer-aided method to predict how a chemical behaves based on its structure. QSAR is a theoretical method widely used in medicinal chemistry and recently was found to be appropriate to be employed either in food research. This method increasing interest in the mid-1980, and was implemented in a computer-aided rational approaches in drug design, representing an attractive method to estimate theoretical data as well to validation of any statistical model that seems to be reasonable in describing an interaction between a bioactive chemical constituent and the respective biological activity. The technique can be used to investigate toxicity, potency, stability and functionalities of food ingredients. One of the principal applications of QSAR method in food research is to understand better toxicology data, in order to inform risk assessments and to support risk management decisions that are protective of human health. Ideally, a risk assessor would have available all of the relevant information about the toxicity of the compound; their interactions with living systems; and the possible exposure conditions. Advances in the development of computational methods have available additional resources for safety assessment such as structure similarity searching and quantitative structure - activity relationship models. The purpose of this chapter is to discuss how a QSAR analysis can be used to predict important information from chemical structure and to review the application of this technique in food research.

INTRODUCTION

Quantitative structure-activity relationships (QSAR) are mathematical relationships linking chemical structure and pharmacological activity for a series of compounds. Is a multi-variant statistical correlation between a property and the geometric molecular structure. Thus, QSAR studies emphasize the important characteristics in a group to occur the biological activity.

QSAR models are developed through the computed property data and a series of *descriptors* - terms representing the system characteristics. Typical descriptors include thermodynamic properties (such as system energies), electronic properties (value of the LUMO (Lowest Unoccupied Molecular Orbital) or HOMO (Highest Occupied Molecular Orbital)), or functions representing molecular shape (molecular shape area, number of routable bonds and others).

Faster innovation of novel materials, at reduced cost, improve performance is market success. Additionally, patent positions may also accelerate the search for alternative materials. In the industry is not feasible to experimentally test the millions of chemicals in industry combinatorial databases, and QSAR screening can provide an alternative. Thus, this theoretical method can be used with advantages in several studies, including with foods, not only in the research of new substances, but could be used to investigate toxicity, potency, stability and functionalities of known food ingredients.

An effective QSAR model depends on a number of factors, and one the most critical is a training set with high-quality biological data. It is desirable that the training set has the biological data coming from the same assay protocol and contains a sufficiently large number of chemicals with diverse structure. Most importantly, both the biological activity/potency data and structural characteristics in terms of various descriptors are evenly distributed as far as possible in a range reflecting the domain in which chemicals to be predicted are located.

A proliferation of QSAR software's in recent years partly driven by practical economic forces and need as well as advances in chemo informatics and computer technology. The advance of these programs is challenged by the reality that few empirical data are available for the tens of thousands of commercial substances that require evaluation. Programs generate equations (models) by statistically identifying molecular descriptors and/or substructural molecular attributes that are correlated with activity.

Jacbson-Kram and Contrera, 2007 remembered Tropsha *et al.*, 2003 and discussed the utility and accuracy of a model. The model is a mathematical function of the molecular characteristics of the molecules in the training data set. If a test molecule is not well represented in the training data molecular library, the test molecule will be outside of the domain of the model and will have a poor statistical probability of an accurate prediction. Various metrics have been developed to define the position of a test chemical relative to a model's chemical space.

FDA AND QSAR

Recently, QSAR analysis in food research is very used to the investigation of the toxicity associating to the molecular similarity. FDA (Food and Drug Administration) Center for Drug Evaluation and Research (CDER), Office of Pharmaceutical Science (OPS), Informatics and Computational Safety Analysis Staff (ICSAS) offer an electronic database on toxicology, facilitating the research. Collaborating with this research ICSAS develops and it makes available programs capable to extract information from the toxicity activity of the compounds.

An interesting paper of Kruhlak *et al.*, 2006, did a review about computational methods being applied at the US Food and Drug Administration. This paper discussed the classification of the some toxicities substances with "structural alerts". They are defined as molecular functionalities to cause toxicity, and their presence in a molecular structure alerts the investigator to the potential toxicities of the test chemical. It is very complicated and expensive for experimentally test the millions of chemicals in industry combinatorial databases. Thus computational analysis are used in the screening to identify structural alerts statistically correlated with toxicity ("in silico first approach"), with smaller costs and time, reducing the need for standard experimental testing in some instances. A test compound that has limited or is lacking experimental data, such as a pharmaceutical impurity, is a probable candidate for screening by computational methods.

Major QSAR softwares currently used by the pharmaceutical and chemical industry include MC4PC (MultiCASE Inc.), MDL-QSAR (MDL Information Systems), and TOPKAT (Accelrys, Inc., Accelrys.com).

MC4PC and MDL-QSAR are two softwares developed by Cooperative Research and Development Agreements (CRADAs) between FDA/CDER and MultiCASE, Inc. and between FDA/CDER and MDL Information Systems, Inc., respectively.

Through the molecular fragment-based and topographical descriptors approach, both of these programs provide decision support information goes safety assessment of pharmaceutical impurities. MDL-QSAR software has been found to produce predictions with over 70% specificity and sensitivity for rodent carcinogenicity and bacterial mutagenicity and MC4PC software have been optimized by FDA/CDER to provide high specificity (>85%), high predictive value (>85%), and low false positive rates (<15%) for carcinogenicity and *Salmonella* mutagenicity. MDL-QSAR uses also E-state descriptor-based similarity employing the widely used Tanimoto and Cosine. Structure similarity searching for related chemical analogs that have experimental data can provide potential toxicity of a test set. These very useful programs were used in structure similarity searching in assessing the toxicity of compounds with little or no available experimental toxicology data clearly indicates the value and the need for toxicological databases which are chemical structure enabled. One of the challenges of modeling a dose relationship is that toxicity must be accounted for by considering the cumulative effect of multiple molecular features present in a chemical.

Substances with genotoxic and carcinogenic properties may be acceptable for some drugs such as antineoplastic and immunosuppressant chemotherapeutics, but the presence of these substances in daily ingestion offer serious risks to the health. Guidance recommend to manufacturers to reduce impurities to the lowest concentration levels that are technically feasible or that convey no significant increase in cancer risk.

Computational software programs and toxicological prediction modules created using these databases have been developed and validated by ICSAS that are:

1) designed to predict potential toxicities of thousands of test organic chemicals at multiple toxicological endpoints in batch mode;
2) made available to FDA/CDER without cost as part of Cooperative Research and Development Agreements (CRADAs);
3) commercially distributed by CRADA partners (MultiCASE, Inc. and MDL Information Systems, Inc.) for use by the pharmaceutical and general chemical industry as well as other regulatory agencies.

International Council of Chemical Associations (ICCA) and the European Chemical Industry Council (CEFIC), which included contributions from the US EPA and FDA, created a set of regulations to establish the applicability and validity of QSAR models:

1. Be associated with a defined endpoint of regulatory importance;
2. Take the form of an unambiguous algorithm;
3. Have a defined domain of applicability;
4. Be associated with appropriate measures of goodness of fit, robustness, and predictivity (In general, acceptable predictions should have a probability value greater than 65%);
5. Have a mechanistic basis.

The prediction of carcinogenicity in rodents is based upon results of toxicology studies from the FDA/CDER, National Institute of Environmental Health Sciences/National Toxicology Program (NIEHS/NTP), International Agency for Research on Cancer, and L. Gold CPDB, as well as the published literature for 2-year carcinogenicity studies in four types cells of the rodent bioassay (male rats, female rats, male mice, and female mice) rats and mice.

The scores ranged from 10 to 80 activity units and were assigned in decreasing order as follows: Scores of 80–50 activity units were assigned to chemicals causing trans-species, trans-gender, multiple site tumors; scores of 49–30 activity units were assigned to compounds causing trans-gender, single site tumors; scores of 29–20 were assigned to equivocal, weak or inconsistent findings or a single site tumor in a single study cell; and inactive chemicals were assigned activity scores of 19–10 units.

The modules used for the prediction of genetic toxicity are based upon results of toxicology studies conducted by the NIEHS/NTP, studies in FDA/CDER archives, and study data collected by the EPA and presented, in part, in the National Institutes of Health/National Library of Medicine (NIH/NLM) GENETOX database.

The maximum recommended daily dose (MRDD) for pharmaceuticals is a limit beyond which a drug's efficacy is not increased or undesirable adverse effects. The estimation of the no observed adverse effect level (NOAEL) (in mg/kg/day) can be an important additional factor for evaluating the relative risk and safe level of an impurity. A database was compiled by ICSAS of over 1300 pharmaceuticals with MRDD, using two software platforms, MC4PC and MDL-QSAR. Chemicals with low MRDDs were classified as high-toxicity compounds and chemicals with high MRDDs were classified as low-toxicity compounds. It was reported in Martindale: The Extra Pharmacopoeia and The Physicians'. The MRDD/NOAEL modeling help a decision support tool for evaluating the relative safe level of untested contaminants or degradents in drug products (Matthews and Machuga, 1995).

In an example a compound (CHEM1234) with three of its metabolites (figure 1), was submitted by an FDA reviewer. Four compounds were analyzed using a MC4PC and one MDL-QSAR modules for rodent carcinogenicity and for genetic toxicity. The results of this investigation are reported in Tables I to IV.

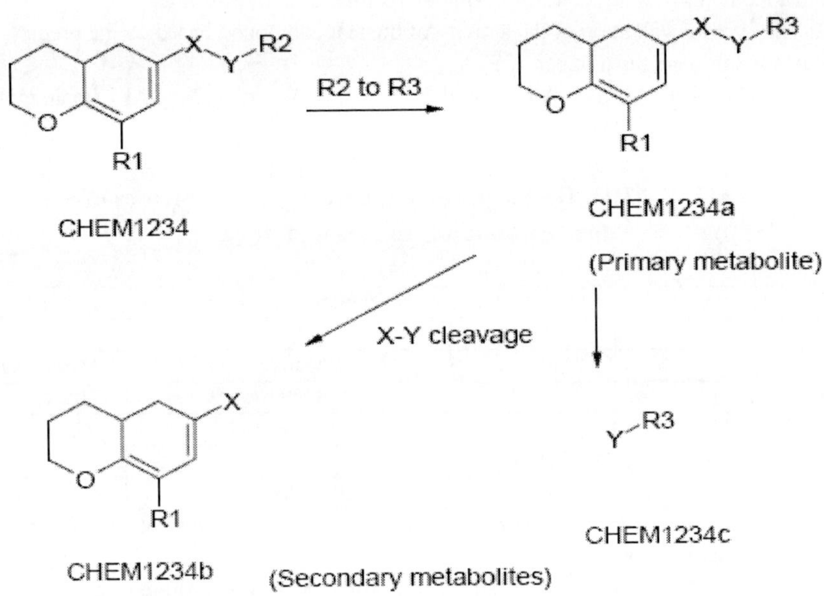

Figure 1. Structural relationship between the four compounds presented in the example.

The MDL-QSAR and MC4PC carcinogenicity predictions are in agreement with each other, with the partial exception of CHEM1234, where the MDL-QSAR positive prediction was assigned a lower level of confidence and considered a "no call". The positive carcinogenicity predictions for the first three compounds are reinforced by the fact that they contain a common structural feature, but the fourth compound prediction is negative suggesting a minimal toxicity contribution when it is a substructure of the other test compounds. Both software, through different approaches, identified molecular attributes associated with biological activity, and can be used as complementary systems. To successfully apply consensus predictions users need to have a comprehensive knowledge of the functional aspects of the software algorithms of each software program for each toxicological endpoint.

Table 1. MC4PC-predicted carcinogenic activities of four compounds in rats and mice

Compound	Structural alerts/carcinogenicity modules							
	AFV Ra	AF3 MR	AF4 FR	AFW Mi	AF1 MM	AF2 FM	No. SSA	Overall call
001 CHEM1234	+B	-Bd	+Bd	-bd	-b	-	3	+
002 CHEM1234a	+B	-Bd	+Bd	-bd	-bd	-	3	+
003 CHEM1234b	+B	+Bd	+B	+Bd	-b	-	3	+
004 CHEM1234c	-D	-D	-Dd	-d	-d	-	0	-

Structural alerts/carcinogenicity modules: “B", significant structural alert, b", non-significant structural alert; “D", significant fragment (fragment associated with a lack of activity); “d", non-significant fragment.

No. SSA: The total number of structurally similar alerts identified by MC4PC.

Overall call: The overall evaluation of the activity of the test compound based on the predictions for the individual modules and the number of SSA.

AFV (rats, Ra), AF3 (male rat, MR), AF4 (female rat, FR), AFW (mice, Mi), AF1 (male mouse, MM), and AF2 (female mouse, FM).

Table 2. MDL-QSAR-predicted carcinogenic activities of four compounds in rats and mice

Compound name	Discriminant analysis model		
	Probability		
	Positive	Negative	Overall call
001 CHEM1234	0.55508	0.44492	NC
002 CHEM1234a	0.78301	0.21699	+
003 CHEM1234b	0.78814	0.21186	+
004 CHEM1234c	0.24122	0.75878	-

Discriminant analysis model: The test compound was assigned a probability that is positive or negative for carcinogenicity in rodents.

Overall call: A “+" or “–" is assigned based on the probability of a positive or negative prediction. ‘NC’, or no call, is presented for compounds with probabilities less than 0.65. Table III - MC4PC estimated genetic toxicity activities of four compounds.

For estimation of the potential toxicological activities of pharmaceutical impurities, a compound must be submitted to the Computational Toxicology Consulting Service (CTCS). The structure must be represented as a single molecular entity in molfile format, with charged moieties neutralized and salts and counter ions removed. The test compound structure is compared to existing commercial databases of pharmaceutical molecules, such as the Derwent World Drug Index and Pharmaprojects, to identify a cluster of structurally similar compounds. The use of a digital representation of chemical structure (e.g., the MDL molfile or Simplified Molecular Input Line Entry System code) as the primary substance identification in the training database makes possible the identification of clusters of substances having similar chemical structure/substructural features and similar pharmacological or toxicological activities.

Table 3.

Compound	Structural alerts/genetic toxicity modules										
	A7A	A7B	A7C	A7D	A7E	A7F	A7G	A7H	A7I	A7J	A7K	
	Salm.	Salm.	E. coli	E. coli	Fungi	Fungi	Dros.	Dros.	Dros.	Rod.	Rod.	
001 CHEM1234	-	-D	-	-4w	-B?w	-w	-	-	-bd5w	+B5w	-5w	
002 CHEM1234a	-	-D	-	-3w	-w	-w	-	-	-d4w	+B4w	-4w	
003 CHEM1234b	-	-	-d	-d	-	-	-	-	-w	-B2w	-2w	
004 CHEM1234c	-	-	-	-d3w	-w	-w	-	-	-d3w	-d3w	-3w	
Compound	Structural alerts/genetic toxicity modules											
	A7O	A7S	A7T	A8J	A8A	A8B	A8C	A8K	A7P	A7R	No. SSA	Overall call
	hgprt	Micro.	Micro.	Micro.	UDS	UDS	UDS	UDS	C. Abs.	C. Abs.		
001 CHEM1234	-bd	-D	-D	-w	-	-w	-dw	-B4w	-d	-x2w	1	-
002 CHEM1234a	-bd	-D	-D	-w	-	-	-dw	-B4w	-d	-w	1	-
003 CHEM1234b	-b	-	-	-d	-	-	-	-w	-	-	0	-
004 CHEM1234c	-d	-B?D	-D	-w	-	-	-w	-B2w	-d	-	0	-

No. SSA: The total number of structurally similar alerts (SSA) identified in the test compound, where the SSAs must be identical or embedded significant structural alerts, across the following subsets of toxicologically related modules: A7C–A7D, A7E–A7F, A7G–A7I, A7J–A7K, A7S–A8J, A8A–A8K, and A7P–A7R. A7A, A7B, and A7O are standalone modules where a significant structural alert in one is considered sufficient evidence to result in a positive prediction for genetic toxicity.

The number "1" denotes a significant structural alert identified in a single module.

Structural alerts/genetic toxicity modules: "B", significant structural alert, "B?", marginally significant structural alert, or biophore; "b", non-significant structural alert; "D", significant deactivating fragment (fragment associated with a lack of activity); "d", non-significant deactivating fragment; "w", warning that an unknown fragment is present in the test compound; "x", unknown fragment that is similar to a known structural alert.

Overall call: The overall evaluation of the activity of the test compound based on the predictions for the individual modules and the number of SSA.

Table 4. MDL-QSAR-estimated Salmonella mutagenicity activities of our compounds

Compound name	Discriminant analysis model		
	Probability		
	Positive	Negative	Overall call
001 CHEM1234	0.00000	1.00000	-
002 CHEM1234a	0.00000	1.00000	-
003 CHEM1234b	0.00000	1.00000	-
004 CHEM1234c	0.00000	1.00000	-

Discriminant analysis model: The test compound was assigned a probability that is positive or negative for carcinogenicity in rodents.

Overall call: A "+" or "–" is assigned based on the probability of a positive or negative prediction. 'NC', or no call, is presented for compounds with probabilities less than 0.65.

Environmental Protection Agency (EPA) developed a strategy for screening and testing a large number of chemicals found in drinking water and food additives for their endocrine disruption potential. EPA established the Endocrine Disruptor Screening and Testing Advisory Committee (EDSTAC).

QSAR models for estrogen receptor (ER) binding; these models yield good statistical results in the training and cross-validation steps and explain some structural determinants for ER binding. The Figure 2 depicts the three structural alerts, i.e., the steroid, DES, and phenolic skeletons, selected to identify potential ER binders (Tong *et al.*, 2003).

Structural alerts are key 2D structural fragments associated with (ER) binding. Each alert independently characterizes a unique structural feature important for the ER binding. Any chemicals containing any one of these structural alerts are considered to be a potential ER binder (Tong *et al.*, 2003).

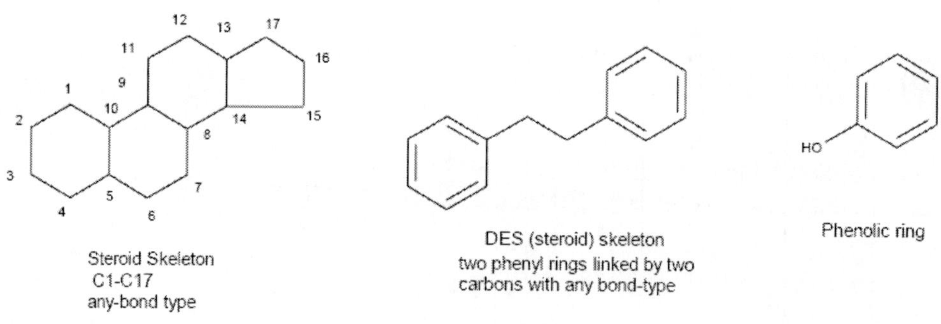

Figure 2. Three structural alerts defined by 2D substructural features commonly observed for ER ligands.

QSAR Analysis of Mutagenic Activity

The ability to repair the initial adducts or damage is an important factor for determining a compound's mutagenic potency.

Heterocyclic amine formation and the impact of structure on their mutagenicity were discussed in several papers. With objective of the goal was an improved understanding of the chemical basis of mutagenicity for this class of heterocyclic amines, Hatch *et al.*, 1996 studied a set of 16 mutagenic aminoimidazo-azaarene. The study included molecular orbital energies and other electronic properties of these compounds, calculated ted using Huckel, semiempirical AM1, and *ab initio* quantum mechanical methods. Factor interrelationships were studied by multiple linear regression and canonical correlation analyses. Hatch *et al.*, concluded that mutagenic potency of heterocyclic amines is related to the size of the aromatic ring system; potency was enhanced by the presence and location of an N-methyl group by addition of ring nitrogen atoms in pyridine, quinoline, and quinoxaline configurations. The potency was inversely related to the energy of the LUMO (lowest unoccupied molecular orbital) of the parent amines. The calculated thermodynamic stability of the nitrenium ions (relative to the parent amine) showed the potency was directly correlated with nitrenium LUMO energy and with the negative charge on the exocyclic nitrogen atom. Hatch and Colvin, 1996 reported a similar study with 66 aromatics and 99 heterocyclic amines for which mutagenic potency data available. The methodology and conclusions were seemed.

Felton *et al.*, 1999 studied a class of imidazopyridines. QSAR analysis correlated the potency of these compounds and chemical properties. A low dipole moment is found to be a qualitative predictor of high mutagenic potency.

Recently, Lau *et al.* investigated the ability of various heterocyclic amine reactive intermediates to fit into the *N*-acetyltransferase (NAT2) active site, using docking studies and quantum mechanical calculations of hydroxylated heterocyclic amines and observed differences mutagenic of the set.

Differences in the stability of the reactive intermediates, specificity for base targets in the gene, have impact the mutagenic potency. The Molecular Modeling study (computer docking of metabolite intermediates into the enzyme active sites) is very important to understand how small structural changes mutagenic potential of the compound. But QSAR analysis could be elucidation because in the Lau *et al.* investigation, for the PhIP isomers (Figure 3), it only explains 20% of the difference of mutagenic activity.

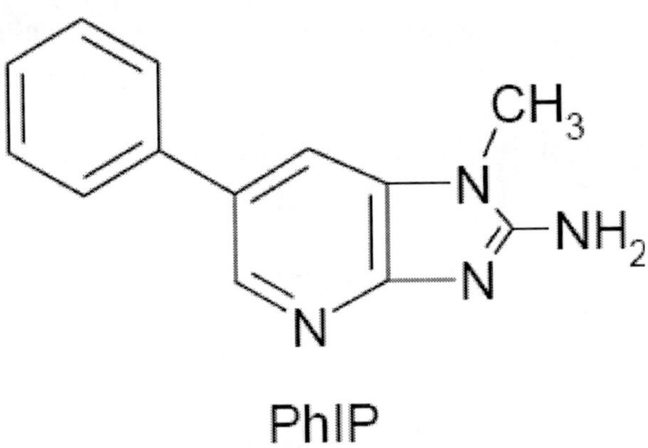

Figure 3. Skeletal type of PhIP isomers.

Thus, Felton *et al.,* 2007, in reported work "Mutagenic potency of food-derived heterocyclic amines", for each compound the optimized structure, calculated LUMO energies using *ab initio* quantum chemical methods. Using the linear relationship between LUMO energy and log mutagenic potency it was possible to extrapolate and predict the potencies of novel compounds. A lower LUMO energy means a higher electron affinity. The results showed a strong correlation between LUMO energy and observed mutagenic potential of several heterocyclic amine mutagens.

Knize *et al.,* 2006 studied the mutagenic potency of twelve 2-amino-trimethylimidazopyridine isomers and summarized the main conclusions of the previous works: the principal determinants of higher mutagenic potency in amines are:

1) a small dipole moment;
2) the combination of b-face ring fusion and N3-methyl group;
3) a lower calculated energy of the p electron system;
4) a smaller energy gap between the amine HOMO and LUMO orbitals (Pearson ''softness'');
5) a more stable nitrenium ion.

The mutagenic activity of polyaromatic hydrocarbons, their amino derivatives and heterocyclic analogues, appears to be related to frontier orbital parameters within the molecules concerned. Lewis *et al.,* 2003 related the mutagenicity of series of chemical carcinogens and specific structural and electronic parameters and discussed the importance of frontier orbital energies to overall mutagenicity in diverse polyaromatic hydrocarbons, benzidines and aminobiphenyls, benzonitrofurans, nitrogenous cooked-food mutagens, benzanthracenes, and chrysenes. Lewis *et al.* concluded that enzymes of the cytochrome P4501 (CYP1) family are closely associated with the metabolic activation of polyaromatic mutagens and carcinogens via the generation of reactive intermediates (usually electrophilic in nature) that attack DNA.

Heterocyclic amines are promutagens and require metabolic activation to become highly mutagenic which are formed during the cooking of foods. Phytochemicals are candidates for antimutagens/anticarcinogens and among them, the flavonoids. Hatch *et al.*, 2000 through quantum chemical calculations, evaluation of molecular planarity via the dihedral angles between the B and C rings (Figure 4), and additional structural and hydropathic variables; applied statistical analyses, (correlation and multiple regression) to develop the QSAR models. This study observed the interference by the flavonoids with cytochrome P450 activation of the promutagens is the probable mechanism for inhibition of mutagenesis.

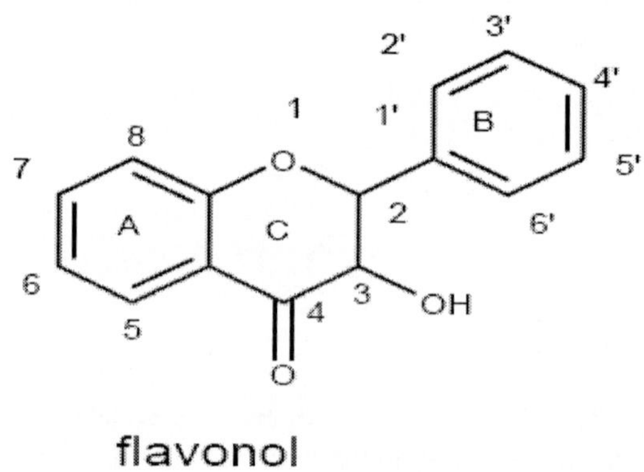

Figure 4. The generic structure of flavonoids (e.g., flavonol itself).

Aldehydes are important industrial compounds that are used for the synthesis of chemicals and pharmaceuticals and as solvents, food additives, and disinfectants. However, because of their reactivity,this compounds are able to interact with electron-rich biological macromolecules and adverse health effects have been reported, including toxicity, allergenic reactions, mutagenicity and carcinogenicity.

QSAR method is an adequately screen these compounds and investigate the risks associated with the use of aldehydes. Benigni *et al.,* 2004 reported an example of the investigation with two aldehydes sets. In first study, an investigation was computed in simple aliphatic aldehydes (Figure 5) and it was involved Physical, Chemical, and Biological Descriptors (Table V). A second QSAR analysis were computed with α-β unsaturated aldehydes and the parametrization also involved the energy value of the lowest unoccupied molecular orbital (LUMO). It parametrizes the ability to accept electrons, the energy value of the highest occupied molecular orbital (HOMO), the partial charges on the carbonilic carbon atom (C-carb) and on the β carbon atom (C-β).

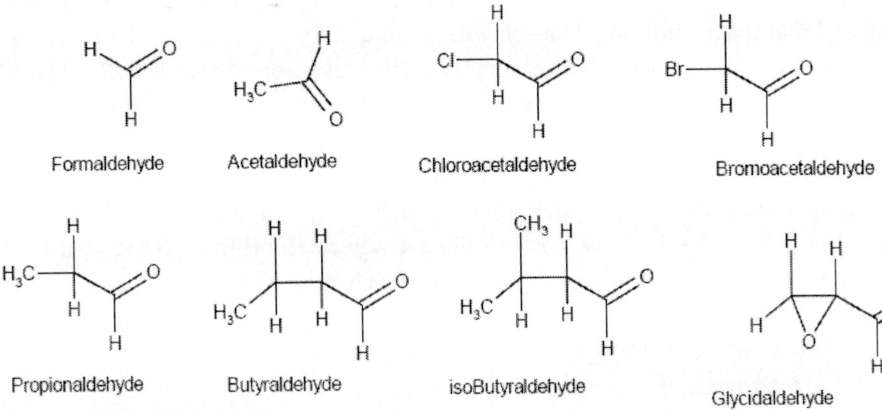

Figure 5. Chemical structures of simple aliphatic aldehydes.

Table 5. Simple Aldehydes: Physical, Chemical, and Biological Descriptors

Code	Compound	LogP	MR	σ	Canc	Sty
1	Formaldehyde	0.35	0.6769	0	+	+
2	Acetaldehyde	_0.224	1.1407	-0.04	+	?
3	Chloroacetaldehyde	-0.111	1.6321	0.17	+	+
4	Bromoacetaldehyde	0.029	1.9177	0.2	-	
5	Propionaldehyde	0.59	1.6045	-0.01		-
6	Butyraldehyde	0.88	2.0683	-0.01		-
7	isoButyraldehyde	0.834	2.0683	0.01	-	-
8	Glycidaldehyde	_0.251	1.5802	0.07	+	+

Hydrophobicity was parametrized by the logarithm of the octanol/water partition coefficient (logP), bulkiness was parametrized by the molecular refractivity (MR), positive values of σ represent electron withdrawal by the substituent; negative values represent electron release, Canc: rodent carcinogenicity. Sty: Salmonella typhimurium mutagenicity, TA100 strain.

LogP and MR discriminated the two groups with almost the same importance (F= 7.15 and F=7.02), whereas σ did not differentiate between the two groups (F= 0.0). The squared canonical correlation of the model based on logP and MR was 0.77 (77% variance explained).

QSAR models for the mutagenicity and carcinogenicity of simple aldehydes and α-β unsaturated aldehydes involved electrophilicity, bulkiness and hydrophobicity in the genotoxic activity of the aldehydes and lend themselves to the prediction of the activity of other untested chemicals of the same class.

BIOACCUMULATION AND COMPUTATIONAL METHODS

The North America Annual Meeting of the Society of Environmental Toxicology and Chemistry (SETAC) 11–12 November 2005 in Baltimore was focused on fish *in vivo* bioaccumulation databases was to explore the sources and state of empirical fish bioaccumulation data. Weisbrod *et al.* 2007, in theirs paper, do a review about that workshop and discussed that the assembling data sets of known quality would enable better assessments of bioaccumulation as well as the development of improved predictive models. The SETAC was focused on fish data because regulatory assessments predominantly focus on the bioconcentration of substances from water into fish, as measured using in vivo tests or predicted using computer models. Quantity, features, and public availability of bioconcentration, bioaccumulation, and biota–sediment accumulation data were reviewed too.

Arnot and Gobas, 2003 discussed how the activity relationship (QSAR) can be use for assessing the bioaccumulation potential of organic chemicals in aquatic food webs. BAF (Chemical's bioaccumulation factor)-QSAR model requires very few input parameters and can also be used in the derivation of water quality guidelines and total maximum daily loadings by relating internal concentrations of organic chemicals in upper trophic fish species to corresponding concentrations in the water.

Persistent Organic Pollutants (POPs) like polychlorinated naphthalenes (PCNs), polychlorinated biphenyls (PCBs), dichlorodiphenyl-trichloroethane (DDT) and hexachlorobenzene (HCB) can contaminate natural ecosystems and accumulate at sizeable levels in aquatic organisms and in the tissues of animals and man (Shüürmann and Klein 1988; Horii *et al.*, 2004).

Experimental determinations capable of detecting these POPs at low concentration are time-consuming and very expensive (Ivanciuc *et al.* 2006). On the other hand, Quantitative Structure Activity Relationships (QSARs) equations can play an important role to make predictions of the bioaccumulation risks before they develop. It can be done using experimental determinations, as octanol-water partition coefficient, or employing physical-chemical parameters. The octanol-water partition coefficient is a good descriptor in assessing the bioaccumulation in the aqueous environment. An important difference between terrestrial and aquatic organisms is that the respiring medium is air rather than water. In this context, the octanol-air partition coefficient must be better than octanol-water partition coefficient, and can be describe the organism-to-air exchange more correctly (Gobas *et al.* 2003).

Employing QSAR methodologies, Puzyn and Falandysz (2005) have studied 75 congeners of chloronaphthalene. They have used 190 descriptors obtained by quantum-chemistry, thermodynamical and topological calculations as independent variables and the logarithm of n-octanol-water partition coefficient and subcooled liquid vapor pressure as dependent variables. Using the backward stepwise regression, the best equation obtained to describe the logarithm of n-octanol-water partition coefficient (K_{OA}) was:

$$\text{Log } K_{OA} = 8.26(0.03)+1.11(0.03)V1+0.15(0.02)V2+0.15(0.02)V4$$
$$n=27,\ r^2 = 0.999,\ Q^2_{CV} = 0.988,\ s = 0.15,\ F = 736$$

where V1 is a linear combination of 133 descriptors connected with compounds molecular size, V2 describe the atomic position and the symmetry of zero and first order neighborhood of chloronaphthalene congeners and V4 describes the molecular properties depending on sigma electrons.

In another study, Ivanciuc *et al.* (2006) have studied the bioconcentration factor (BCF) and the bioaccumulation factor (BAF) for polychlorinated biphenyls using quantitative super-structure-activity relationship (QSSAR) models. In this approach the splinoid poset and cluster expansion models were applied for the modeling of bioconcentration factors and bioaccumulation factors of PCBs for various fish species. This two models are specifically developed for a network of chemicals compounds that present a parent skeleton. The predictive ability evaluated with the leave-one-out cross validation, for 20 QSSAR models, shows that the splinoid model are better than the cluster expansion model. The best splinoid model, obtained using 58 PCBs, have the following statistical parameter values: $r = 0.958$ and $s = 0.245$ and the best cluster-expansion model, obtained using either 58 PCBs, have the following statistical parameter values: $r = 0.908$ and $s = 0.372$. The best model was used to predict the bioconcentration factor for the remaining PCBs.

Dimitrov *et al.* have studied either the bioaccumulation potential of some chemicals using the K_{ow} and the experimental bioconcentration factors (BCF) values as dependent variables. The obtained models have been compared, with respect to predict the bioaccumulative and the very bioaccumulative chemicals, with other models previously published. In order to reduce the false positive predictions showed in other studies, the effect of molecular weight and the geometry was analyzed. Additionally, the maximum potential of bioaccumulation was either considered in the analysis. The maximum bioconcentration factors and maximum diameter threshold reduced significantly the false positive predictions (Dimitrov *et al.* 2003).

These kinds of studies can be applied, for example, to categorize chemicals present on domestic substances in terms of their persistence, bioaccumulation potential and toxicity.

CONCLUSION

The QSAR procedures are applied extensively to a wide range of scientific disciplines including chemistry, biology, and toxicology. In drug discovery and environmental toxicology, QSAR models are now regarded as a scientifically credible tool for predicting and classifying the biological activities of untested chemicals.

QSAR models are developed scientifically and statistically valid. They can be applied to further chemicals of the same class to predict their genetic toxicity, potency, bioaccumulation and several activities of structure chemicals (provided that the chemical descriptors of the chemicals to be predicted are in the same range of those used to build the models). QSAR models are used prospectively to define and rationalize a set of chemicals that may further improve the model's robustness and predictive capability. These new chemicals are assayed, and the data are then used to challenge and refine the QSAR model. Thus, the process results in the iterative increase of the chemistry space of the training set.

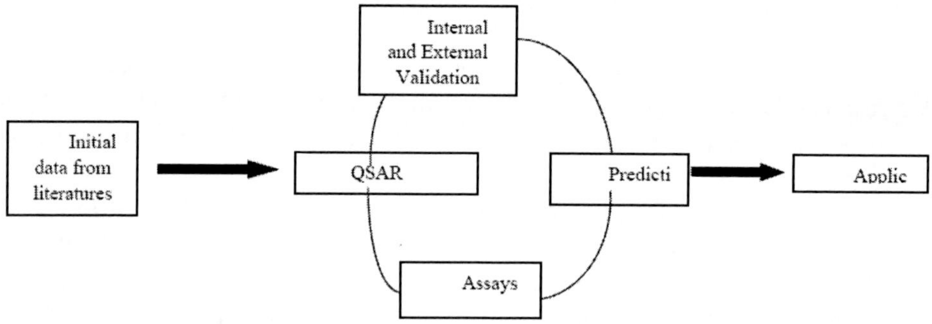

Figure 6. The recursive process to develop QSAR models.

REFERENCES

Arnot J. A. and Gobas F. A. P. C. (2003) A Generic QSAR for Assessing the Bioaccumulation Potential of Organic Chemicals in Aquatic Food Webs, *QSAR Comb. Sci.* 22 337-345

Benigni R., Passerini L. and Rodomonte A. (2003) Structure–Activity Relationships for the Mutagenicity and Carcinogenicity of Simple and α-β Unsaturated Aldehydes, *Environmental and Molecular Mutagenesis*, 42, 136-143.

Dimitrov, S. D. , Dimitrova, N. C., Walker, J. D., Veith, G. D and Mekenyan, O. G. (2003) *QSAR Comb. SCi*., 22, 58-68.

Elton J. S., Knize M. G., Hatch F. T., Tanga M. J. and Colvin M. E. (1999) Heterocyclic amine formation and the impact of structure on their mutagenicity, *Cancer* Letters, 143, 127-134.

Felton J. S., Knize M. G., Wu R. W., Colvin M. E., Hatch F. T. and Malfatti M. A. (2007) Mutagenic potency of food-derived heterocyclic amines, *Fundamental and Molecular. Mechanisms of Mutagenesis Mutation Research*, 616, 90-94.

Gobas, F. A. P. C., Kelly, B. C. and Arnot, J. A. (2003) QSAR Combi. Sci., 22, 329-336.

Hatch F. T., Colvin M. E. and Seidl E. T. (1996) Structural and Quantum Chemical Factors Affecting Mutagenic Potency of Aminoimidazo-Azaarenes. *Environmental and Molecular Mutagenesis,* 27, 314-330.

Hatch F. T. and Colvin M. E. (1997) Quantitative Structure-Activity (QSAR) Relationships of mutagenic aromatic and heterocyclic amines. *Fundamental and Molecular. Mechanisms of Mutagenesis Mutation Research,* 376, 87-96.

Hatch F. T., Lightstone F. C. and Colvin M. E. (2000) Quantitative Structure-Activity Relationship of Flavonoids for Inhibition of Heterocyclic Amine Mutagenicity. *Environmental and Molecular Mutagenesis*, 35, 279-299.

Hatch F. T., Knize M. G. and Colvin M. E. (2001) Extended Quantitative Structure–Activity Relationships for 80 Aromatic and Heterocyclic Amines: Structural, Electronic, and Hydropathic Factors Affecting Mutagenic Potency. *Environmental and Molecular Mutagenesis,* 38, 268-291.

Horii, Y., Okada, M., Amano, K., Naya, T., Hanari, N., Taniyasu, S., Yamashita, N., Falandysz, J., Rostkowski, P. and Puzyn, T. (2004). *Journal of Environmental Science and Health* A, 39, 587-609.

Ivanciuc, T., Ivanciuc and O., Klein, D. (2006) *J. Molecular Diversity*, 10, 133-145.

Jacbson-Kram D. and Contrera J. F. (2007) Genetic Toxicity Assessment: Employing the Best Science for Human Safety Forum Series, Evaluation Part I: Early Screening for Potential Human Mutagens, *Toxicological Sciences* 96, 16–20

Krhlak N. L., Contrera J. F., Benz R. D. and Mathws E. J. (2007) Progress in QSAR toxicity screening of pharmaceutical impurities. *Advances Drug Delivery Reviews*, 59, 43-55.

Knize M. G., Hatch F. T., Tanga M. J., Lau E. Y. and Colvin M. E. (2006) A QSAR for the Mutagenic Potencies of Twelve 2-Amino-trimethylimidazopyridine Isomers: Structural, Quantum Chemical, and Hydropathic Factors. *Environmental and Molecular Mutagenesis,* 47, 132-146.

Lewis D. F. V., Ioannides C. and Parke D. V. (2003) A Quantitative Structure-Activity Relationship (QSAR) Study of Mutagenicity in Several Series of Organic Chemicals Likely to be Activated by Cytochrome P450 Enzymes. Teratogenesis, Carcinogenesis, and Mutagenesis Supplement, 1, 187-193.

Matthews E. J. and Machuga E. J. (1995) Threshold of estimated toxicity for regulation of indirect food additives. *Toxicology letters*, 79, 123-129.

Tong W., Fang H., Hong H., Xie Q., Perkins R., Anson J. and Sheehan D. M. (2003) Regulatory application of SAR/QSAR for priority setting of endocrine disruptors: A perspective. *Pure and Applied Chemistry* 75, 2375–2388.

Puzyn, T. and Falandysz, J. (2005) *Atmospheric Environment*, 39, 1439-1446.

Shüürmann, G. and Klein, W. (1988). *Chemosphere,* 17, 1551-1574.

Weisbrod A.V., Burkhard L.P., Arnot J., Mekenyan O., Howard P. H. and Russom C. (2007) Workgroup Report: Review of Fish Bioaccumulation Databases Used to Identify Persistent, Bioaccumulative, Toxic Substances. *Environmental Health Perspectives,* 15,255-261.

INDEX

A

B

C

D

E

F

G

H

I

N

O

P

Q

R

S

T

U

V

W

X

Y

Z